Systems Biology - Theory, Techniques and Applications

nova
science publishers
www.novapublishers.com

Systems Biology - Theory, Techniques and Applications

Transcriptome Analysis and Why it Matters
Sagarika Mishra, PhD
2023. ISBN: 978-1-61728-298-0 (eBook)

From Systems Biology to Systems Medicine
James A. Marcum (Editor)
2020. ISBN: 978-1-53617-960-6 (Hardcover)
2020. ISBN: 978-1-53617-961-3 (eBook)

Recent Trends in 'Computational Omics: Concepts and Methodology'
Pramod Katara (Editor)
2020. ISBN: 978-1-53617-941-5 (Hardcover)
2020. ISBN: 978-1-53617-942-2 (eBook)

Proteomics: Advances in Research and Applications
Ricardo Parker (Editor)
2019. ISBN: 978-1-53616-440-4 (Softcover)
2019. ISBN: 978-1-53616-441-1 (eBook)

More information about this series can be found at
https://novapublishers.com/product-category/series/systems-biology-theory-techniques-and-applications/

James A. Marcum

The Conceptual Foundations of Systems Medicine

nova
science publishers
www.novapublishers.com

https://doi.org/10.52305/LUOY0764

NOTICE TO THE READER

The Publisher has taken reasonable care in the preparation of this book but makes no expressed or implied warranty of any kind and assumes no responsibility for any errors or omissions. No liability is assumed for incidental or consequential damages in connection with or arising out of information contained in this book. The Publisher shall not be liable for any special, consequential, or exemplary damages resulting, in whole or in part, from the readers' use of, or reliance upon, this material. Any parts of this book based on government reports are so indicated and copyright is claimed for those parts to the extent applicable to compilations of such works.

Independent verification should be sought for any data, advice or recommendations contained in this book. In addition, no responsibility is assumed by the Publisher for any injury and/or damage to persons or property arising from any methods, products, instructions, ideas or otherwise contained in this publication.

This publication is designed to provide accurate and authoritative information with regards to the subject matter covered herein. It is sold with the clear understanding that the Publisher is not engaged in rendering legal or any other professional services. If legal or any other expert assistance is required, the services of a competent person should be sought. FROM A DECLARATION OF PARTICIPANTS JOINTLY ADOPTED BY A COMMITTEE OF THE AMERICAN BAR ASSOCIATION AND A COMMITTEE OF PUBLISHERS.

Library of Congress Cataloging-in-Publication Data

ISBN: 979-8-89113-495-9

Published by Nova Science Publishers, Inc. † New York

Contents

Preface ix

Acknowledgments xiii

Chapter 1 **Biomedicine and Systems Medicine** 1

Abstract 1

1. Biomedicine and Evidence-Based Medicine 1

1.1. Biomedicine *2*

1.2. Evidence-Based Medicine *5*

1.3. COVID-19 Challenge *8*

2. Systems Medicine 10

2.1. Defining Systems Medicine *11*

2.2. Systems Biomedicine *12*

2.3. Molecular Systems Medicine *14*

2.4. Personalized Medicine *15*

2.5. Precision Medicine *18*

2.6. Network Medicine *20*

2.7. From P3 to P7 Systems Medicine *21*

Conclusion 26

Chapter 2 **Mechanism and Organicism** 27

Abstract 27

1. Introduction 27

2. Mechanism and Organicism 29

2.1. Mechanism *29*

2.2. Organicism *34*

3. Reductionism and Wholism 39

3.1. Reductionism *40*

3.2. Wholism *49*

4. Materialism and New Materialism 59

4.1. Materialism *59*

4.2. Physicalism *62*

4.3. New Materialism ... *64*
5. Upward and Downward Causation ... 66
5.1. Upward Causation ... *67*
5.2. Downward Causation ... *69*
Conclusion ... 72

Chapter 3 **Resultant and Emergence** ... 75
Abstract ... 75
1. Introduction ... 75
2. Resultant and Emergence ... 76
2.1. Resultant ... *76*
2.2. Emergence ... *78*
3. Synthesis and Emergent Synthesis ... 89
3.1. Synthesis ... *89*
3.2. Emergent Synthesis ... *91*
4. Geneticism and Epigeneticism ... 93
4.1. Geneticism ... *94*
4.2. Epigeneticism ... *98*
5. Determinism and Stochasticity ... 103
5.1. Determinism ... *103*
5.2. Stochasticity ... *106*
Conclusion ... 110

Chapter 4 **Homeostasis and Robustness** ... 113
Abstract ... 113
1. Introduction ... 113
2. Homeostasis and Robustness ... 115
2.1. Homeostasis ... *115*
2.2. Robustness ... *124*
3. Linear and Nonlinear Dynamics ... 131
3.1. Linear Dynamics ... *131*
3.2. Nonlinear Dynamics ... *134*
4. Stasis and Evolvability ... 137
4.1. Stasis ... *137*
4.2. Evolvability ... *138*
Conclusion ... 143

Chapter 5 **Challenges Facing Systems Medicine** ... 145
Abstract ... 145
1. Introduction ... 145
2. Methodological Challenges ... 146

2.1. Technological Challenges *147*
2.2. Computational Challenges *149*
3. Conceptual and Theoretical Challenges 153
4. Social and Political Challenges 156
5. Ethical Challenges 160
6. COVID-19 Pandemic 164
Conclusion 166

Glossary 169

Annotated Bibliography 177

References 203

Index 281

About the Author 289

Preface

Medicine has made significant advances over the past several centuries, especially from humoral pathology in which the etiology of disease was articulated with respect to the four humors of blood, phlegm, and yellow and black bile, then to solidest pathology in which disease was explained with respect to dysfunctional organs, tissues, and cells, and finally to contemporary genetic pathology in which disease is expounded in terms of mutated genes (Van Den Tweel and Taylor 2010, Zhang et al. 2008). Within the past couple decades, medicine has undergone another significant advance, particularly with respect to systems pathology (Costa 2012, Faratian et al. 2009). Part of that advance includes the incorporation of epigenetic mechanisms, such as DNA methylation and histone modifications, in understanding the etiology of disease (Egger et al. 2004, Zoghbi and Beaudet 2016). For example, these epigenetic mechanisms are intimately involved in carcinogenesis and metastasis, and they constitute, along with epigenomics, the cancer epigenome (Marcum 2019). More generally, medicine is undergoing a revolutionary shift from the biomedical model to a systems medicine model (Marcum 2020). A large part of that shift involves a transformation in the conceptual foundation and framework of medicine and its practice. This book represents an inquiry into and examination of that conceptual transformation.

To that end, the notion of systems medicine is explored in the first chapter, especially in terms of introducing P7 systems medicine (Marcum 2021)—a derivative of Leroy Hood's P4 medicine (Hood 2013)—after exploring the biomedical model and evidence-based medicine (EBM). Then in the next three chapters, the conceptual foundations of systems medicine, especially P7 systems medicine, are examined to provide a conceptual and theoretical framework. In the first chapter, the concept of organicism is explored, along with the associated concepts of wholism, new materialism, and downward causation. In the next chapter, the concept of emergence is examined, including other related concepts such as emergent synthesis, epigenesis, and stochasticity. In the last chapter, the concept of robustness is investigated, along with the affiliated concepts of nonlinear dynamics, evolvability, and fragility. The relationship among these concepts is crucial for grounding systems medicine—for it reflects an ontology of the organism qua whole, which then results in its emergence, or in terms of P7 medicine the personal P, which displays a robust state for maintaining health and wellbeing.

Importantly, throughout these three chapters (Chapters 2-4) the conceptual foundation of systems medicine is compared and at times contrasted with biomedicine's mechanistic ontology in which the patient is reduced to resultant and material parts and the maintenance of those parts through homeostasis (Table 1). Specifically, the concepts of organicism and mechanism are originally examined and contrasted, along with the associated concepts of wholeness and reductionism, new materialism and materialism, and downward and upward causation. Next, the concepts of emergence and resultant are explored and compared, including the related concepts of emergent synthesis and synthesis, epigenesis and geneticism, and nonlinear and linear dynamics. And finally, the concepts of robustness and homeostasis are considered and juxtaposed, along with the affiliated concepts of stochasticity and determinism, and evolvability and stasis. Crucially, the contrast between these concepts is critical for addressing the problems facing the biomedical and evidence-based approaches to medicine and healthcare. In a concluding chapter, the challenges facing the implementation of systems medicine, particularly P7 systems medicine, are addressed in terms of advancing medicine and its practice in the twenty-first century—especially as the coronavirus disease 2019 (COVID-19) pandemic wanes and disappears from the public consciousness over the next few years.

Table 1. Comparison of conceptual foundations between biomedicine and systems medicine (see text for details)

Biomedicine	**Systems Medicine**
Mechanism	Organicism
Reductionism	Wholism
Materialism	New materialism
Upward causation	Downward causation
Resultant	Emergence
Synthesis	Emergent synthesis
Geneticism	Epigeneticism
Determinism	Stochasticity
Homeostasis	Robustness
Linear dynamics	Nonlinear dynamics
Stasis	Evolvability

The present book, then, represents a sustained analysis of the conceptual foundations of contemporary systems medicine in contrast to the biomedical model and its associated EBM. Although the conceptual foundations of contemporary systems medicine are at best complex and highly nuanced, clinicians and other healthcare professions must need to have a firm grasp of these foundations of their field in order to navigate better the myriad changes that are currently taking place in contemporary medicine, as well as in the healthcare system in general, and the challenges facing it today (Marcum 2017a). To that end, this book attempts to introduce the reader to the fundamental concepts that are animating the development of contemporary systems medicine. Finally, it represents a sequel to a book (Marcum 2020) in which the path from systems biology to system medicine is charted and a revision of a book (Marcum 2009) in which the conceptual foundations of systems biology are examined.

Acknowledgments

Throughout the research and writing of this book, I was indebted not only to numerous colleagues, including especially Patrick Daly, Michael Loughlin, Andrew Miles, Cristian Saborido, Daniel Sulmasy, Felix Tretter, and Sona Vasudevan, but also to my students since I used part of the book's material to teach a course on the philosophy of medicine. Finally, I dedicate the book to the memory of my grandparents, William James and Martha (née Krause) Marcum, who instilled in me a passion for education and hard work.

Chapter 1

Biomedicine and Systems Medicine

Abstract

The biomedical model is currently the predominant approach to healthcare within the industrialized world, and it gave rise to evidence-based medicine (EBM) and its practice during the latter part of the twentieth century (Au 2021, Borck 2020, Lock and Nguyen 2018, Straus et al. 2019, Valles 2020). The model's conceptual foundation consists of reductionist mechanisms in which physiological and pathological processes are the homeostatic resultant of these mechanisms. Moreover, biomedicine is chiefly molecular in its approach to health and disease and is responsible for the current genomic approach to healthcare. Besides EBM, it also serves as a basis for approaches to systems medicine itself, particularly systems biomedicine (Liu 2010, Wolkenhauer et al. 2009) and molecular systems medicine (Tretter and Löffler-Stastka 2019, Tretter et al. 2021). However, systems medicine, especially as developed over the past several decades, represents a radical or even revolutionary shift from the biomedical model because of the latter's failure to address the deluge of chronic diseases plaguing the Western lifestyle (Gaines and Davis-Floyd 2004, Mykhalovskiy and Weir 2004). In this chapter, the biomedical model and its offspring EBM are initially discussed, followed by several types of systems medicine and culminating in P7 systems medicine.

Keywords: biomedicine, evidence-based medicine, network medicine, personalized medicine, precision medicine, systems medicine

1. Biomedicine and Evidence-Based Medicine

During the latter half of the twenty century, biomedicine, along with EBM, was the predominant model of healthcare in terms of education, research, and clinical practice (Cambrosio and Keating 2001, Marcum 2020).[1] The term biomedicine emerged between the two world wars and was associated with the U.S. military and civil research, although its immediate historical foundation was set in the nineteenth century (Marcum 2020). "From somewhere in the mid-nineteenth century," as Ilana Löwy claims, "doctors did not just evoke 'science;' they increasingly relied on laboratory sciences" (2011, p. 117). According to the biomedical model, health is the resultant or outcome of homeostatic mechanisms that maintain the proper or normal bodily functions, while disease is the consequence of a disruption in these mechanisms that results in abnormal or pathological dysfunctions. Moreover, biomedicine's advent overlaps with the emergence of molecular biology, especially with respect to the reduction of disease to its molecular components and mechanisms (Boniolo and Nathan 2017). Christopher Boorse's biostatistical theory is an excellent example of biomedicine's understanding of health and disease (Boorse 2014), as well as its limitations (Valles 2020). In this section, what constitutes biomedicine is explored, along with EBM, as well as critiques of both models and the impact COVID-19 has had on them.

1.1. Biomedicine

Biomedicine represents the culmination of the scientification of Western medicine during the twentieth century and is often identified as scientific medicine (Fangerau and Badura-Lotter 2019, Gaines and Davis-Floyd 2004, Valles 2020). Biomedicine is the outcome of the convergence of both the biomolecular and biological sciences with medicine in terms of medical knowledge and clinical practice for diagnosing and treating disease at the molecular and cellular level or scale. Moreover, Lani Russell points out the impact biomedicine had on understanding the nature of health and disease. Russell writes, biomedicine is "an approach to health and illness which defines health as the absence of disease, portraying the human organism as either functioning 'normally' or else dysfunctional and therefore diseased" (2014, p. 7). And as Bruno Strasser stresses, "biomedicine and biomedical research were understood as a kind of medicine that was closely associated with experimentation and the laboratory rather than doctor's knowledge and the clinic" (2014, p. 11).

---

[1] Personally, biomedicine was the model that I was taught as a student in the 1970s and then practiced throughout the 1980s and 1990s as a biomedical research scientist (Marcum et al. 1982, Marcum et al. 1984, Marcum and Rosenberg 1989, Torok et al. 1993).

Biomedicine exhibits several key features, including a dependence on the natural sciences, especially experimental sciences, and a reductionist stance towards biological processes (Krieger 1994, Valles 2020). The last feature results in the reduction of the patient to simply a body part—often a mechanical part (Marcum 2004). Moreover, Howard Stein has identified four tenets to biomedicine:

> (1) the "basic sciences": anatomy, physiology, biochemistry, microbiology, pathology; (2) the belief that medical science is and should be based upon rational, scientific, dispassionate, objective, professional judgment; (3) the belief that disease and its attendant suffering are ultimately to be understood in terms of pathological entities, organic in nature, and that treatment optimally consists of a technological procedure or intervention that results in a cure; (4) the belief that medical knowledge and skills are best organized by creating specialties around "organ systems" (1990, p. xiv).

Both health and disease then are defined and classified in terms of molecular, cellular, and organismic components and mechanisms (National Research Council 2011).

The biomedical model was certainly responsible for a variety of medical advances during the twentieth century, and its advocates claimed that the model is primarily responsible for both the length and quality of modern life in industrialized societies (National Research Council 2011). For example, the discovery of insulin is certainly a poster child for the power of the biomedical model with respect to both basic research and clinical application (Bliss 1982). But biomedicine's greatest success came with antibiotics and the cure of bacterial or infectious diseases, especially with the discovery of penicillin (Magner 2009). The biomedical approach for treating and curing disease was to develop pharmaceuticals drugs and surgical devices and procedures that restored normal mechanistic functioning. Finally, the model's conceptual foundations believed responsible for its success included mechanism, reductionism, materialism, geneticism, determinism, linear dynamics, and homeostasis, among other concepts (Marcum 2008a, Valles 2020). In a very real sense, biomedicine is a molecular approach to health and disease (Strasser and Fantini 1998, Tretter et al. 2021).

Another impact of biomedicine on medicine and society itself is the medicalization of bodily functions, spanning from birth to death (Nye 2003, Szasz 2007, Van Dijk et al. 2020). "Medicalization' describes a process," according to Peter Conrad, "by which nonmedical problems become defined and treated as medical problems, usually in terms of illness and disorders" (2007, p. 4). Examples of medicalization include sleep disorders, menopause, obesity, and erectile dysfunction; and, of course, it generates incredible revenues of the healthcare industry, as well as ethical problems (Blackburn 2011, Conrad et al. 2010). And the impact has led to overmedicalization, overdiagnosis, overtreatment, and polypharmacy (Brodersen 2017, Petrazzuoli et al. 2022, Treadwell and McCartney 2016). Overmedicalization has also led to the biomedicalization of society itself, along with the healthcare system (Clarke 2014, Clarke et al. 2021). "Biomedicalization is our term," as Adele Clarke and the other members of "the gang of five" originally described it, "for the increasingly complex, multisited, multidirectional processes of medicalization that today are being both extended and reconstituted through the emergent social forms and practices of a highly and increasingly technoscientific biomedicine" (Clarke et al. 2003, p. 162). Its impact ranges from bodily diseases and psychological disorders to social and lifestyle ills (Clarke et al. 2021).

The biomedical model, however, is not without its critics and detractors (Foss 2002, Fuller 2017, Hewa and Hetherington 1995, Kirkengen et al. 2016, Longino et al. 1995, Wade and Halligan 2004), especially from an anthropological and a sociological perspective and the charge that biomedicine resulted in a biomedicalization of society (Clarke et al. 2003, Lock and Gordon 1988). However, the most notable critic of biomedical model was George Engel (1977). Engel's criticism of the model focused on its reduction of illness to the molecules and mechanics of disease pathology and etiology. To replace the model, he introduced a biopsychosocial model of medicine and healthcare, which situated the biological elements of disease processes within the psychological and social dimensions of the patient's illness experience. Engel also situated his model within systems theory, which emphasizes the interrelatedness of component parts. His goal was for the patient to be treated as an autonomous and a whole person, with dignity, rather than simply as a diseased body part, which often adds to the patient's suffering (Cassell 2004).

The impact of Engel's biopsychosocial model, however, was generally restricted to psychiatry and primary care; and it was not adopted widely across medical disciplines and specialties (Ghaemi 2017). Engel's critics claimed that his model was simply too eclectic and lacked conceptual coherence for integrating the biological, psychological, and social dimensions of illness, primarily because it failed to incorporate general systems theory sufficiently

(Benning 2015, Kontos 2011). Engel (1977), as noted earlier, did cite literature on the application of systems theory to medicine, such as Ludwig von Bertalanffy (1974) and Ervin Laszlo (1972), but he did not incorporate systems theory in any significant detail. Although Engle's biopsychosocial model has attracted those who continue to defend it (Bolton and Gillett 2019, Farre and Rapley 2017, Tretter et al. 2021), the biomedical model has remained the standard for biomedical research and clinical practice, especially in terms of its current form as EBM (Rahim et al. 2012).

1.2. Evidence-Based Medicine

EBM is an offshoot of the biomedical model, even though the latter stresses the importance of pathological mechanisms for understanding and treating diseases, while the former appeared on the medical landscape towards the end of the twentieth century with the Evidence-Based Medicine Working Group at McMaster University in Canada (Claridge and Fabian 2005, Falzer 2021, Guyatt et al. 2015, Sur and Dahm 2011).[2] It was chiefly in response to the deluge of medical knowledge and information that was being published annually. Since then, it has become the predominant model for conducting biomedical research, for teaching not only physicians but also other healthcare professionals, and for practicing clinical medicine and healthcare—often known as evidence-based practice (Greenhalgh 2018, Houser and Oman 2011). In what now has become the standard definition of EBM, David Sackett and colleagues wrote, "Evidence based medicine is the conscientious, explicit, and judicious use of current best evidence in making decisions about the care of individual patients" (Sackett et al. 1996, p. 71). The assumption behind EBM and evidence-based healthcare is that by grounding clinical practice on solid research evidence, especially from randomized controlled trials, the best clinical outcome is possible if not guaranteed, given both the clinician's expertise and the patient's values and preferences.

The practice of EBM consists of five steps (Straus et al. 2019). The first involves asking pertinent questions concerning the disease's etiology and about the patient's diagnosis, prognosis, and possible treatments and interventions, or even prevention. The standard protocol for this step is captured in the acronym, PICO (Leonardo 2018). "P" stands for the patient

[2] Besides EBM, the biomedical model has also spawned other approaches to medicine, including translational medicine, precision and/or personalized medicine, stratified medicine, and genomic medicine (Au 2021).

who seeks medical attention and to which population the patient belongs, while "I" stands for the interventions and their comparison for diagnosing or treating the patient or population. "C" represents the comparison groups or populations undertaken for interventions, while "O" represents the sought after clinical outcome. The next step is to utilize the relevant literature to obtain the necessary evidence and information to answer the questions. The third step involves critically evaluating and appraising the evidence and information in terms of its soundness with respect to its veracity, its impact with respect to the magnitude of its effect, and its applicability in the clinical setting for the patient. In the penultimate step, the critical appraisal conducted in the previous step is integrated with both the clinician's expertise and the patient's values, preferences, and circumstances. The last step involves the clinician pondering and evaluating how well the first four steps were implemented to provide the best quality care possible.[3] In sum, EBM provides healthcare based on, as well as informed by, evidence from the professional literature, clinician, and patient.

EBM is (in)famous for the evidence pyramid in which the quality of the evidence for making sound clinical decisions presumably increases during ascension along the pyramid (Brighton et al. 2003, Pinkston 2020). At the base of the pyramid is expert opinion, along with theoretical and background information (Figure 1). The next level consists of observational studies, followed by case and case-controlled studies. The subsequent level consists of randomized controlled clinical trials, which are considered the "gold" standard of evidence (Barton 2000, Hackshaw 2009),[4] followed by systematic reviews of the trials. The pinnacle consists of meta-analyses, such as the Cochrane Reviews.[5] The pyramid has been heavily criticized and even pronounced "dead" (Tugwell and Knottnerus 2015), but it has continued to evolve even into the early twenty-first century (Murad et al. 2016, Rosner 2012, Shaneyfelt 2016). Although the pyramid remains a topic of discussion and debate, especially for philosophers of medicine, it has been abandoned by clinical practitioners for the GRADE system of determining the quality of the evidence—but still the various levels of evidence continue to guide the

---

[3] The five steps can be summarized as ask, acquire, appraise, apply, and audit (Rosenberg and Donald 1995).

[4] Several pundits challenge the "gold" standard ranking of randomized controlled trials (Cartwright 2007, Grossman and Mackenzie 2005, Kaptchuk 2001).

[5] Meta-analysis represents "a formal, epidemiologic, quantitative statistical technique that analyzes the results of different studies on the same topic and integrates the evidence into a single conclusion" (Mahmood et al. 2021, p. 2556).

evaluation of evidence (GRADE Working Group 2004).[6] In response to criticism, EBM has evolved to include both clinical expertise and patient values. In the most recent version of EBM, it is defined as "the integration of the best research evidence with our clinical expertise and our patient's unique values and circumstances" (Straus et al. 2019, p. 1).

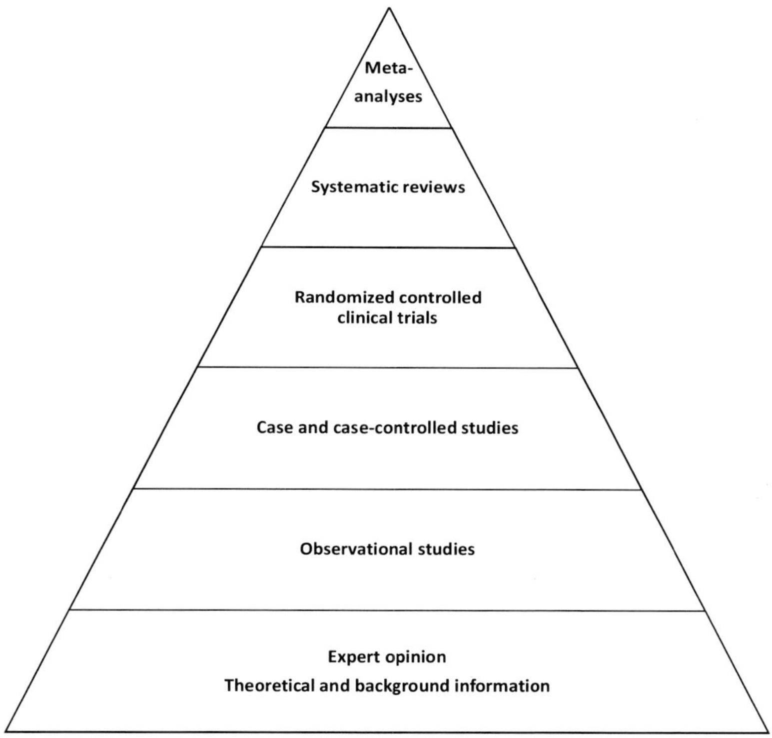

Figure 1. Evidence-Based Medicine pyramid of evidence.

EBM since its introduction has been criticized with respect to numerous issues and concerns (Cohen et al. 2004, Sehon and Stanley 2003). One of the more contentious issues has been the notion and nature of evidence itself (Greenhalgh et al. 2014, Martini 2021, Mebius et al. 2016, Worrall 2002). One criticism in particular charges that the evidence is too narrowly confined to the

[6] GRADE stands for "Grading of Recommendations, Assessment, Development and Evaluations" and consists of four levels—very low, low, moderate, and high—which are used to evaluate the evidence's quality (Guyatt et al. 2008).

statistical evidence from random controlled trials, systematic reviews, and meta-analyses and that additional types of evidence must be included for a robust evidence-based approach to medicine. Specifically, a group of over forty clinicians and philosophers made a clarion call for an expanded notion of evidence to include mechanistic evidence, i.e., evidence provided by the disease mechanism itself (Anjum et al. 2020). This robust EBM reflects the evidential pluralism of Federica Russo and Jon Williamson (2007), which has become known as the Russo-Williamson Thesis (Illari 2011). Although the notion of mechanistic evidence does have its critics (Howick 2011, Solomon 2015), it has become an important part of the biomedical landscape, especially during the COVID-19 pandemic (Aronson et al. 2021, Greenhalgh et al. 2022).

Besides the debate over evidence, other contested issues associated with and criticisms of EBM include its strictly myopic empirical approach to clinical outcomes based on randomized clinical trials; difficulty of implementing such trials for individual patients; prohibiting clinician and patient autonomy; its cookbook approach; time constraints and unrealistic expectations placed upon clinicians; and most importantly EBM itself is not evidence-based (Cohen et al. 2004, Dopson et al. 2003, Trinder and Reynolds 2000). Given the debate throughout the twenty-first century, Trisha Greenhalgh and colleagues claim that EBM is undergoing a crisis, particularly in terms of the quality of the evidence in the published literature; the marginal benefits or effect size reported for many clinical trials; and difficulties in mapping evidence-based guidelines onto complex multimorbid clinical cases (Greenhalgh et al. 2014).[7] Moreover, Joachim Sturmberg (2019) contends that EBM's philosophical foundation is limited to simple linear causation when most diseases and illnesses represent complex nonlinear causation. Finally, in homage to Sackett, John Ioannidis (2016) argues that commercial interests and conflicts of interests are hijacking EBM.[8]

1.3. COVID-19 Challenge

Although the COVID-19 pandemic startled the global community, still the emergence of viral and other infectious diseases has been presaged to plague humanity with possibly no relief in sight (Garrett 1994). COVID-19 has

---

[7] The crisis is rather ironic since EBM was initially hailed as a Kuhnian paradigm shift (Guyatt et al. 1992), although this claim too has been contested (Sehon and Stanley 2003).

[8] Jeremy Howick (2019) also raises the issue of cooperate sponsorship and funding of clinical research, which he calls the financial bias.

revealed the serious challenges facing the biomedical model, especially in terms of therapeutics (Rehman et al. 2021). Although several drugs have been repurposed or repositioned, such as azithromycin, bevacizumab, chloroquine and hydroxychloroquine, favipiravir, interferons, ivermectin, lopinavir, remdesivir, ribavirin, and ritonavir, to treat severe acute respiratory syndrome coronavirus 2 (SARS-CoV-2) infection, few if any have been effective to date (Ng et al. 2021, Grundeis et al. 2023, Popp et al. 2022, Singh et al. 2021). However, the one challenge biomedicine met was the production of effective and safe vaccines, especially the mRNA vaccines, although the current challenge is to develop a universal vaccine (Morens et al. 2022).

Basically, the challenges of the COVID-19 pandemic for biomedicine are two-fold. The first is understanding the biology of SARS-CoV-2 and the host's response to the virus, as well as genetic variants of the virus (Catanzaro et al. 2020, Guilger-Casagrande et al. 2021, Shereen et al. 2020). An associated challenge to the first is the restraint the pandemic has placed on conducting biomedical research (Smith and Goodhew 2021). The second challenge is performing clinical trials to show the efficacy and safety of repositioned or innovative drugs. Generally, such trials can take years if not decades to conduct (Brown et al. 2022). This latter challenge is also one that faces EBM directly.

The basic premise of EBM is for the clinician to incorporate the best evidence, especially from randomized controlled trials, with the patient's values and preferences to provide the best quality care. Unfortunately, given the speed by which the coronavirus spread during the early 2020s, time was of essence for obtaining quality evidence to treat patients suffering from coronavirus infection (Landucci and Volpe 2020). Since such trials cannot necessarily be expedited unreasonably, a clinician treating infected patients is forced to make a judgment on how best to proceed, given uncertain or no evidence. The challenge of COVID-19 to EBM has Greenhalgh (2020) fearing that the pandemic is a nemesis for EBM. Her fear is that the principles upon which EBM is founded, which include certainty, linear causality and predictability, are no match for a complex pandemic, which exhibits uncertainty, nonlinear causality, and unpredictability. Simon Carley and colleagues summarize their assessment of the COVID-19's challenge to EBM accordingly,

> The principles of EBM are more important now than at any other time in our careers. We must collectively do all that we can to ensure that our response to the pandemic is based on the science and not on the

emotional, political or economic issues that challenge it (Carley et al. 2020, p. 574).

Finally, Felix Tretter and colleagues note that the pandemic has exposed the lack of integration of medical specialties that are associated with EBM, including molecular systems medicine, and they propose an organismal systems medicine approach to address the challenge of integrating these specialties to tackle the complexities associated with the COVID-19 pandemic (Tretter and Franz-Balsen 2020, Tretter and Marcum 2022, Tretter et al. 2021).

2. Systems Medicine

With the initial completion of the Human Genome Program in the early 2000s (International Human Genome Sequencing Consortium 2004), the way was paved for the emergence of a systems biology approach to investigating the complexity of biological organisms (Ferrell 2009, Galperin and Ellison 2006, Marcum 2009, Palsson 2006, 2015, Russell and Superti-Furga 2005, Westerhoff and Alberghina 2005), which eventually gave rise to the emergence of systems medicine (Marcum 2020, Morel et al. 2004). The current high-throughput technologies of genomics, epigenomics, proteomics, metabolomics, and microbiomics, in particular, provide vast amounts of data about the dynamic states of cells and tissues, whether normal or pathological (Aggarwal and Lee 2003, Ballereau et al. 2013, Bruggeman and Westerhoff 2007, Fanos 2016). Research in systems medicine today employs systems biology, computational analyses, and formal models to gain insights into omics data, especially for developing safe and effective therapeutics as well as preventive medicine (Assmus et al. 2006, Davidov et al. 2003, Hood et al. 2004, Schmitz and Wolkenhauer 2016). Before launching into the conceptual and theoretical foundations of systems medicine in this section, what systems medicine is exactly needs to be examined, which also brings up the various types of systems medicine.[9] Systems medicine is not a single entity but includes a variety of configurations such as systems biomedicine, molecular systems medicine, personalized medicine, precision medicine, network medicine, and P4, P5, P6, and P7 systems medicine.

---

[9] For a more detailed discussion on the nature of systems medicine and its various types, see Marcum (2020).

2.1. Defining Systems Medicine

Unfortunately, no consensus definition for systems medicine exists within the literature, although there are several astute and helpful definitions. For example, Gilles Clermont and colleagues from a workshop on systems medicine defined it "as the application of systems biology to the prevention of, understanding and modulation of, and recovery from developmental disorders and pathologic processes in human health" (Clermont et al. 2009, p. 2). Although systems biology is an important discipline for understanding systems medicine, they acknowledge that systems biology pertains more to the molecular scale while systems medicine must "incorporate mesoscale clinical information into its models; in particular, classic clinical variables, biomarkers, and medical imaging data" (Clermont et al. 2009, p. 2). Moreover, systems medicine also involves multiscale modeling from the molecular to organisms, populations, and ecosystems, and they give the example of malignant tumors and their complexity. Besides systems biology, systems medicine also relies on other disciplines such as clinical medicine and population epidemiology.

Joseph Loscalzo and colleagues also define systems medicine in terms of systems biology. Accordingly, "systems medicine is defined as an emerging discipline that integrates comprehensively computational modeling, 'omics data, physiological data, clinical data, and environmental factors to predict model disease expression (the pathophenome)" (Wang et al. 2015, p. 142). Besides systems biology, systems pharmacology, personalized medicine, and environmental factors are also important constituents that compose a systems approach to medicine and healthcare. As the authors claim, wholistic integration of these various disciplines is key to implementing systems medicine and to understanding how it differs from the biomedical reductionistic approach. Indeed, such integration is viewed as a "guiding principle" of systems medicine that "provides a more comprehensive and coherent picture of complex research problems" (Wolkenhauer et al. 2013, p. 505).

After reviewing several definitions of systems medicine within the literature, Marc Kirschner (2016) distinguishes between a strategic definition and a scientific definition of systems medicine. Kirschner defines systems medicine strategically as "an interdisciplinary approach to improve diagnosis, prognosis, and therapy, through the integration of multiple data and the integration of expertise from all relevant disciplines including biostatistics, bioinformatics, health informatics, and Systems Biology into clinical research" (2016, p. 4). He then defines scientific systems medicine as "the science that studies how physiological functions emerge from the interactions between cells and tissues and how this influences the behavior of these components in the human body" (2016, p. 4). In sum, systems medicine utilizes systems biology and systems thinking to investigate bodily and pathological functions and complexity from a systems theoretical approach and to improve clinical outcomes.

Finally, Sebastian Schleidgen and colleagues offer a "précising" definition of systems medicine in terms of providing a clear definition that adheres to specific criteria (necessity, non-circularity, non-redundancy, consistency, non-vagueness, and coherence) in an attempt to eliminate definitional vagueness. After mining the literature for around 100 definitions of systems medicine, they define it as

> an approach seeking to improve medical research (i.e., the understanding of complex processes occurring in diseases, pathologies and health states as well as innovative approaches to drug discovery) and health care (i.e., prevention, prediction, diagnosis and treatment) through stratification by means of Systems Biology (i.e., data integration, modeling, experimentation and bioinformatics) (Schleidgen et al. 2017, p. 1)

In sum, systems medicine involves the incorporation of systems biology into medical research and clinical practice, as Clermont and colleagues assert, to improve clinical outcomes. But as they admit, their "definition is *not* a 'consensus definition'...[since] consensus was neither a goal nor a criterion" (Schleidgen et al. 2017, p. 14). Rather their goal was simply to articulate a definition that could be used effectively to address the clinical advantages of systems medicine.

2.2. Systems Biomedicine

In the early 1990s, Takenobu Kamada (1991, 1992) originally introduced systems biomedicine in an attempt to combine systems science, molecular biology, and engineering with biomedicine. The goal of systems biomedicine is to treat the patient as a whole person and not simply as a diseased body part. According to Kamada, "a disease is not only the malfunction of an organ, but that of the mechanism of a human body, a 'holon'" (1991, p. 1). Arthur Koestler coined the term "holon" several decades earlier to resolve the divide between atomism and holism and "to supplant the dualistic way of thinking in terms of 'parts' and 'wholes,' which is so deeply engrained in our mental habits, by a multi-levelled, stratified approach" (1970, p. 136). According to Koestler, holons represent sub-wholes along a hierarchical continuum from the micro-level to the macro-level. "The organism," then for Koestler, "is to be regarded as a multi-levelled hierarchy of semi-autonomous sub-wholes, branching into sub-wholes of a lower order, and so on" (1970, p. 148). And as Kamada concludes, "understanding of human being under the holonism theory…will unify directions in molecular biology, medical engineering and medicosociology to provide the new paradigm, '*systems biomedicine*'" (1991, p. 1).

Systems biomedicine is a multifaceted discipline that integrates the biomedical sciences with systems theory and thinking, systems biology, and other sciences and systems sciences, along with medical informatics, nanobiotechnology, omics technology, and computational technology (Kim et al. 2013, Liu 2010, Medina 2013, Wolkenhauer et al. 2009, Wu et al. 2016, Zhang et al. 2013). "Systems biomedicine," according to Xiangdong Wang and colleagues, "is an interdisciplinary field of study that looks at the systems of the human body as part of an integrated whole, incorporating biochemical, physiological, and environmental interactions" (Wu et al. 2016, p. 324). Although it strives to improve clinical outcomes, its emphasis is more on biomedical, big data, and translational research rather than on clinical practice (Capobianco and Lió 2014, Turanli et al. 2017). As Depei Liu and colleagues write, systems biomedicine's chief "aim is to reveal the patho-physiologic mechanism of disease" (Zhang et al. 2013, p. 140). However, one of its major aims is "to apply mechanistic insights to clinical application and to improve patients' quality of life" (Antony et al. 2012, p. 604).

Systems biomedicine relies heavily upon computational modeling of vast omics data for both basic research and clinical application (Aurich and Thiele 2016, Batra et al. 2022, Dubitzky 2016). In terms of basic research, Liu and colleagues champion the integrated personalized omics profiling or iPOP for determining the disease phenotype, not simply to treat the disease but also to prevent its future expression (Zhang et al. 2013). In other examples, a systems biomedicine approach is taken to investigate and explain protein-protein interactions or PPIs in various disease processes and networks (Sevimoglu and Arga 2014, Slater et al. 2020). In terms of clinical application, for example, systems biomedicine provides the resources, especially in terms of bioinformatics, for treating cancer metastasis based on the clinical data for the individual patient (Singh 2022, Wu et al. 2016). Other examples include rabies (Azimzadeh Jamalkandi et al. 2016) and lung diseases (Zeng et al. 2018).

Finally, systems biomedicine is a discipline with respect to institutional organizations and professional literature. In terms of institutions, the best known is Luxembourg's Centre for Systems Biomedicine (https://wwwen.uni.lu/lcsb). Part of the Centre's mission is to conduct basic systems research to "analyse the mechanisms of disease pathogenesis" and to "identify and validate new targets for disease prevention and intervention" (https://wwwen.uni.lu/lcsb/vision_mission). University of California at Los Angeles is another institution that has a vibrant Center for Systems Biomedicine (https://www.uclahealth.org/gastro/csbm). "Systems biomedicine," according to its website, "can be described as an emerging approach to biomedical science that seeks to integratively infer, annotate, and quantify multi-variate complexity of the molecular and cellular processes of living systems, with ultimate aim of constructing formal algorithmic models for prediction of process outcomes from component input" (https://www.uclahealth.org/gastro/csbm/systems-biomedicine).

Besides institutions, systems biomedicine also enjoys a robust professional literature. For example, Edison Liu and Douglas Lauffenberger (2010) edited a book on the systems biomedicine and its conceptual foundations, computational modeling, and research and clinical applications. Moreover, the journal *Systems Biomedicine* was founded in 2013 and published by Taylor & Francis. In an editorial introducing the journal, Sol Efroni, editor-in-chief, wrote that systems biomedicine "is about embracing methods from systems biology for their practical uses in biomedicine" (2013, p. 1). Although only two volumes of the journal were published, its aim was to publish articles that investigated the molecular networks underlying diseases of the immune and central nervous systems, as well as cancer. One example of such an article was on the disease network or diseasome (Emmert-Streib et al. 2013).

2.3. Molecular Systems Medicine

As biomedicine and EBM continued to develop during the twentieth century, it focused on the molecular components of pathophysiological processes and eventually gave rise to molecular medicine (Runge and Patterson 2006, Trent 2012). "Molecular medicine," according to Jens Kurreck and Cy Aron Stein, "is a discipline dedicated to understanding normal and pathological cellular processes at the molecular level" (2016, p. 2). Molecular medicine's origins are rooted in Linus Pauling's pivotal paper on sickle cell anemia in which the disease's etiology was defined strictly in molecular terms (Pauling et al. 1949). And molecular medicine continued to grow in reputation and influence until it was touted by the end of the twentieth century as medicine's future "in a changing world" (Culliton 1995, p. 1). Although molecular medicine's future seemed unbridled, problems soon appeared on the horizon—especially in terms of gene therapy (Marcum 2005, Steel 2005).

After the appearance of molecular systems biology, molecular systems medicine soon emerged to tackle the problems challenging molecular medicine from a systems perspective (Boogerd et al. 2013, Latterich 2005, Tretter 2019). As for molecular medicine, it too has been championed as the future of medicine in the twenty-first century. "Molecular systems medicine," as Mingyu Liang and colleagues claim "is the future of medicine and biomedicine. One must understand humans as molecular systems to truly understand human health and disease" (Liang et al. 2022, p. 2). However, molecular systems medicine faces a major issue in that it is too reductionistic to explain complex diseases and comorbidities, particularly from a wholistic viewpoint. For example, Felix Tretter and Henriette Löffler-Stastka charge that "it ignores emergence in multi-level systems: emergence of life from abiotic matter, emergence of consciousness from biotic matter, and emergence of culture from conscious systems" (2019, p. 4). Finally, besides its challenging issues molecular systems medicine has been instrumental in the rise of both personalized and precision medicine (Almeida et al. 2013).

2.4. Personalized Medicine

With the completion of the Human Genome Project in the early part of the twenty-first century, the biomedical community was enthralled with the possibility of tailoring treatment to fit a patient's uniquely individual therapeutic needs, based on genomics and other omics technologies (Jain 2021, Prainsack 2017, Snyder 2016). Although personalized medicine became fashionable among biomedical scientists and clinicians, confusion emerged in the literature as to exactly what it is. To clarify that confusion, Schleidgen and colleagues identified three major types of personalized medicine, through exploring the literature (Schleidgen et al. 2013). The first type is traditional in the sense that a clinician engages a patient personally in the clinical encounter. The next type involves stratifying patients into groups and subgroups based on specific genomic and other omics markers. The final type pertains to treating the patient as a whole person, who is embedded within a social and culture context. Based on these three types, they concluded that personalized medicine

> seeks to improve tailoring and timing of preventive and therapeutic measures by utilizing biological information and biomarkers on the level of molecular disease pathways, genetics, proteomics as well as metabolomics (Schleidgen et al. 2013, p. 9).

Unfortunately, the debate over the nature of personalized medicine has not subsided, especially in terms of its humanistic dimensions (Giroux 2020). For instance, Nathan Cherny and colleagues insist that "Biological Personalized Therapeutics" is a better designation for personalized medicine (Cherny et al. 2014), while alternative designations like stratified medicine and individualized medicine continue to surface in the professional literature (March and Schott 2017. Pokorska-Bocci et al. 2014).

The pharmaceutical industry certainly became invested in the personalized medical approach to pharmaceuticals by tailoring drugs in terms of their efficacy and safety for individual patients (Bates 2010, Ginsburg and McCarthy 2001, Shastry 2007). During the end of the twenty century and at the beginning of the twenty-first century, around a dozen pharmaceutical firms formed "The SNP Consortium" in which the firms planned to map genetic variations associated with sundry diseases (Holden 2002, Thorisson and Stein 2003).[10] SNPs stands for a single-nucleotide polymorphisms within DNA sequences. These polymorphisms can be in protein coding sequences or exomes of the genome but need not be in the exomes (Edwards et al. 2007). SNPs occur on average around every 500-600 base pairs, and they often serve simply as markers for particular diseases (Taylor et al. 2001, Weiner and Hudson 2002). Moreover, SNPs can be grouped together into inherited haplotypes (Shastry 2003, Voisey and Morris 2008). The SNP Consortium's goal is not only to develop new drugs for treating genetic diseases but also to tailor those drugs in terms of their efficacy and safety. Thus, personalized medicine's slogan has become "the right drug, for the right patient, at the right time" (Annas 2014, p. 159).

[10] The International HapMap Project was established in the early twenty-first century to generate a database of common SNPs associated with various disease phenotypes (The International HapMap Consortium 2003, 2005, Thorisson et al. 2005).

Although enthusiasm for personalized medicine was high at the beginning of the twenty-first century, its development was rather stunted because of technical, political, and ethical challenges (Ginsburg and McCarthy 2001, Goetz and Schork 2018, Hood 2003). With respect to technical challenges, SNP identification and mapping take time and are expensive, even though new technologies with respect to biochips and microarrays are advancing mapping efforts (Jain 2021, Nair 2010). Although technical advances are happening frequently, such as next generation sequencing, the immensity of the genomic data is hampering the analysis of such data (Fernald et al. 2011, Kilpinen and Barrett 2013). In terms of political challenges, institutional infrastructure is sorely required to support research and is being supplied but not quickly enough (Alyass et al. 2015, Bates 2010). However, a number of funding initiatives, such as the U.S. National Center for Advancing Translational Sciences (https://ncats.nih.gov/), are facilitating transfer of basic genomic technology to the bedside. Finally, ethical challenges include the privacy and confidentiality, as well as ownership, of genomic and other omics data, the gap between informed consent and understanding omics data, and genetic discrimination, especially in terms of employment and health insurance (Joly et al. 2014, Salari and Larijani 2017).

Finally, one of the more major problems or challenges confronting personalized medicine is its precision with respect to identifying the exact genetic defect and its relationship to the disease phenotype (Ibrahim et al. 2016). What is particularly problematic is that SNPs and haplotypes are not exact or specific enough in terms of explaining causally disease etiology. What is needed is greater precision in terms of genomic sequencing, and next-generation DNA sequencing is championed to provide the needed precision (Hu et al. 2021, Kchouk et al. 2017). The success of next-generation sequencing is best illustrated in the clinical case of Nicholas Volker, who developed inflammatory bowel disease before his second birthday and underwent over 100 unsuccessful surgical procedures during the next three years to treat the disease (DeWeerdt 2016, Johnson and Gallagher 2016). Next-generation sequencing revealed that Volter was suffering from a rare immunological disease, X-linked lymphoproliferative syndrome 2, due to an *XIAP* gene deficiency (Longoni et al. 2014). The Volter case attracted considerable media attention, and it not only established personalized medicine (Feero and Guttmacher 2014), but it also heralded the rise of precision medicine in that disease etiology could now be identified in terms of the patient's precise genomic sequence (Juengst et al. 2016, Katsnelson 2013).

2.5. Precision Medicine

In his 30 January 2015 State of the Union address, then President Barack Obama announced the U.S. Precision Medicine Initiative (Ashley 2015, Collins and Varmus 2015, Vegter 2018). In that address, Obama defended the initiative accordingly,

> Doctors have always recognized that every patient is unique, and doctors have always tried to tailor their treatments as best they can to individuals… And that's the promise of precision medicine—delivering the right treatments, at the right time, every time to the right person (The White House 2015).

The initiative was originally based on the U.S. National Research Council's 2011 report, *Toward Precision Medicine* (National Research Council 2011, Olson 2017). And the term, precision medicine, was introduced earlier within the healthcare literature by Clayton Christensen and coauthors: "Only when diseases are diagnosed precisely can therapy that is predictably effective for each patient be developed and standardized. We term this domain precision medicine" (Christensen et al. 2009, p. xxii).

To implement precision medicine nationally in the U.S., the National Institutes of Health launched in 2016 the Precision Medicine Initiative Cohort Program, "All of Us" (National Institutes of Health 2016). The program consists of an ongoing longitudinal study to collect behavioral, clinical, environmental, omics, and physiological data on over one million participants and to address ethical, legal and social issues associated with the initiative (Sankar and Parker 2017). In a 2019 special report on the program, over 175,000 participants had contributed biospecimens to date of which greater than 80% were collected from historically underrepresented people in biomedical research (All of Us Research Program Investigators 2019). Both the public and professional communities have been enthusiastic about the program, especially in terms of its diversity (Fox 2020, Mapes 2020, Ramirez et al. 2022).

Although precision and personalized medicine share much in common, precision medicine, in contrast to personalized medicine, strives for a finer-grained stratification of patient subpopulations, i.e., subpopulations that have an n = 1, and their different susceptibility to therapy (Ashley 2016, Kosorok and Laber 2019). This finer-grained stratification is defined by the committee responsible for the *Toward Precision Medicine* report as "the tailoring of medical treatment to the individual characteristics of each patient" (National Research Council 2011, p. 125). Based on the report's definition, "the power of precision medicine," according to Geoffrey Ginsburg and Kathryn Phillips, "lies in its ability to guide health care decisions toward the most effective treatment for a given patient and, thus, improve care quality while reducing the need for unnecessary diagnostic testing and therapies" (2018, p. 694). Finally, precision medicine strives not only for reproducibility of omics and clinical data but also for the data's accuracy with respect to their facticity, especially in terms of the data's precision for diagnosing and treating diseases (Ashley 2016, Jameson and Longo 2015). To that end, one of the more immediate goals for the precision medicine initiative is to support genomic research on carcinogenesis, which has begun to yield considerable advances into detecting and understanding cancer (Nassar et al. 2020, Saulsberry and Olopade 2021, Shin et al. 2018). Indeed, a recent report on analysis of participants in the *All of Us* Research Program revealed the detection of cancer in a significant portion of the participants (Aschebrook-Kilfoy et al. 2022).

An important longer-term goal of precision medicine is developing a new taxonomy or classification of diseases or what is historically called nosology (Berman 2018, National Research Council 2011). Traditionally, nosology was founded on correlating clinical symptoms and signs with the patient's pathological state. However, precision medicine's disease taxonomy is based on the disease's genetic or genomic composition. This new disease taxonomy has important implications for the reference class problem, i.e., no patient reference class is ever complete (Boniolo et al. 2021, Dahabreh et al. 2016, Hájek 2007). In other words, precision treatment for the unique patient avoids dangerous heterogeneous side effects of therapy often associated with large reference classes.

Although precision medicine has gained notoriety among biomedical scientists and clinicians, critics have raised technical, practical, political, social, and ethical concerns and challenges about its clinical implementation (Duffy 2016, Sankar and Parker 2017, Verma and Barh 2017). For example, one of the more pressing challenges is technical in terms of developing the technology not only with respect to obtaining sufficient omics data required for practicing precision medicine but also the computation power for analyzing and understanding those data (Vlahou et al. 2018). Another challenge is practical in terms of incorporating precision medicine technology within the clinical encounter, especially when such technology can often be disruptive for the clinician (Hilty et al. 2021). Finally, ethical concerns emerge over genetic essentialism in which people are categorized in terms of their genomes (Heine et al. 2017). Despite these concerns and challenges, precision medicine is certainly viewed as an integral part of medicine's future (Denny and Collins 2021).

2.6. Network Medicine

Another approach to analyzing complex phenomena besides systems theory and science is network theory and science (Barabási 2016, Estrada and Knight 2015, Lewis 2011, Meidanis 2021, Newman 2018). Network theory and science involve graphing the relationships and interactions among various components of a network or system. And the fundamental structure of a network consists of nodes, which are discrete elements within the network, and edges, which represent the relationships or connections among the various nodes. In terms of network topology, a node can represent a hub if it has multiple connections with other nodes, especially with peripheral nodes. Networks also display particular dynamics in how different nodes function with respect to their edges, which can explain the overall performance of networks (Newman et al. 2006). Network dynamics, especially in the biological and biomedical sciences, are contingent on the topological arrangements and starting concentrations of nodal elements, as well as the strength and direction of nodal connections and interactions (Junker and Schreiber 2011, Zhang 2018).

Network medicine is an extension of systems biomedicine, molecular systems medicine, and precision medicine with respect to implementing network or graph theory in analyzing disease mechanisms, and it represents the current application of network theory and science to twenty-first century medicine (Barabási et al. 2011, Loscalzo et al. 2017). Specifically, it is used to analyze and model the various components responsible for disease etiology in terms of PPIs, gene-protein interactions, and even disease-phenotype interactions (Chan and Loscalzo 2012, Ivanov et al. 2016, Silverman et al. 2022). The fundamental unit for network medicine is the interactome, which consists of a ~25,000 protein-coding gene network, along with RNA networks, PPI networks, metabolic networks, and regulatory networks (Sonawane et al. 2019, Vidal et al. 2011).

From analysis of different interactomes, various genes have been identified to be involved in chronic diseases and many of them represent hub genes that are associated with a modular core of genes within a genomic network or interactome (Geronikolou et al. 2016, Maiorino et al. 2020). In other words, sets of essential genes are highly connected with one another, in contrast to non-essential genes that are located within a network's modular periphery and are not highly connected with one another. Moreover, many diseases share genes such that mutation or alteration of a particular gene in one functional network module can lead to expression of a different disease within another functional network module and thereby account for comorbidities (Akram and Liao 2019, Belling et al. 2017).

An important outcome of mapping the interactome for various diseases in terms of network medicine has been the introduction of the diseasome, which consists of a modular network composed of specific interacting genes and proteins involved in the mechanism of disease etiology (Goh and Choi 2012, Hosseininejad and Hashempour 2017). Additional investigation of these diseasomes, especially with respect to PPIs, resulted in the discovery of the "core diseasome" (Janjić and Pržulj 2012). This core is homogenous in its composition and consists of driver genes that are responsible for expression of disease phenotypes. The cancerome is an example of such a diseasome, which is assembled through the analysis of integrative molecular components and factors constituting a tumor (Jalili et al. 2016). Moreover, the assemblage of the cancerome network consists of molecular, functional, and clinical factors involved in the various components and processes of carcinogenesis. Finally, the goal of network medicine, especially with respect to therapeutics, is the development of the drugome in which pharmaceutical drugs are designed to treat individual patients in a personalized and precise way (Boran and Iyengar 2010, Chen et al. 2014, Zhou et al. 2016).

2.7. From P3 to P7 Systems Medicine

With the completion of the Human Genome Project in the early part of the twenty-first century, systems biology emerged to analyze the vast amounts of data obtained from the various omics technologies (Marcum 2009, Trewavas 2006). Systems medicine soon followed in the footsteps of systems biology (Marcum 2020). In the early twenty-first century, Hood and colleagues initially introduced P3 systems medicine that was predictive, preventive, and personalized and then expanded it to P4 systems medicine with an additional P for participatory. P4 systems medicine was then expanded by other advocates of systems medicine even further with additional Ps, such as psycho-cognitive, population, and political, to yield P5 and P6 systems medicine. Finally, a P7 systems medicine has been recently proposed that includes additional Ps, especially in terms of humanizing systems medicine. Each of these systems medicine is briefly introduced in the remainder of this section.

2.7.1. P3 and P4 Systems Medicine

Hood and colleagues proposed a notion of systems medicine, which they initially called P3 systems medicine and then expanded it to P4 systems medicine (Hood et al. 2004, Hood et al. 2012, Hood 2013, Marcum 2020). The first P stands for predictive and involves the identification of SNPs associated with disease etiology. The second P stands for preventive and involves the development of drugs and other therapeutic interventions to block or prevent the disease's expression or to mitigate its damage if expressed. The third P stands for personalized and entails the patient's individual omics and clinical data, as well as illness experience. And finally, the fourth P stands for participatory and pertains to the patient's full and active participation in either treating and managing or preventing the disease. In sum, P4 systems medicine for Hood and colleagues is not so much reactive in treating the disease as it is proactive in preventing it.

2.7.2. P5 and P6 Systems Medicine

Hood's P4 systems medicine has served as a scaffolding upon which other clinicians have appended additional Ps (Marcum 2020). For example, Muin Khoury and colleagues added a population P to P4 medicine to develop a P5 systems medicine in which each of the four Ps is viewed through a population or public health perspective (Khoury et al. 2012). Santo Davide Ferrara (2017) introduced another example of P5 medicine that adds a political P to P4 medicine, particularly with respect to tackling bio-medicolegal injustices and thereby protecting the patient's dignity and values from being compromised. A third type of P5 medicine incorporates a psycho-cognitive P into P4 medicine to include both the patient's behavioral and cognitive dimensions (Pravettoni and Triberti 2020). Nicola Bragazzi (2013a) has introduced the notion of psychiatome to denote this P. Finally, proponents of this latter P5 medicine have enlarged it to include a public P, to devise a P6 medicine (Bragazzi and Del Puente 2013). Bragazzi (2013b) illustrates this type of systems medicine with the clinical case of Salvatore Iaconesi, who was diagnosed with a brain tumor and decided to make his clinical records public to challenge the proscriptions and isolation that cancer patients often suffer.

2.7.3. P7 Systems Medicine

Recently, a P7 systems medicine was introduced to humanize systems medicine (Marcum 2021). The proposed P7 medicine builds off the diverse types of P3-6 systems medicine not only in terms of including the various Ps proposed so far, but also with respect to differentiating between two Ps—the physico-biomolecular P and the personal P. These two specific Ps are often conflated as the personalized P in other approaches to systems medicine. Importantly, the personal P, which involves the notion of personhood, addresses especially the criticism of Hood's P4 medicine as impersonal (Horwitz et al. 2013, Vogt et al. 2016), in order to render P7 medicine as personal in a humanistic manner rather than simply in a technical way. Specifically, the personal P is developed in terms of traditional personalism and contemporary new materialism. The proposed P7 systems medicine, which includes both precision and personalized medicine via the personal P, is composed of seven Ps, which can be divided into two major categories. The first category consists of four P-components, the physico-biomolecular P or P1 component, the psycho-cognitive P or P2 component, the populational-public P or P3 component, and the personal P or P4 component, along with their associated biomes and systems sciences (Table 2). The first three P components are integrated or entangled to generate the personal P (Figure 2).

Table 2. P7 medicine's P-components, with associated biomes/omics and systems sciences (see text for details)

P-Components	Biomes/omics	Systems Sciences
P1 (Physico-biomolecular P)	Genomics/Epigenomics	Systems genetics
	Transcriptomics/Proteomics	Systems cell biology
	Metabolomics/Nutrigenomics	Systems nutrition
P2 (Psycho-cognitive P)	Connectomics	Systems neuroscience
	Cognomics	Systems psychology
	Psychiatome	Systems psychiatry
P3 (Population-public P)	Exposomics	Systems epidemiology
	Microbiomics	Systems microbiology
	Enviromics/Environomics	Systems ecology
P4 (Personal P)	Physiome	Systems physiology
	Pathome	Systems pathology
	Personome	Lifestyle science

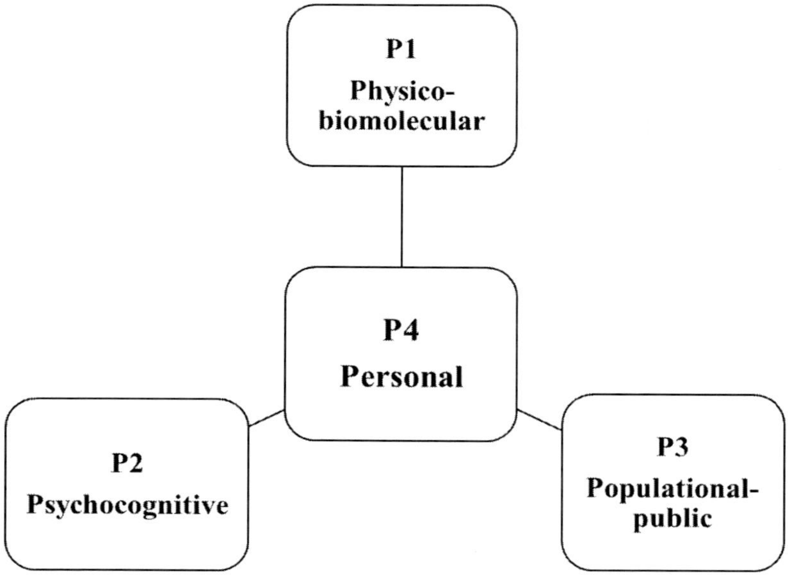

Figure 2. Integration of the P1-3 components to form the personal P4 (see text for details).

The second category of Ps composing P7 medicine consists of the three P-actions, which consists of the predictive P or P5, the participatory P or P6, and the preventive P or P7. The interactions of the P-actions conform to a specific configuration, which is important for operationalizing and implementing P7 medicine clinically. To that end, both prediction (P5) and participation (P6) are integrated with one another for the prevention (P7) of an illness (Figure 3). Importantly, the three P-actions must be carried out for each of the first three P-components or insufficient information is obtained to make a clinical decision and can mislead the clinician and patient as to the best course of action. When the first three P-components have been actionized through P5-7, then they are entangled materially to create the personal P4 (Figure 4). Once created, P4 is actionized through the three P-actions and the patient can thereby be treated in both a personalized and precise manner. In other words, possible health risks are more precisely predictable based on the data and information obtained from the various P-components and the patient can be motivated to participate optimally either in preventing the health risk and thereby maintaining health or in treating or managing the disease. In sum, P7 medicine as a robust type of systems medicine through both the P-components and P-actions, which provide the means for both personalized and precision medicine to optimize health and to minimize illness—whether physical or mental.

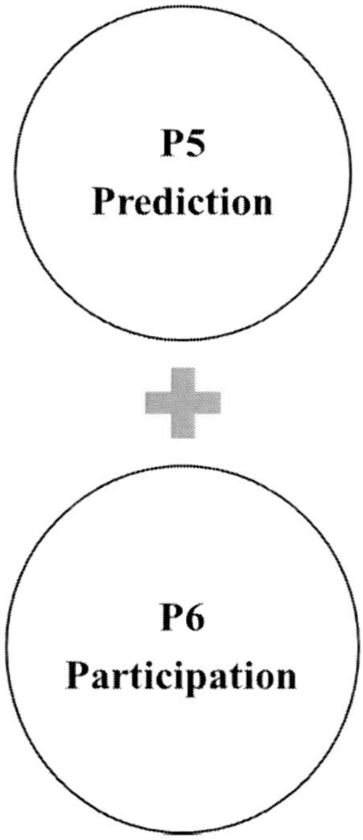

Figure 3. Integration of the three P-actions (see text for details).

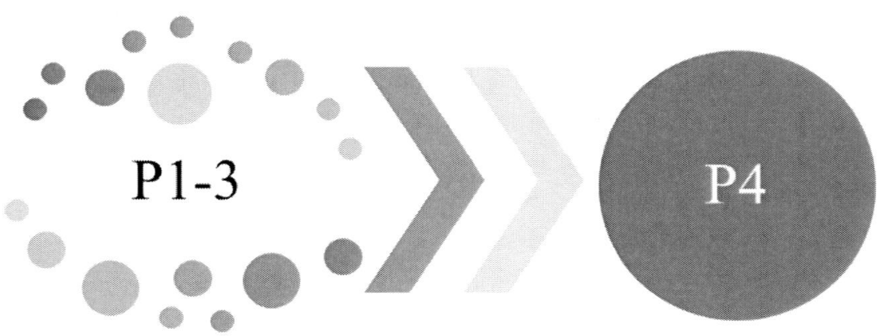

Figure 4. Entanglement of the P1-3 components to create the personal P4 (see text for detail).

Conclusion

Systems medicine regardless of its type—whether its systems biomedicine, molecular systems medicine, personalized medicine, precision medicine, or one of the P3-7 systems medicine—certainly represents the future of medicine. The biomedical model and molecular medicine, along with EBM, although powerful in terms of introducing science into medicine during the twentieth century, lacks the conceptual and theoretical foundation or framework for implementing the genomic and other omics into the clinic for the twenty-first century. Systems medicine provides that framework, especially in terms of technological advances for obtaining and analyzing omics data and with respect to a paradigmatic shift in conceptual and theoretical foundations. The present book represents an attempt to explore both the conceptual and theoretical foundations of systems medicine and the challenges facing it in an effort to advance its implementation in both the laboratory and clinic.

Chapter 2

Mechanism and Organicism

Abstract

In this chapter, the concept of organicism, along with other affiliated concepts including wholism, new materialism, and downward causation, are examined in terms of providing an ontological framework for systems medicine. Specifically, organicism provides the necessary conceptual foundation for viewing the patient as a person, especially in terms of personal health and not simply as a diseased body part, as is often common in the biomedical sciences, but also with respect to public or political health. And these concepts are contrasted throughout the chapter with traditional biomedical model's mechanism concept and its associated concepts of reductionism, materialism, and upward causation.

Keywords: causation, materialism, mechanism, organicism, physicalism, reductionism, wholism

1. Introduction

The biomedical model relies heavily on the concept of mechanism, especially in terms of portraying the body as a machine. Although mechanism and its associated mechanical philosophy have a long history, beginning with the ancient Greeks, the scientific revolution represents mechanism's contemporary origins (Cohen 1985, Dijksterhuis 1986, Gaukroger 2006, Shapin 1996). René Descartes is probably the best-known person espousing a mechanical philosophy. Descartes explained natural phenomena in terms of their mechanical parts (Garber 2002). However, other early modern philosophers also developed robust mechanical philosophies, including Robert Boyle, Pierre Gassendi, Galileo Galilei, Thomas Hobbes, Robert Hooke, Christiaan Huygens, and of course Isaac Newton, to name but a few (Glennan 2017, Westfall 1977). Each of these natural philosophers developed a mechanical philosophy that differed from the other on some critical points. Although mechanical philosophy reached its zenith in the seventeenth century, its influence is still apparent in the contemporary natural sciences and their practices—especially the biological and biomedical sciences (Darden et al. 2018, Sheldrake 1980)[11]

In contrast to biomedicine's mechanism, systems medicine relies conceptually on the notion of organicism or organism (Ayers and Day 2015, Boissel 2015, Rosslenbroich 2016, Tretter 2019, Zanin 2021).[12] Organicism is a term popularized in the first half of the twentieth century, with its roots in the nineteenth century (Phillips 1970). Although the American biologist William Ritter is generally credited with coining the term in 1919 (Mayr 1998, Verschuuren 1995), Joseph Needham (1928) notes that the French zoologist, Yves Delage, championed the term in his 1903 *l'Hérédité et les grands Problèmes de la Biologie*. Delage defined life in terms of organicism as

> the form of the body, the properties and characters of its diverse parts, as resulting from the reciprocal play or struggle of all its elements, cells, fibres, tissues, organs, which act the one on the other, modify one the other, allot among themselves each its place and part, and lead all together to the final result (Needham 1928, pp. 29-30).

The living organism, then, is the integration of its parts and this integration is crucial for understanding life itself, as well as the organism's relationship to its environment.

Throughout the twentieth century, the concept of organicism was broadened in its reference to include eventually the natural world as living—analogous to a living organism. Alfred North Whitehead particularly developed in detail, through his reading of Plato's *Timaeus*, a philosophy or doctrine of organism, especially in terms of Whitehead's process metaphysics in contrast to the substance metaphysics of mechanism (Herrick 1929, Whitehead 1979). For Whitehead, the world was "comparable to an organism, in which all the components are interrelated to one another and function within a common order" (Marcum 2008b, p. 145).

Organicism is often contrasted with mechanism but the relationship between the two concepts is rather complex in that both concepts share the belief that the material or physical substrate is necessary and sufficient for

[11] The early twentieth-century revolutions in quantum and relativity theories severely limited mechanical philosophy's use, especially the Newtonian version, in modern physics.

[12] The concepts of organicism and organism are often used interchangeably; but they differ in that organicism is a broader concept that includes living organisms while organism is a narrower concepts that is restricted to living beings.

understanding the world but organicism rejects the mechanistic belief that such substrate is sufficient (Gilbert and Sarkar 2000, Ruse 2013). Finally, the concept of organicism was in response not only to mechanism but also to vitalism in which a nonmaterial component or force—such as *élan vital*—is a critical ontological element for constituting and explaining higher-level or living phenomena (Allen 2018, Marcum and Verschuuren 1986, Sheldrake 1981a, b).

2. Mechanism and Organicism

Mechanism is the founding intuitive concept of the biomedical sciences and of a mechanical philosophy in general in which the universe and natural phenomena are reducible to matter and motion. In this section, the concept's historical roots are initially explored and then explicated in terms of contemporary mechanists' understanding of it, especially as it relates to biomedicine and evidence-based medicine (EBM). Next the historical roots of organicism are discussed and the concept is then contrasted with mechanism. The section concludes with exploring not simply the relationship between the two concepts but also with how mechanism and organicism are in some sense complementary with one another as foundational concepts to systems medicine.

2.1. Mechanism

The concept of mechanism has a long history in which natural phenomena are compared to machines composed of matter in motion. According to the historian of science, Richard Westfall, the concept can be defined such that "all the phenomena of nature are produced by particles of matter in motion" (1977, p. 33). In terms of matter, many early mechanists thought that natural phenomena are composed of atoms or corpuscles. For example, Robert Boyle used the notion of corpuscles to explain the *prima naturalia* of natural phenomena (Anstey 2000). In terms of motion, Boyle, as a natural philosopher, utilized atomic or corpuscular movement, in which the atoms or corpuscles collide with and modify each other, to explain the various activities and changes of natural phenomena. Moreover, he contended that local motion causes generation and corruption of natural phenomena. And with the naturalization of phenomena, the elimination of occult forces—such as the soul or vital force—from explanations of natural events was another important intuition for the conceptualization of mechanism (Craver and Darden 2005).[13]

Natural philosophers, then, were fiercely committed to the analogy of natural phenomena with machines or automata (Craver and Darden 2005, Dijksterhuis 1986, Westfall 1977). Moreover, the rise of modern science reflected the history of mechanism, given the similarity between machines and natural phenomena (Berryman 2003, De Solla Price 1964). In general, a machine is defined as "a contrivance, with organized parts whose interconnected workings can be easily understood" (Craver and Darden 2005, p. 234). The machine analogy was important in establishing mechanistic philosophy, since the analogy's heuristic promise was that natural philosophers could control and manipulate natural phenomena qua machines via their component parts. The machine analogy was also apt because the functions of machines are often deterministic and follow fundamental engineering rules and principles. The chief assumption in the analogy between machines and natural phenomena was the inherent intelligibility of nature itself. A major part of that intelligibility centered on temporally and spatially extended causal processes. In other words, mechanisms are processes that connect within a particular location "a cause (or beginning state) to an effect (or end state)" (Craver and Darden 2005, p. 236).

Mechanical philosophy had a profound effect, beginning in the sixteenth and seventeenth centuries, on the history of both biology and medicine (Hall 1975a). For example, Descartes wrote in the *Treatise on Man*, after bracketing the soul from the body, "I suppose the body to be just a statue or a machine made of earth" (1998, p. 99). According to Descartes, the concept of mechanism was not simply a research strategy in assuming that the body is a machine but more importantly it was a doctrine as well. As a doctrine, he believed "bodies have only those properties that follow upon their being extended substances, and perhaps a few additional properties like impenetrability" (Des Chene 2001, p. 14). For Descartes, bodily changes

---

13 The concept of mechanism offers an alternative explanatory scheme to the traditional explanatory scheme based on the deductive-nomological model (Bechtel and Abrahamsen 2005, Hempel 1965). The basis of mechanistic explanations is not any generalized law; rather, it is the family resemblance with respect to their schematization or modeling of a phenomenon's component parts and operations. A major advantage of such mechanistic explanations over deductive-nomological explanations is that the former provide scientists with a heuristic guide for discovering novel phenomena and for testing proposed mechanisms. In other words, mechanisms are especially open to investigation particularly through experimentation, which is at the heart of the biomedical sciences (Craver and Darden 2005).

reflected the interaction of these extended substances. The Cartesian mechanism continued to have a major impact on the development and eventual institutionalization of the biological and medical sciences and was instrumental in vanquishing vitalism in the early twentieth century (Allen 2018). Biologists, such as Jacques Loeb (1912) and his physico-chemical approach to biological and medical phenomena, were persuasive in overcoming the vitalistic approaches of both Hans Spemann and his notion of organizer and Hans Driesch and his notion of entelechy. The impact of mechanism bears its greatest fruit in the development of molecular biology, which was to convert contemporary medicine into a molecular discipline and practice (Darden 2006, Marcum 2020).

2.1.1. Molecular Biology

The success of molecular biology, especially during the twentieth century, was due to the ability of biomedical scientists to reduce complex biological phenomena, like diseases, into their mechanistic parts and to demonstrate how these parts interact with one another (Bechtel 2006, Darden 2006, Marcum 2020, Tretter 2019). The interaction of these parts accounts for or explains the entity's resultant or mechanistic properties. Stuart Glennan provides a well-known definition for this type of mechanism. "A mechanism for a behavior," according to Glennan, "is a complex system that produces that behavior by the interaction of a number of parts, where the interactions between parts can be characterized by direct, invariant, change relating generalizations" (2002, p. S344). The important notion associated with this definition is interaction, which Glennan defines as "an occasion on which a change in a property of one part brings about a change in a property of another part" (2002, p. S344). The interactions of a system's or network's component parts are sufficient to account for its resultant or mechanistic properties. In addition, natural laws or generalizations, which describe how two or more variables relate such that a change in one variable accounts for change in another, govern these interactions.[14]

Peter Machamer, Lindley Darden, and Carl Craver (MDC) proposed another definition of mechanism, in which they stressed a mechanism's process-like nature. "Mechanisms," according to MDC, "are entities and activities organized such that they are productive of regular changes from start

[14] Earlier, Glennan (1996) defined mechanism with respect to natural laws but latter contrasted the "new mechanism" with traditional scientific explanations by emphasizing mechanisms over laws (Glennan 2017).

or set-up to finish or termination conditions" (2000, p. 3). They illustrated the concept as follows:

$$A \rightarrow B \rightarrow C$$

The letters A, B, and C, represent entities or agencies, while the arrows activities. Whereas activities are producers or processes of change, entities are the agents involved in the change. MDC claimed that their concept of mechanism exhibits ontic, descriptive, and epistemic adequacy. As for ontic adequacy, MDC's concept of mechanism combines both substantive and process ontology such that ontology is neither eliminable nor reducible to the other. Their concept also exhibits a descriptive adequacy by illuminating the initial and final conditions, as well as the intermediate conditions, for change. Finally, MDC's concept of mechanism is epistemically adequate since it renders complex phenomena intelligible in terms of mechanistic explanations.[15] Although many examples of mechanism are available from the biomedical sciences, such as intermediate metabolism, MDC cited the central dogma of molecular biology as the prime example for their notion of mechanism.

The central dogma is *the* paradigm of molecular biology, and molecular biologists have used it to guide their research since its introduction (Thieffry and Sarkar 1998). In the late 1950s, Francis Crick proposed publicly the central dogma at a symposium in London.[16] According to Crick's version of the dogma, a polymerase transcribes DNA into RNA, which is then translated into protein, and both DNA and RNA can replicate themselves. In MDC's terms, DNA, RNA, and protein represent entities or agents; while transcription, translation, and replication are activities in which the agents participate, and through which change occurs.

Finally, Crick's notion of the central dogma also represents what MDC call a mechanism schema, since the agents and activities described in abstract form are instantiated in concrete detail. Indeed, Crick's version of the dogma was an abstract schema in which biologists had yet to discover most of the mechanistic details, and it illustrated the incompleteness of knowledge in the late 1950s and early 1960s. For example, actual transfers of genetic

---

[15] MDC claim that Glennan's account of mechanism focuses simply on the epistemic. However, James Tabery (2004) demonstrates that Glennan's notion of interaction is equivalent to MDC's notion of activity.

[16] Interestingly, MDC use James Watson's figure, first published in his textbook on molecular biology, for illustrating the dogma.

information included DNA → RNA → protein, while possible or probable transfers included RNA → DNA and DNA → protein. However, transfers of genetic information from protein → DNA or RNA or protein represented prohibited transfers. In fact, Crick claimed that "the discovery of just one type of present day cell which could carry out any of the three unknown transfers would shake the whole intellectual basis of molecular biology" (1970, p. 563). Although Crick prohibited the flow of genetic information from protein to other biological macromolecules, he did not prohibit other types of information from regulating the expression of genetic information, such as involved in epigenetic control of gene expression (Allis and Jenuwein 2016, Delcuve et al. 2009).[17]

2.1.2. Biomedicine

The central dogma of molecular biology was the dominant paradigm for biomedicine, during the twentieth century, especially as biomedicine became an information science (Lenoir 1999). Indeed, the dogma eventually led to the bioinformatics revolution in the biological and biomedical sciences (Searls 2010). In other words, DNA contains the genetic information that shapes living organisms through the production of proteins and other macromolecules, i.e., genotype dictates phenotype—which has important implications for biomedicine. Specifically, diseases could now be explained and thereby treated as aberrant or dysfunctional genetic mechanisms (Claussnitzer et al. 2020). For example, human aging itself, along with the "hallmarks of aging" (López-Otín et al. 2023), and the various diseases associated with it, especially cancer, can be explained in terms of "genetic factors" and the mechanisms accompanying those factors (Melzer et al. 2020, Perls et al. 2002).

Mechanism, therefore, is the central concept of the biomedical model (Clarke and Russo 2017, Moss 2012, Nicholson 2012). Thus, diseases can be investigated and explained mechanistically in terms of macromolecular entities like genes and proteins, which has led to the field of "biomedical ontology" (Röhl 2012). Philosophically, ontology refers to the kinds or types of "furniture" that occupy the "world of systems" (Bunge 1977, 1979).

[17] Several systems biologists utilize mechanistic explanations to account for systems phenomena (Bechtel 2007, Boogerd et al. 2007a, Brigandt et al. 2017, Richardson and Stephan 2007a). Although mechanistic systems biology and biomedicine represents a legitimate approach to biomedical research, without a wholistic context, biological and biomedical scientists cannot adequately or sufficiently explain a system since the parts in isolation do not provide enough relevant information (Soto and Sonnenschein 2018).

Biomedical ontology, then, is concerned with the material entities and processes that make up living bodies and the types of diseases and illnesses from which patients suffer. With the rise of computational analysis, biomedical ontologies have evolved to cover a vast diversion of healthcare activities from patient data to biomedical research data (Alexander 2006). In the U.S. in particular, for example, the National Center for Biomedical Ontology (https://www.bioontology.org/) provides resources, known as BioPortal, for advancing the development of tools and web repositories for best medical practices (Musen et al. 2012).

Besides biomedicine, mechanism is also an important concept for EBM+, which is based on the Russo-Williamson Thesis (Parkkinen et al. 2018). According to Williamson, EBM+ "motivates the systematic evaluation of mechanistic studies alongside association studies when assessing a causal claim in medicine" (2021, p.193). Although EBM itself relies strictly on randomized controlled trials and does not rely on pathophysiological mechanisms for providing the best approach to effective therapies, EBM+ accommodates the mechanistic entities and their relationships to one another from association studies as significant evidence for determining whether a causal relationship exists. In other words, a mechanism, such as A → B → C, provides evidence that supports clinical trials and prohibits developing therapies that might simply operate from a "black box" perspective. Consequently, EBM+ incorporates the mechanisms of disease etiology for developing best practices for treating patients.

2.2. Organicism

What made mechanism such a powerful concept for supporting the biomedical sciences was that it vanquished vitalism (Allen 2018, Hein 1969, Peterson 2016). The main problem with vitalism was not so much its anti-mechanism or anti-materialism stance but rather its overemphasis of or overreliance on metaphysics (Marcum and Verschuuren 1986). According to Elena Gagliasso, vitalism "represents more a metaphysics than a methodology of research, the living world is radically separated from the inorganic for its peculiar vital properties" (2003, p. 342). Organicism, on the other hand, not only avoids this problem by including the material or physical as necessary for defining living organisms, but it also avoids the problem associated with mechanism. According to organicists, just as a vital force is insufficient as an ontological category to investigate adequately or to manipulate effectively living organisms, so are mechanical parts alone as advocated by mechanists. In other words, what organicists argue is that mechanical parts are necessary they are insufficient for explaining the whole. What mechanism fails to consider when causally explaining biological or biomedical phenomena from a mechanistic stance is what Daniel Nicholson calls the "*organismic context*" (2012, p. 159).[18] Moreover, mechanism represents a metaphor that, according to Lenny Moss, has "run out of steam" in terms of accounting for living processes (2012, p. 170).

2.2.1. Organismic Biology

Organicism is often championed as a third approach, in contrast to vitalism and mechanism, for twentieth and twenty-first century organismic biology, especially developmental biology (Gilbert and Sarkar 2000, Haraway 1976, Peterson 2016).[19] The term has its origins, however, in the nineteenth century, particularly in Parisian medicine in which organicism referred to locating diseases to particular organs (Cawadias 1952, Hall 1975b, Hannaway and La Berge 1998). René Laennec was especially instrumental in founding the organismic approach to clinical etiology and practice. According to Jacalyn Duffin, by the time of Laennec's death in 1826 "many doctors refused to admit that diseases could exist without associated organic lesions" (1986, p. 195). Indeed, members of the Parisian School, such as Léon Rostan and Jean Bouillaud, were very influential in promoting organicism. "Rostan," as Harris Coulter notes, "permitted each organ in the body to be an autonomous and spontaneous generator of disease" (2000, p. 527). And Coulter goes on to quote Rostan, "Never at the sick bed do you hear them [physicians] talk about vital properties...such talk is only for the books. In practice, they are all organicists" (2000, p. 530).[20]

---

[18] As Nicholson goes on to elaborate, "mechanismic explanations specify only those features of the underlying causal networks that biologists deem *most relevant* for manipulating and controlling the phenomena whilst at the same time presupposing a great deal of the organismic context that makes them possible" (2012, p. 159).

[19] Interestingly, Hilda Hein (1969) claims that organicism is not particularly a third distinct approach or position in the mechanism-vitalism debate but rather represents a vitalistic position in the molecular biology-organicism debate. For further discussion of the history of organicism, see Peterson (2016).

[20] The Parisian organicists faced severe challenges from the medical community, especially Rudolf Virchow and his mechanistic approach to disease. Virchow's position was that "those who rejected the 'life force' as an outmoded idea but wanted to replace it with an 'idea of the organism' having the same legislative power in the body were deceiving themselves" (Rather 1988, p. 108).

In the first half of the twentieth century, several prominent biologists and philosophers continued to champion organicism in contrast to mechanism and vitalism (Haraway 1876, Peterson 2016). As noted earlier, Ritter was especially active in promoting organicism. Along with Edna Bailey, they claimed that organisms as "wholes are so related to their parts that not only does the existence of the whole depend on the orderly cooperation and interdependence of its parts, but the whole exercises a measure of determinative control over its parts" (Ritter and Bailey 1928, p. 308). John Scott Haldane was another champion of organicism, especially as he contrasted the living organism to a machine. Whereas a machine can be separated into its individual parts, "if one thing was certain about the parts of a living body," as Needham interpreted Haldane, "it was that they were not independent, they went together in such a manner that after separation they ceased entirely to be themselves" (1928, p. 31). Finally, the most influential advocates of organicism were members of the Theoretical Biology Club, which was composed of biologists such as Needham, Joseph Woodger, Dorothy Winch, and Conrad Waddington, among others (Peterson 2016).

Although certain biologists continued to champion organicism, the mechanistic view of life eventually overwhelmed the organicistic view (Nicholson and Gawne 2015, Peterson 2016). What was problematic for advocates of organicism was an inability to develop the requisite technology to investigate living organisms as intact entities, and so organicism eventually faded from the scene by the second half of the twentieth century. However, at the beginning of the twenty-first century organicism has had a revival, especially after the completion of the Human Genome Project (Botz-Bornstein 2020, Nicholson 2014). An important reason for its revival in the post-genomic era is the development of omics technology, which has permitted biomedical scientists to gather large amounts of data on patients, to use these data to treat patients specifically as individuals, and finally to predict possible diseases to which patients are susceptible based on their omics data (Chen and Snyder 2013, Loscalzo and Barabasi 2011). And Michael Snyder has championed iPOP for advancing personalized medicine (Babu and Snyder 2023, Li-Pook-Than and Snyder 2013).

According to contemporary organicists, system properties are independent of the system's parts and the properties of those parts. For example, Gagliasso contends for a living organism:

> the particular properties are given by the relationships between the parts and the characteristics considered as defining of any living entity (an

> organ, an organism, an organic and environmental system) and are determined by all the relationships that interconnect the diverse entities and that transform both the entities and the relations (2003, p. 344).

In other words, as a concept organicism envisions only a single whole of which all other entities are parts. For example, Morton Beckner recognizes a form of organicism in which "higher level processes…are autonomous with respect to lower levels" (1974, p. 171). According to Robert Wilson (2005), the world of organisms is well structured and sufficiently complex to defy reductionistic mechanism. Moreover, the whole, according to organicists, can be an atom or the universe itself. Each of the entities that comprise the world qua whole are alive in the sense that life is a fundamental property of the world. Life is simply not attributable to any one thing since life itself is a process that animates the system and not just its parts (Dupré 2020). For example, although viruses lack the physical apparatus for replication, they still contain the essential genetic information for replication. In other words, they are alive since they exhibit an important feature of life—replication or reproduction—which allows them to undergo Darwinian evolution (Chodasewicz 2014).

Contemporary organicism is a relational concept and depends on the interrelated relationships of the parts that make up the organic whole (Beckner 2006, Botz-Bornstein 2020, Elsassar 1998, Nicholson 2014). Further, an organism's composition is not necessarily what determines it; rather, an organism depends upon the organization or structure of its components (Brooks et al. 2021). For structure is critical for promoting specific interactions of the components. As Michel Morange stresses, the organism's ontological complexities "lay not in the nature of the macromolecular components, but in the way these components associate and interact to generate complex [and ontological distinct] structures and functions" (2006, p. 357). Ernst Mayr makes a similar plea for organicism:

> The basis for organicism is the fact that living beings have organization. They are not just piles of characters or molecules, because their function depends entirely on their organization, their mutual interrelations, interactions, and interdependencies (1998, p. 19).

For contemporary organicists, the structure-function relationship is what defines the organism and not necessarily its resultant material composition or an animating force or agency. In other words, life can be made of different materials as long as it reflects living processes.[21]

2.2.2. Organismic Systems Medicine

The concept of organicism is foundational for systems medicine since it encompasses not simply the diseased parts of the patient qua organism but the patient's illness experience qua person. Felix Tretter (2019) credits Ludwig von Bertalanffy's organismic biology as the foundation for an organismic systems medicine approach to clinical knowledge and practice (Bertalanffy 1974). Tretter goes on to contrast organismic systems medicine to a molecular systems medicine in that the former takes into consideration the patient's developmental stage within an ecological and environmental context, which includes the molecular or omics data, while the latter considers only such molecular data. Ana Soto and Carlos Sonnenschein (2018) also champion an organismic foundation for both medical research and clinical practice, and they identify three principles towards that end. The three principles concern the agency of the organism in terms of the principle of proliferation, the principle of variation, and the principle of organization.

Bernd Rosslenbroich (2016) also identifies five principles for implementing organismic biology into medicine.[22] The first is that the patient qua organism is organized on or at different systems levels, while the next two closely related principles are that each system level is regulated by rules specific for that level and that the various levels are interdependent such that no one level is privileged causally. The final two principles pertain to organismic autonomy, i.e., the patient qua organism is self-regulatory, robust, independent, and flexible, and to phenotypic plasticity, i.e., changes are in response to perturbations to the patient qua system. "Health," as Rosslenbroich concludes, "can be described in medicine and psychology as the capacity for dynamically balanced systems autonomy" (2016, p. 10). And such health is systems medicine's goal.

In sum, organicism is the concept that life is a fundamental property of the world. And it is certainly the foundational concept of P7 systems medicine. Specifically, the personal P (P4) is composed not simply of three specific integrated P1-3 components (Figure 2), but these components also interact

---

[21] Unfortunately, what constitutes the fundamental properties of life or what life is essentially is a highly contested issue (Weber 2018).

[22] These principles owe their inspiration to Denis Noble's ten principles of systems biology (Kohl and Noble 2009), which both Soto and Sonnenschein (2018) and Tretter (2019) also use to ground their organismic systems medicine.

with one another to constitute the personal P (Figure 5). The first is the P1 component or the physico-biomolecular P, which is composed of the patient's material and physical substrate that gives rise to the other components. The next component is P2 or the psycho-cognitive P, which constitutes the patient's conscious, cognitive, and behavioral dimensions. This component then gives rise to the P3 component or the populational-public P, which involves the patient's social, cultural, and political, as well as ecological, dimensions. These three components together are then responsible for the emergence of the final component, P4 or the personal P, which represents the patient's personhood. As shown in Figure 5, components P1-3 combine interactively to form the personal P, and life is distributed throughout these components such that disruption in the dynamics of any one component can result in illness. Finally, health and illness are not particular states privileged to any one particular component, especially in terms of causing either health or illness, but rather they are an integrated and interactive property of the various entangled Ps, which constitute the patient (Figure 4).

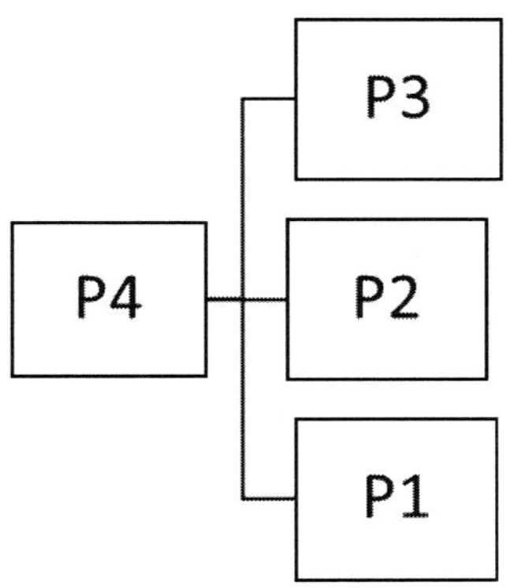

Figure 5. The integration of the P1-3 components to constitute P4 (see text for details).

3. Reductionism and Wholism

The concept of reductionism enjoys a privileged position in the development and history of the modern natural sciences, especially the biomedical sciences. The chief idea behind the concept of reductionism is that scientists can investigate and explain natural phenomena or systems and their properties in terms of their component parts and their properties. While reductionism focuses on lower levels and parts to investigate an organism's functional properties, wholism focuses on higher levels of organization—such as the tissue or organism—and function to examine and explain living processes. In this section, reductionism is initially examined followed by wholism and the two concepts are discussed in terms of their role in contemporary medicine.

3.1. Reductionism

Beginning in the seventeenth century, natural philosophers reduced complex natural phenomena to their component parts in an attempt to explain and manipulate these phenomena (Bowler and Morus 2020). For example, they investigated and explained the nature of light in terms of corpuscles and rays (Sabra 1981). Newtonian physics, in particular, established reductionism in modern science (Crowell 2003, Jones 2000, 2013). Reductionism proved extremely successful and became the standard conception or assumption by which to determine a discipline's scientific nature and by which to unify the natural sciences, especially the biological and biomedical sciences (Chibbaro et al. 2014, Kaiser 2015, Schaffner 1967).[23] Thus, it is no surprise that the chief concept of twentieth-century molecular biology was reductionism (Van Regenmortel 2004). For example, George Church and collaborators believed that through reductionist biology "the complete determination of a biological system becomes a concrete, achievable goal" (Selinger et al. 2003, p. 254).

According to the concept of reductionism, natural phenomena and their properties can be investigated, described, and explained in terms of their component parts and their properties. As John Dupré elucidates, reductionism is "the view that the ultimate scientific understanding of a range of phenomena is to be gained exclusively from looking at the constituents of those phenomena and their properties" (1993, p. 88). In other words, the whole is equal to the synthesis or sum of its parts. With respect to the standard hierarchy model of natural phenomena, reductionism claims that the analytic relationship between the different hierarchical levels is a downward movement from higher to lower levels, as higher-level entities are

[23] An important issue in the philosophy of science is the unity of science (Looijen 2000). Philosophers and scientists alike utilize reductionism to support this unity, especially the reduction of the special sciences to the physical sciences, and a Theory of Everything that in turn explains all natural phenomena. Wholism, on the other hand, supports a pluralistic view of nature in which ontologically distinct entities exist at higher levels of organization, which are not completely reducible to or explainable in terms of lower-level parts.

methodologically (sub)divided into their individual parts (as represented by the downward direction of the arrows in Figure 6). In other words, phenomena at the higher levels, such as biological organisms, can be investigated and explained in terms of phenomena at the lower levels, such as cells, since phenomena at the lower levels give rise to or cause phenomena at the next highest level, i.e., causation is from the bottom to the upper levels. For example, the genes, or genotype, determine or control characteristics and behavior of an organism, or its phenotype (Figure 6). In sum, the downward analytic approach or method is based on a synthetic upwards causal relationship among lower-level parts.

Ecosystem

↓

Populations

↓

Organisms

↓

Organ systems

↓

Organs

↓

Tissues

↓

Cells

↓

Organelles

↓

Macromolecules

Figure 6. Hierarchical relationships involved in biological reductionism. The Figure is not complete or exhaustive since non-represented phenomena exist at both ends; rather, it is simply illustrative of hierarchical reduction.

3.1.1. Ontological, Methodological, and Epistemological Reductionism

Reductionism, especially in the biological or biomedical sciences, often comes in at least three types: ontological, methodological, and epistemological (Andersen 2017, Ayala 1974, Boogerd et al. 2007a, Brigandt and Love 2017, Verschuuren, 2017). Ontological reductionism refers to the material or physical components that make up natural phenomena, in that the material composition of complex phenomena are reducible to simpler material components. For example, the body is composed of cells that are composed of subcellular organelles and macromolecules. Methodological reductionism involves the strategy or method and protocols or techniques by which to investigate higher-level phenomena in terms of lower-level phenomena. For example, the body can be investigated with respect to its cellular composition. Epistemological reductionism refers to the description and explanation of higher-level phenomena in theoretical terms and laws used to describe and explain lower-level phenomena. For example, the body can be explained with respect to its cellular makeup.

Moreover, the relationship among ontological, methodological, and epistemological reductionism is important. Ontological reductionism serves as an assumption about the material components that make up natural phenomena. For the biomedical sciences, it is assumed that the body is composed of basic parts, such as cells and tissues. Based on that assumption, scientists invent and develop methods and technology to investigate these phenomena in terms of their elemental components. Of course, the development of the microscope was very instrumental in identifying the body's cellular composition (Wilson 1995). In turn, scientists then utilize the observations and results obtained from these investigations to reduce theoretical explanations for complex phenomena to the theoretical explanations for the elemental components constituting complex phenomena. In sum, these three reductionisms are related in the sense that ontological reductionism serves as a guiding assumption for conducting scientific investigations, and the results from those investigations serve to explain higher-level phenomena in terms of lower-level phenomena.

Ontological reductionism is the notion that complex phenomena are reducible to or determinable by simpler entities and forces that compose them (Brigandt and Love 2017, Looijen 2000, Sachse 2007). Although several forms of ontological reductionism exist, the most radical form is atomism, in which "the entities of the 'lowest' level of organization…are somehow 'fundamental,' that they have an ontological 'surplus value' over entities at higher levels" (Looijen 2000, p. 15). Higher-level entities, then, are derivatives of lower-level atoms or subatomic particles, which exhibit an ontological richness to account for complex phenomena. In other words, higher-level phenomena are nothing more than the complexification or coalescence of lower-level phenomena. For the biological and biomedical sciences, the cell is, as it were, the atom of the organism's body. Roughly put, complex entities like cells are nothing but aggregations or accretions of simpler entities.[24] In more analytical terms, cells supervene on subcellular entities or, in other words, changes in cellular properties reflect changes in subcellular properties. Although higher-level phenomena appear to be ontologically distinct, they are really manifestations and compilations of lower-level phenomena. For example, the mind is not an ontological entity distinct from the brain's function—regardless of how complex that function may be.

Moreover, besides the actual material comprising the higher-level phenomena, the properties of those phenomena are nothing more than the expression or the result of lower-level properties. In other words, "any property token of the special sciences is identical with a configuration of physical property tokens" (Sachse 2007, pp. 21-22).[25] As for higher-level entities, their properties also appear to be ontologically distinct from the properties of lower-level entities, but they are not; rather, they are simply determined by or derived from them. For example, changes in a cell's genotype and the expression of its mutated genes determine the phenotypic behavior of a cancer cell, such as for the somatic mutation theory (Hanahan and Weinger 2000).[26] Moreover, the causal chain is again one-way, so that higher-level phenomena and their properties are a causal outcome or result of lower-level entities and their properties (Figure 6).

Methodological reductionism generally refers to how scientists conduct or should conduct themselves in exploring or investigating experimentally natural phenomena and it can be divided into two types (Brigandt and Love 2017, Looijen 2000).[27] The first involves "reducing wholes to parts and explaining of higher levels in terms of lower ones as the ultimate direction for all scientific research" (Jones 2000, p. 140). This type of reductionism refers

---

[24] Donald MacKay (1974) called the notion that all natural phenomena are nothing but physical entities, "nothing-buttery."

[25] Such reduction is often labelled token-token reductionism (Brigandt and Love 2017).

[26] The somatic mutation theory originally explained cancer in terms of genomic alterations, although the theory now includes epigenomic changes (Marcum 2019).

[27] Wimsatt (2006) complains that methodological reductionism fails to provide adequate guidance for precisely how to conduct scientific or experimental investigations from a reductionist stance.

to a "research strategy of trying to understand complex systems by studying their parts" (Boogerd et al. 2007a, p. 10). Moreover, it claims, "the best strategy for obtaining knowledge of higher levels of organization is to study lower-level entities and their interactions between them" (Looijen 2000, p. 20). As such, methodological reductionism itself serves as a rule or principle for guiding and conducting research. As a methodological principle, its claim is that the individual component parts are the only proper means to investigate complex phenomena (Verschuuren 1995, 2017). Thus, investigating subcellular parts is the best means for understanding cellular structure and behavior.

The first type of methodological reductionism leads to the second type. If the strategy of research is to analyze complex entities in terms of simple entities, then scientific methods or protocols should permit such an analysis.[28] Methodological reductionism thereby involves "reducing the methods in the different sciences to those of physics" (Jones 2000, p. 140). But there are two ways to view such a reduction: either a common method for the natural sciences or the use of techniques that disclose the component parts of an entity or event. Contemporary philosophers of science reject the notion of a common method for the natural sciences; rather pluralism, with respect to experimental techniques and protocols, is the order of the day (Looijen 2000). However, methodological reductionism as practiced by most biological and biomedical scientists involves experimental protocols utilized to investigate complex living phenomena at the level of their components, such as macromolecules and cells, rather than at the level of the organism. This type of methodological reductionism realizes and supports the first type.

Epistemological reductionism is the reduction of scientific knowledge, whether in terms of theories, laws, or explanations, from a higher level of organization to that of a lower or more basic level (Beckner 1974, Brigandt and Love 2017, Jones 2000). In other words, biologists can reduce, without loss of information, the theories and laws used to explain biological phenomena to, or derive them from, the theories and laws used to explain chemical phenomena. In turn, chemists can reduce, again without loss of information, the theories and laws used to explain chemical phenomena to, or derive them from, the theories and laws used to explain physical phenomena. "Ultimately," according to epistemological reductionists, "there will be no hierarchy of theories [laws, and explanations]" (Jones 2000, p. 27). Rather, the

[28] Jones notes that advocates of methodological reductionism claim, "the analytic method is ultimately the only legitimate method for studying reality, regardless of how it is composed" (2000, p. 28).

hierarchy collapses onto the physical level. Thus, all scientific—if not all human—knowledge is fundamentally physical knowledge.

Ernest Nagel formulated the traditional model of epistemological reductionism in a 1949 essay entitled, "The Meaning of Reduction in the Natural Sciences," and further developed his model in a book entitled, *The Structure of Science*. According to Nagel (1961), theories and laws used to explain phenomena at a higher or secondary level, such as biology, are straightforwardly reducible to, or derivable from, theories and laws used to explain phenomena at a lower or primary level, such as chemistry. Importantly, the reduction is possible as long as the terms of the secondary theories or laws are also present in the primary theories or laws. These reductions Nagel termed homogeneous. Symbolically, philosophers illustrate these reductions accordingly:

T_2 or $L_2 \rightarrow T_1$ or L_1

Where T_2 or L_2 is the reduced theory or law, and T_1 or L_1 is the theory or law to which scientists reduce T_2 or L_2. In contrast, heterogeneous reductions are cases in which terms present in T_2 or L_2 are not present in T_1 or L_1. For these reductions, Nagel postulated bridge principles or laws to connect the vocabulary of the theories and laws being reduced and the vocabulary of the theories and laws doing the reducing. To that end, the bridge laws contain the terms present in both T_2 or L_2 and T_1 or L_1.

Critics have raised a number of issues and problems with Nagel's account of epistemological reductionism, especially with his notion of bridge principles (Batterman 2002, Brigandt and Love 2017).[29] For example, Paul Feyerabend (1962) argued that philosophers cannot reduce the term of a secondary theory or law to, or derive it from, that of a primary theory or law because the secondary and primary theories or laws are incommensurable with one another. Hence, bridge principles cannot connect the terms from the secondary and primary theories or laws because the terms refer to different phenomena. In other words, no overlap exists between the two theories or laws; rather, these laws and theories do not share a common measure to connect them without loss of information. Contrary to epistemological reductionism, the relationship between various levels in a hierarchy is not simple identity (Dupré 1993). According to critics, the relationship is not even

[29] Nagel's reductionism continues to be debated within the literature (Dizadji-Bahmani et al. 2010, Schaffner 2012, Van Riel 2011).

as straightforward as epistemological reductionists allege it is because of the complexity of higher-level phenomena. The basis for incommensurability is the complexity of higher-level phenomena and their irreducibility to lower-level phenomena, which is ultimately the sticking point between reductionists and antireductionists.

3.1.2. Biomedicine and Evidence-Based Medicine

The biomedical community accepts and promotes reductionism for several reasons. The first is that reductionism is highly successful for identifying the mechanisms underlying a patient's pathophysiology (Brigandt and Love 2017, Robinson 1992). Part of reductionism's success is its simplification and analysis of complex processes into their constitutive parts. By isolating and identifying the various components of complex entities and their properties, reductionists claim they can then piece together or synthesize the underlying mechanisms, especially for diseases.

Reductionism, then, provides the opportunity for a simple and consistent narrative about biomedical phenomena, which allows biomedical scientists to manipulate and control such phenomena. In addition, it provides a robust causal relationship between higher-level phenomena and their component parts such that "causality entails reductionism" (Dupré 1993, p. 99). In other words, lower-level entities and their properties are causally efficient, if not sufficient, in producing higher-level entities and their properties. Thus, a method of reductive analysis and synthesis is adequate for investigating and explaining complex phenomena. Finally, reductionism provides universal statements about complex phenomena, like patients and their pathophysiological processes. For example, a reductive strategy is instrumental in identifying the molecular entities involved in tumorigenesis, which is comparable in various—if not all—patients.

An example of the success of modern biomedical reductionism is the reduction (or replacement) of classical genetics to (or with) molecular genetics or molecular biology and eventually to (or with) genomics (Brigandt and Love 2017, Hull 1974, Ruse 1971, Sachse 2007, Sarkar 1998).[30] Historically, the reduction began with Gregor Mendel in the nineteenth century and his experiments on the hereditary transmission of specific phenotypic traits in the common garden pea plant, *Pisum sativum*. Mendel was responsible for the reduction of heredity to discrete factors. His research goal was to demonstrate

[30] Molecular biology, although later in historical origin, includes molecular genetics, which focuses on the molecular basis of heredity, while molecular biology on the molecular basis of biological phenomena.

that transmission of the specific traits in this plant was not due to the blending of hereditary factors but to the transmission of discrete factors (Olby 1985). In other words, Mendel assumed that hereditary traits are due to separate factors that do not mix with one another. To that end, Mendel (1950) conducted experiments that supported this assumption. He interpreted the evidence obtained from these experiments in terms of two laws or principles: segregation of factors and independent assortment of factors. The first law states that the hereditary factors are separate from one another or not connected to each other physically, while the second law states that the factors sort independently of each other during gamete formation.

At the beginning of the twentieth century, biologists rediscovered Mendel's two laws and called his hereditary factors genes and the study of them, vis-à-vis inheritance, genetics (Bateson 1909, Johannsen 1909, Sturtevant 1965).[31] A second reduction occurred during the twentieth century, in which biologists assumed macromolecules compose genes. Biologists then used this assumption of ontological reductionism to conduct experiments to isolate the macromolecules responsible for hereditary transmission. Initially, they thought proteins constituted genes, but the experiments of Oswald Avery and colleagues with specific strains of bacteria demonstrated that DNA was responsible for the transmission of phenotypic traits (Avery et al. 1944, Lederberg 1994). Ultimately, hereditary information was reducible to DNA nucleotide sequence (Olby 1974, Watson and Crick 1953). This latter reduction is identified as a strong type, which "assumes a spatial basis for a hierarchical reduction, that is, quite literally, the behavior of the wholes is supposed to be explained by those of their constituent parts" (Sarkar 1998, p. 136). In other words, an organism's, as well as a patient's, phenotypic characteristics are the consequence of or caused by the sequence of DNA nucleotide bases or genotype.

With respect to a patient's phenotype (the behavior of the whole, i.e., its character traits) and genotype (the constitutive genetic parts of the whole, i.e., its genes), the former reduces to the latter (Brigandt and Love 2017, Sachse 2007, Sarkar 1998, Strohman 2002). For example, a cell's phenotype is reducible to its subcellular parts such as the ribosomes, membranes, and organelles (Figure 7).[32] These parts are further reducible to the nongenetic

---

[31] Biologists also modified Mendel's laws to include phenomena such as linkage of genes to each other on a chromosome (Rheinberger and Gaudillière 2004).

[32] Organelles, such as chloroplasts and mitochondria, are also cells that contain their own subcellular parts, such as ribosomes, membranes, and more significantly a circular chromosome.

macromolecules, like lipids, carbohydrates, and proteins. In turn, these macromolecules are reducible to genes in that the latter are causally responsible for the former, i.e., genes are ultimately responsible for the production of these macromolecules.[33] This reduction represents the first type of phenotype to genotype reduction (R_1, Figure 7).[34] And, it corresponds to the reduction of heredity to classical genetics. The molecular genetics/biology and genomic revolutions, with the reduction of genes to DNA, represents a second type of reduction (R_2, Figure 7).[35] Importantly, R_2 is physical in nature rather than functional as for R_1 (Sarkar 1998).

Cell (phenotype)

↓

Subcellular parts

↓

Nongenetic (macro)molecules

↓

Genes (genotype, R_1)

↓

DNA (genotype, R_2)

Figure 7. Reduction of cell phenotype to genotype. The arrows show the direction of reduction, which is reversed with respect to causal efficacy.

Interestingly, the reductionist approach of the molecular biology paradigm is still a viable metaphysics for some systems biologists—but not without modification (Bose 2013, Gatherer 2010). For example, Peter Sorger (2005) defends a reductionist approach to systems biology. For Sorger,

---

[33] Even though genes do not encode for lipids or carbohydrates, they do encode for the proteins that are responsible for their synthesis.

[34] The physical components directly involved in the reduction include a subcellular compartment (the nucleus), chromosomes, and then genes.

[35] Chromosomes and genes are not simply composed of DNA but also contain other macromolecules, such as histones.

molecular biology provides the component parts necessary for explaining and controlling biological phenomena. He cites, for instance, the benefit of the molecular biology paradigm for drug discovery. What is important for him, however, is not simply the reductive analysis of a biological organism into its molecular parts but also the synthesis of those parts into a functional whole, especially in terms of reaction engineering. "The well-developed field of reaction engineering," confesses Sorger, "suggests a future program for a 'reductionistic systems biology' that should be more congenial to those of us with molecular training" (2005, p. 9). What he finds appealing about reaction engineering is its emphasis on mathematical modeling, which represents for him the means by which to synthesize the whole from its parts. But he recognizes drawbacks to the application of reaction engineering to systems biology and proposes multiscale modeling strategies. These strategies, according to Sorger, "integrate information at different length and time scales, from proteins to cells and cells to organisms, while capturing both continuum processes (e.g., an abundant kinase phosphorylating a substrate) and discrete stochastic processes (the eventual effect on cell proliferation)" (2005, p. 10). Finally, as noted earlier, a molecular approach is also taken towards systems medicine (Tretter and Löffler-Stastka 2019, Tretter et al. 2021).

In sum briefly, for the biomedical model and EBM the patient is a machine that can be reduced to its component parts. Disease, then, represents a malfunction of the patient qua machine in which some part has become broken or dysfunctional and thereby compromises the patient's bodily integrity and function. The goal of biomedicine and EBM is to restore as best as possible the patient's bodily integrity and function. EBM in particular relies on reduction in terms of identifying through clinical trials and meta-analysis of the clinical evidence pharmaceutical drugs and surgical devices that may restore the patient to normal or near-normal functioning.

3.2. Wholism

Although reductionism is a popular concept among scientists, especially biological and biomedical scientists, it has its limits and critics (Brigandt and Love 2017, Buzzoni et al. 2022, Kaiser 2011, Rocca and Anjum 2020, Valles 2020). To that end, a number of holistic positions have been espoused over the last century (Delker and Mann 2017, Gallagher and Appenzeller 1999, Gilbert and Sarkar 2000, Koestler and Smythies 1969, Verschuuren 2017, Wolfe 2012). Although holism, a term coined by Jan Smuts (1926), is found throughout the literature, its cognate wholism is the preferred term.[36] Smuts used the concept in terms of creative evolution to account for whole making, which is rather too vitalistic in terms of transcendent ontology, i.e., "whole-making" represents an independent agency apart from the whole itself (Jörgenfelt and Partington 2019).[37] Wholism, however, is a naturalist or physicalist concept but not in a reductionist sense since the parts of the whole are necessary for constituting but not sufficient for determining the whole, and agency is embedded or entangled within the material or matter itself qua whole (Chong and Ray 2002, Placek 2004, Polanyi 1968). This is particularly worked out in terms of new materialism in which agency is embedded or entangled within the material or matter itself.

In the remainder of this section, wholism is initially defined and then examined in terms of its metaphysical, methodological, epistemological, and ontological dimensions, as well as its implications for P7 systems medicine (Esfeld 2009, Marcum 2021). The sequence here is important in that wholism functions as a metaphysical assumption by which methodological questions concerning natural phenomena are addressed experimentally and theoretically. Through this process the whole is understood and explained epistemically, and its ontological nature is categorized in terms of integrated levels. The nature of the patient, especially in terms of the personal P (P4) for P7 medicine, is also discussed throughout the rest of this section, particularly in contrast to the biomedical model's reductionist approach. Finally, although wholism is often contrasted with materialist and mechanistic reductionism, the relationship between them is much more complex than simply an oppositional dualism; rather, the two concepts can be complementary to one another.

3.2.1. Defining Wholism

The concept of wholism relies on the notion of wholeness or unity, which entails an irreducible and a dynamical totality that is complete and undivided (Piechocinska 2004). The main idea behind the concept is that the investigation and explanation of natural phenomena or systems and their properties only in terms of their component parts and their properties are deficient and incomplete; rather, the whole must be investigated and explained

---

[36] Both holism and wholism share a common etymology of the Greek term *holos* (Sorbel 2010).

[37] Another reason for preferring wholism is that Smuts' impetus for coining holism was political in that he sought unity for South Africa based on holistic British imperialism but a unity that unfortunately excluded native South Africans (Crafford 1946, Dubow 2008). Even though wholism does represent another "ism," hopefully it represents one that entangles and includes rather than separates and excludes.

on its own terms. In other words, "the whole is fundamental, not any one level" or part (Jones 2000, p. 337). As Denis Noble (2006) claims, no one level is privileged causally. In short, the whole and its properties are greater than the sum of its parts or levels and their properties (Hanson 1995, McDaniel 2010). Although the component parts that compose natural phenomena do provide the basis from which phenomena at higher levels materialize (Chisholm 1973, Findlay and Thagard 2012), the component parts do not entirely cause or account for the whole (Boogerd et al. 2007a). Consequently, natural phenomena at lower levels must be investigated and explained in terms of phenomena at higher levels, since phenomena at higher levels regulate or control phenomena at the lower levels.

In *Wholeness and the Implicate Order*, David Bohm (2005) provides an insightful discussion of the wholism concept in terms of the notion of wholeness. According to Bohm, wholeness is a dynamic totality or the whole, which processes or progresses across space and over time. He contrasts wholeness to fragmentation in which the totality of natural phenomena is split into individual shards of matter that lose their implicate order or pattern and integrity. For Bohm, wholeness qua implicate order

> is not to be understood solely in terms of a regular arrangement of *objects* (e.g., in rows) or as a regular arrangement of *events* (e.g., in a series). Rather, a *total order* is contained, in some *implicit* sense, in each region of space and time (2005, p. 188).

By implicit or implicate, he means an enfolding in which order is deeply structured or patterned within the whole. He goes on to contrast implicate order with explicate order in which implicate order is unfolded as explicate order, especially in terms of scientific laws and abstractions. In other words, natural phenomena qua wholeness are fundamentally monistic but when investigated through a reductionist scientific method, the whole is pluralized into fragments.[38] The challenge for modern science and medicine, then, is two-fold vis-à-vis wholism: how to reassemble the unfolded parts to understand the whole and how to investigate or analyze the whole without unfolding it.

---

[38] See Nancy Cartwright (1999) on the notion of dappled world and its associated metaphysical wholism (Esfeld 2008).

3.2.2. Ontological, Methodological, and Epistemological Wholism and P7 Systems Medicine

Philosophically, the concept of wholism has important metaphysical, methodological, epistemological, and ontological dimensions, as well as implications for systems medicine—especially P7 systems medicine. Metaphysically, wholeness represents an assumption about how to view patients and understand them, especially in terms of their integral unity as personal P or P4 agents. To investigate that unity with respect to higher levels requires a methodology that does not simply reduce or fragment them into component parts, as true for reductionist biomedicine, but maintains their integrity as a whole. Epistemologically, wholism implies that patients as higher-level entities are to be understood in terms appropriate for that level or component and not just in terms for explaining lower-level components. For example, the patient's populational-public P or P3 component requires social, cultural, political, and ecological terms that explicate disease etiology and treatment. Finally, patients as higher-level or whole entities are ontologically distinct from their lower-level parts. In other words, as higher-level entities they are not just composites of lower-level parts; rather, they are entities in their own right, with their own unique properties. In sum, wholism serves as an assumption about the material components that make up patients as natural phenomena; and, based on this assumption, methods and technology must be employed to investigate them in terms of their ontological integrity. The observations and results obtained from these investigations are used to formulate and confirm explanations of complex higher-level phenomena like illnesses and what they are ontologically.

Wholism is metaphysically assumed in order to ask scientific questions about the natural world and thereby to construct a scientific worldview and its repository of scientific facts and truth (Piechocinska 2004, Seager 2018). As an assumption, it presupposes that a higher-level entity constitutes an entangled and a dynamically interacting and intra-acting whole—according to new materialist Karen Barad (2007)[39]—that is complete in itself and irreducible to its parts or components both functionally and causally. But at the same time, the higher-level entity qua a dynamic whole can be partially analyzed in terms of its interacting and intra-acting parts. And so, the reductive analysis must give way to an emergent synthesis (Ueda 2001), which is driven primarily by downward and not simply by upward causation. Finally, as an

---

[39] By intra-acting, Barad (2007) locates agency within the processes of the whole regardless of scale or level.

assumption, wholism is not verifiable or even empirically justifiable. In Collingwoodian phraseology, it is an absolute presupposition (Collingwood 1998).[40] In other words, wholism is something that is taken for granted and not justified empirically so that apposite questions can be formulated for investigating the world.[41] As an absolute metaphysical presupposition, wholism is neither an answer to a question nor a proposition; rather, it provides the conceptual scaffolding, or what Collingwood calls the "logical efficacy" (1998, p. 32), upon which a scientific worldview and knowledge are hung and structured.

Wholism as a metaphysical assumption for systems medicine, especially in terms of P7 systems medicine (Marcum 2021), is critical for moving from a biomedical reductionist approach and understanding of the patient to a systems wholistic approach and understanding (Federoff and Gostin 2009, Sturmberg 2016, Vogt et al. 2016, Yuan 2019). By assuming wholism, the integrity of the personal P (P4) for P7 systems medicine remains intact even though it is comprised of the physico-biomolecular P (P1), psycho-cognitive P (P2), and populational-public P (P3). Through its assumption of reductionism, biomedicine has a rather myopic and fragmented view of the patient qua person; and such a view can often lead to medical errors that can either harm or even kill the patient (Levins 2014). Indeed, the assumption may blind the clinician to obvious clinical facts and prevent an accurate diagnosis.[42] Finally, wholism undergirds the healthcare profession in that the profession assumes that healing is a return to an integral whole or as close to achieving wholeness as possible or even creating a new robust wholeness. For wholeness denotes a sense of soundness in body as good health.

Whereas methodological reductionism concentrates on lower levels to investigate an organism's component parts, such as the biomolecular components of the cell, methodological wholism focuses on higher levels of organization—such as the tissue, organ, organism, or even the ecosystem—as illustrated as the personal P (P4) in P7 systems medicine. In other words, methodological wholism "claims that life can only be understood by studying it as a *whole*" (Verschuuren 1995, p. 40). Just as methodological reductionism functions both as a regulative principle for research strategy and for designing the actual procedures for conducting research, so does methodological

---

[40] In contrast to absolute presuppositions are relative presuppositions, which, according to Collingwood (1998), are verifiable.

[41] But these assumptions must be questioned philosophically, which is the task of the present volume.

[42] For an example of such blindness, see Marcum (2017).

wholism for systems medicine. As a principle for research strategy, methodological wholism directs systems research towards the whole phenomenon, as a system embedded in its environmental context. Rather than being monistic, however, in its investigation of natural phenomena, methodological wholism is pluralistic (Jones 2000, 2013). In other words, this methodological wholeness holds that the world is "dappled" (Cartwright 1999) or "disordered" (Dupré 1993). And it recognizes that each hierarchical level or network requires its own research strategy not reducible to the methodological strategy below it or ultimately to that of the most basic physical level. Consequently, each systemic hierarchical level or network of organization requires a strategy for investigating and understanding natural phenomena at that level.

In terms of the procedures and protocols for conducting systems and clinical research, methodological wholism rejects the notion that one scientific method applies to each natural science; rather, it shares with methodological reductionism the belief that multiple methods are available for each science (Cartwright 1999, Dupré 1993). However, methodological wholism differs from methodological reductionism in that it does not envision the methods of physical science as being foundational for investigating natural phenomena at higher levels. Rather, it advocates methods and protocols that are appropriate for the specific systemic hierarchical level or network under investigation, especially in terms of omics technology. To that end, methodological wholism stresses research methods and procedures that focus on the whole phenomenon appropriate to a specific level or network of organization. As such, wholes qua methodology "is often associated with a descriptive or phenomenological method" (Looijen 2000, p. 21). For P7 systems medicine, the phenomenological is imperative in understanding the patient's illness and it is not bracketed from clinical practice as in the reductionistic biomedical model.

Finally, methodological wholism does not bracket the observer from research strategies and protocols, as is often the case for methodological reductionism—especially in terms of claiming an objective foundation for scientific knowledge. Rather, the observer is a significant part or agent of the technological and experimental set-up and has an impact on the observations and results obtained from the investigation. In other words, the investigator qua agent is part of—or entangled within—the whole, which is being studied or investigated (Barad 2007). This has important implications for clinical research from a P7 systems medicine perspective in that the researcher engages the subjective dimension in an authentic manner. Really, objectivity relies on subjectivity, which Bernard Lonergan (1972) argues for from a methodological perspective. "Genuine objectivity," as Lonergan writes, "is the fruit of authentic subjectivity" (1972, p. 292). What he means is that scientific knowing does not necessarily involve envisioning abstract universals that prescind from the particular; rather such envisioning must include the particular in an authentic manner (Bracken 1984).

According to epistemological wholism, "complex wholes are considered not to be understandable from the mere knowledge of the behaviour of the parts in isolation" (Boogerd et al. 2007a, p. 11). Instead, from a wholistic perspective the whole's properties are knowable and understandable in terms of an integrated system in which the system's integrity is not violated but maintained. In other words, the concepts and terms that constitute theories and laws at higher hierarchical levels are not reducible to concepts and terms of theories and laws at lower levels. Although the laws of physics constrain biological phenomena, yet "they have their own laws that are not reducible to laws covering both inanimate and animate reality; therefore, these phenomena need their own level of theories to explain them" (Jones 2000, p. 32). In other words, as Renzo Morchio (2003) summarizes the concern of wholists or antireductionists: biological laws and theories are not reducible to physical laws and theories without remainder. For P7 systems medicine, the personal P (P4) is not reducible to the P1-3 components but represents a unique epistemic category that requires its own theories and lexical terminology.

Epistemological wholists are not simply interested in the isolation of the parts and the behavior of those parts but in understanding and explicating the relationships or integration of those parts and the behavioral properties of the whole, especially in terms of organizational principles (Kohl et al. 2010, Miller 2018). To that end, they are concerned not only with the system's information but also with the meaning of that information, especially in terms of how the parts constitute a system and how a system imposes order on its parts (Gagliasso 2003). In fact, wholists claim to have every right to construct theories without concern for the lower-level parts and have done so throughout history, although concern for the parts does appear to bring rigor to biological and biomedical theories. However, as Beckner points out, "undue preoccupation on the part of biologists [of an organismic stripe] with lower-level phenomena is likely to stand in the way of discovery and understanding of the higher levels" (1974, p. 171). For P7 systems medicine, the personal P (P4) is dependent on the P1-3 components but not reducible to them epistemologically. Thus, the personal P cannot be explicated in terms of a P1, P2, or P3 component individually, but must be explicated wholistically as the P4 component.

Whereas reductionistic theories are mechanistic in that the whole is explained with respect to the activities of the parts, wholistic "theories are indeed often phenomenological theories" (Looijen 2000, p. 21). "A phenomenological theory," according to Looijen, "is a descriptive theory with respect to a given level of organization" (2000, p. 308). However, phenomenological theories refer not simply to the description of natural phenomena but also to their explanation. However, that explanation does not involve a hierarchically vertical movement in terms of reducing the vocabulary and concepts from higher to lower levels but rather to a horizontal movement in which scientists utilize the vocabulary and concepts appropriate for that hierarchical level to describe and explain natural phenomena. In other words, systems scientists must maintain the integrity of the whole when describing and explaining it theoretically or nomologically. And clinicians vis-à-vis P7 systems medicine must maintain the integrity of patients qua wholeness, when not only describing but also accounting for their illness narratives.

According to Dupré, "reductive explanation is required to account for *how* things of a certain kind do what they do; but they typically do not help us to understand or to predict *what*, among behaviors of which it is capable, a complex thing will do" (1993, p. 106). In other words, reductionism is not as deterministic as reductionists often portray it (Anderson 1972). For wholism, as Gagliasso argues, "the living world consists in a reality that can be understood only in its global and inseparable unity" (2003, p. 344). Generally, higher-level phenomena outstrip the explanatory capacity utilized to account for lower-level phenomena.[43] The world is not as ordered or determined as reductionists believe or assume it is; rather, as noted earlier, the world is "dappled" (Cartwright 1999) or "disordered" (Dupré 1993). And this has important implications for P7 systems medicine, especially in terms of treating each patient qua personal P (P4). Emphasizing one of the P1-3 components at the expense of the others reduces the patient epistemically and prohibits the clinician from obtaining the requisite information for treating the patient effectively and especially humanitarianly.

Ontological wholism contends that a distinct domain or category is not reducible to another (usually a lower-level part) ontologically distinct domain (Andersen 2001, Esfeld 1999). In other words, simply combining or "putting together the parts will not produce the wholes (such as living systems) or account for their properties and behaviors" (Konopka 2007, p. 12). However,

---

[43] An example is the genotype to phenotype gap (Strohman 2002).

wholism does not preclude that the whole is not made up of lower-level parts, which it does share tangentially with ontological approaches such as constitutive reductionism in which systems are constituted causally by lower-level systems (Sachse 2007). What is important ontologically for wholeness is how the parts are configured or structured functionally. Ontological wholism, then, is distinct from ontological reductionism in that the structure or pattern of the material components is crucial. "A cell, or an organism," claims Geert Verschuuren, "is actually a particular, almost unique *organization* of components with a special relationship to each other" (1995, p. 37). Moreover, the two ontologies are distinguishable from each other in that ontological reductionism prohibits any causal agency of the whole upon its parts while ontological wholism demands or requires it. In fact, ontological wholism privies downward over upward causation.

Another important problem with reductionism ontologically from a wholistic perspective is the hierarchical categories and their relationships (Looijen 2000). A higher-level ontological category like organism may not be comprised simply of lower-level categories, such as cells or organs. For example, unicellular organisms like algae are composed of organelles not organs. So, in a broad and unspecific sense the hierarchical categories from a reductionist perspective with a bottom-up orientation fail to capture the diverse ontological relationships in nature. Wholists with a top-down orientation do not have this problem and can focus on higher-level phenomena that act upon or constrain lower-level phenomena, which has important implications for P7 systems medicine in that the patient's integrity must be maintained ontologically as the personal P (P4) and is not simply reduced to its P1-3 components.

In summary, biomedical and systems scientists have discussed and debated the limits of reductionism over the last several decades (Bock and Goode 1998, Dupré 1993, Fang and Casadevall 2011, Looijen 2000, Van Regenmortel and Hull 2002). Antireductionists and wholists view reductionism as just too simplistic, given the overwhelming complexity of natural and especially biological and biomedical systems. For example, the reduction of Mendel's laws to molecular biology terms is not a simple matter of transforming these laws into the latter terms or even replacing the former with the latter (Andersen 2017, Jones 2000, 2013). Rather, the theoretical terms of Mendel's laws and the phenomena they represent and explain are simply irreducible to molecular biology terms, without loss of valuable information about the organism and its behavior. Moreover, no straightforward bridge principles or laws can connect Mendel's laws to molecular biology laws in a complete or even adequate fashion. Rather bridge principles are deeply problematic, given that such principles must be biconditionals incorporating not only the terms from both the reduced theory and the reducing theory but also an ad hoc factor that permits the reducing (Dupré 1993). This latter factor is what antireductionists find so disturbing since it often represents information lost in the reduction. Again, the theoretical terms representing Mendel's laws account for entities that are not part of molecular biology's linguistic landscape. In a very real sense, strict molecular biology terms are inadequate or insufficient to account for the phenomena explained by Mendel's laws.

Wholists are not just concerned only with the digital information (nucleotide sequence) encoded within the genome but also with the meaning of that information, particularly with respect to the construction of a living organism or system from its parts and how meaning imposes order on its parts (Jones 2000, 2013). The gene is not so much a physical entity as it is a conceptual entity and, as such, depends on how biologists define the gene and its hereditary information (Griffiths and Stotz 2006, Kiberstis and Roberts 2002, Moss 2003, Portin and Wilkins 2017). From a wholistic perspective, that information is defined in terms of the whole context rather than the gene's linear sequence of nucleotide bases. In other words, a gene is an artificial construct, and not simply a concrete fact, which functions within a larger theoretical context. That context involves higher levels of meaning that impose informational or epigenetic control, which originates strictly from those higher levels and impinges upon lower levels. Moreover, the physical gene is also problematic from a material reductionist perspective (El-Hani 2007). A gene is not as readily or easily defined physically as a linear sequence of nucleotides. For example, a given linear sequence of nucleotides can function as multiple templates for transcription through frame shifts (Ketteler 2012, Kimbrough 1979).

Finally, one of the main problems associated with reductionism is the genotype to phenotype gap (Gjuvsland et al. 2013, Kim and Przytycka 2013, Morange 2006, Strohman 2002). The relationship between genotype and phenotype for systems biologists is not straightforward. Rather than the genotype being responsible for or determining biological phenomena, the whole organism is responsible for or determines lower-level phenomena. In other words, environmental and other epigenetic factors influence the expression of genes, especially during an organism's development. Genes are simply the substrate through which a biological organism plays out a system's regulatory and developmental processes or a disease's etiology. Moreover, the regulation of phenotypic characteristics is more complex than simply a single regulatory gene. For example, the regulation of the bacterial *lac* operon requires a number of genes working in concert with one another and the environment (Griffiths et al. 1999). The pleiotropic interaction of genes with each other and with their environment represents the components that biological phenomena manipulate and control. Moreover, knockout studies in which biologists delete a single gene during an organism's development do not yield expected or predicted results and observations (Deutscher et al. 2008, Nelson 2015). Utilizing knockout studies, biologists are often incapable of demonstrating the functions of genes identified in isolation. Unfortunately, these studies are unable to realize the potential for mapping phenotype onto genotype. Thus, for P7 systems medicine the phenotype of the personal P (P4) is not simply the outcome of the physico-biomolecular P (P1) but also includes the psycho-cognitive P (P2) and populational-public P (P3).

4. Materialism and New Materialism

Broadly, the concept of materialism states that natural objects ontologically are simply or strictly composed of or reducible to matter, which is not only necessary but also sufficient to account for these objects. However, the problem surfaces as to how to account for change or motion in natural objects, which the concept of physicalism addresses but in a rather controversial way in that the material and efficient case are constitutive to physical matter itself. New materialism has arisen to address the problem in that matter inherently contains or is imbued with the power or agency of change or motion; but again, this concept is rather controversial. In this section, materialism is examined initially, followed by physicalism, and how both are central concepts for biomedicine and evidence-based medicine (EBM). The section ends with a discussion of new materialism as the conceptual foundation for P7 systems medicine.

4.1. Materialism

The concept of materialism has a deep history with its roots firmly planted in ancient Greek philosophy, especially in Democritus' atomism and Aristotle's notion of material causation (Brown and Ladyman 2019, Novack 1965, Wolfe 2016). In *Metaphysics*, Aristotle (1979) distinguished four causes responsible for natural phenomena: material, efficient or artificer, formal, and final or teleological. His list represents a culmination of the Pre-Socratics' and Plato's discussion of causation. The material cause pertains to the substance or matter out of which a physical object is constructed, while the efficient or artificer cause represents the agency or primary source responsible for constructing the object. The formal cause to the plan or design by which the physical object is constructed, while the final or teleological cause the purpose or function for which it is constructed. For example, a table is constructed out of wood by a carpenter. It may have a design of a flat square surface from which four legs are attached at each corner perpendicular to the plane's surface and is used to eat meals or to play cards. In response to scholastic abuses of Aristotle's causes, Francis Bacon (1994) divided the causes into two categories, physical (material and efficient) and metaphysical (formal and final), and he rejected the metaphysical causes at the beginning of the scientific revolution in the sixteenth century, which set the foundation for the emergence of modern materialism (Vickers 1992).

By the seventeenth century moral philosophers debated issues concerning efficient causation, while natural philosophers were interested in material or mechanistic causation (Crane and Farkas 2004). For example, Descartes (1998) unpacked the concept of materialism with respect to natural objects being composed of extended matter or what he called the *res extensa*, i.e., that which occupies space. But this traditional view of the concept has its problems. "Materialism," according to Robin Brown and James Ladyman's interpretation of this view, "is an ontological theory that presupposes an intuitive concept of *space*, and the primary claim of materialism is that the only objects that exist are those that occupy space" (2019, p. 3). And Brown and Ladyman go on to argue that this definition is limited to only *res extensa* and then they revised the concept to include objects that do not occupy space directly, such as thoughts and momentum, but do depend on objects that do occupy space. Thus, the mind qua *res cogitans* depends on the brain qua *res extensa*. And besides the ontological problem, they also point out the epistemological problem of knowing what the material or matter is that makes up an object. In other words, how is materialism epistemically justified? Michael Philips (2003) addresses this question by noting that answering it is the province of physics. But this has been problematic in that the physics community has yet to reach a consensus on how to answer the question.

During the eighteenth century, mechanical materialism emerged in which objects, particularly the human body, were taken to be physical machines like clocks. The French physician and philosopher Julien Offray de La Mettrie extended Descartes' mechanist philosophy of animals qua machines to the human body and argued that the body can be treated as a machine. In *L'Homme-machine*, La Mettrie (1996) claimed that the human body is composed of various springs in which the various parts function in concert to set the human body in motion (Smith 2002). According to La Mettrie, "man is only an animal or a construction made of springs which all wind each other up" and the soul itself is simply the "mainspring of the whole machine" (1996, p. 31). He then proceeded to compare the human machine to a clock, in which the various organs represent the clock's different components. The human body's different components interact with one another to account fully for living processes. For example, the formation of chyle occurs in the digestive system, after which it enters the blood circulatory system and then finally animates the body's various organ systems. Thus, a mechanistic material cause is sufficient to explain the body's different functions. Taken as a whole, the human body is a machine composed of several components that function interdependently.

During the nineteenth century, although scientists from both England and France subscribed to materialism, German scientists were just beginning to develop a scientific materialism, an offshoot of mechanical materialism, which begins with Ludwig Feuerbach's criticism of Hegelian idealism (Bayertz 2015, Gregory 1977). The shift to this type of materialism was particularly evident among biologists. For example, the zoologist Carl Vogt claimed that "thoughts stand in the same relation to the brain in which bile stands to the liver or urine to the kidneys" (Bayertz 2015, p. 612). The mechanistic approach to understanding and explaining biological functions advances during the nineteenth century through investigating the chemistry of these functions. For example, Alexander Schmidt, who studied under Felix Hoppe-Seyler at the Virchow Pathological Institute in Berlin, isolates the ferment or enzyme responsible for fibrin clot formation (Marcum 1998). Continued chemical analysis of thrombosis or blood clotting resulted in a network of enzymes and cofactors, as well as other molecular and cellular components, responsible for it (Marcum 2013). Biological chemistry paved the way for investigating the chemical substances and compounds that compose biological organisms and that are responsible for living processes.

Scientific materialism continued to develop during the twentieth century, particularly with the physicist and philosopher Mario Bunge as one of its chief advocates. In *Scientific Materialism*, Bunge (1981) labored to bring exactness to formulating materialism by making it consistent with the sciences, from physics to the social sciences. He began by establishing that matter is not inert but dynamic and that modern science has not dematerialized matter. Moreover, he acknowledged that as science continues to investigate the physical world its theories are bound to change but still this change does not refute that the world is composed of physical matter. He next weaved into his formulation both systemist and emergentist attributes for matter. For example, the cell is a system of subcellular parts in which the property of life emerges through an evolutionary process. Hence, no immaterial vital forces are required to animate the cell. Bunge concluded that a viable scientific materialism is scientifically exact in that it is consistent with contemporary scientific knowledge, and that its ontology is composed of materially dynamic and evolutionarily emergent systems.

4.2. Physicalism

Throughout the twentieth century, materialism was closely yoked to physics and as physics progressed rather radically, materialism transformed into physicalism (Loewer 2001, Papineau 2001, Stoljar 2010). Besides scientists, philosophers also championed physicalism, especially those of the Vienna Circle (Kraft 1953, Stadler 2001). For example, one of the main members of the Vienna Circle, Otto Neurath (1931) concluded his article entitled "Physicalism: The philosophy of the Vienna Circle"—after rejecting metaphysical theses such as vitalism—accordingly, "the concrete success of human effort which does not make use of *theses devoid of sense* but is rooted in the soil of Physicalism" (1931, p. 623). John Smart was another very influential American analytic philosopher who promoted a physicalist version of materialism: "By 'materialism' I mean the theory that there is nothing in the world over and above those entities which are postulated by physics" (1963, p. 651). And he specifically denied earlier "billiard-ball" physics, opting for contemporary physics in which matter and energy are independent of one another but still interrelated.

Although physicalism remains popular among contemporary philosophers (Bourget and Chalmers 2014), there is little consensus on how to define it (Dove 2018, Elpidorou 2018, Ney 2008).[44] But even though there is little consensus, physicalism is generally identified with the physical, especially in terms of combining material and efficient causes. For example,

[44] Moreover, there are a fair number of vocal critics of both materialism and physicalism (BonJour 2010, Gillett and Loewer 2001, Sheldrake 2013).

as William Seager so succinctly articulated it, physicalism is "the claim that everything is physical" (2000, p. 340). In other words, the world and everything in it is corporal or physical in nature and there is nothing in it that is not physical. Thomas Nagel offers another definition of physicalism with respect to the human person as "the thesis that a person, with all his psychological attributes, is nothing over and above his body, with all its physical attributes" (1965, p. 339). Indeed, philosophers use physicalism to examine the relationship between the mind and the body, in which mind states are simply equated with brain states—known as the identity theory (Wilkes 1978). The problem with this conception of physicalism is its naiveté, in that experience reveals greater complexity than just the physical (Stoljar 2010). However, the concept of physicalism is not as simple as it appears but comes in a variety of forms based on particular assumptions (Tiehen 2018).

A more prevalent definition of physicalism, which avoids the problems associated with its naive form, is in terms of modern physical sciences. For example, as Timothy Crane and David Mellor note, physicalism is traditionally defined as "all entities and, properties, relations, and facts…which are studied by physics or other physical sciences" (1990, p. 394). Engel also claims that physicalism "assumes that the language of chemistry and physics will ultimately suffice to explain biological phenomena" (1977, p. 130). And for Hellman and Thompson (1975), mathematical physics best exemplifies the most "basic" physical science. By defining physicalism thusly, it is grounded in both rationalism and empiricism that confers a sense of authority to physicalism enjoyed by the natural sciences. But the problem associated with this interpretation of physicalism is that what constitutes the physical has changed dramatically throughout science's history, which has led to Hempel's dilemma. Carl Hempel (1980) observed that the corpus of facts within the physical sciences is continually changing so physicalism appears more like a moving target when defining what physical or physicality means. Although there is no solution to the dilemma still physics provides the best means for understanding physicality (Bokulich 2011, Melnyk 1997, Stoljar 2010).

Regardless of the philosophical problems associated with either materialism or physicalism, the concepts are the chief cornerstones of the biomedical model and EBM (Marcum 2004). Accordingly, the human body is perceived as a material or physical and mechanized object that is reducible to an assemblage of parts. From this perspective the patient's body is a machine à la Descartes and La Mettrie composed of individual parts, which can be fixed or even replaced with new ones when lost or broken. Obviously, this model of the body has had a profound impact on how disease is diagnosed and treated. Disease, according to the biomedical model, is interpreted in terms of dysfunctional parts, which are disconnected from the integrity of the patient's body and lived context. Working from such a model of the body, contemporary healthcare practitioners function primarily as mechanics or technicians, whose reductive clinical gaze is focused neither on the patient as a whole nor on the patient's lived context but rather it is almost exclusively if not completely on the diseased body or body part (Ristić et al. 2021). Modern healthcare technology has played a critical role in the development of this model for the patient's body, by providing the necessary instrumentation and techniques for reducing patients to their bodily parts (Moore and Maitland 2014). According to this model, patients' bodies are parts of a healthcare machine-world of interconnected machines used to diagnose and to treat patients qua parts.

4.3. New Materialism

Rather than a materially mechanized body, systems medicine, especially P7 medicine, is contingent on an organically phenomenal body, which depends on the concept of new materialism (Fox and Alldred 2019, Gamble et al. 2019, Lemke 2021). But before launching into the concept, Whitehead's process metaphysics provides the organic backdrop for engaging it fully. Whitehead takes on scientific materialism, which pertains to "irreducible brute matter" (1925, p. 24), in the 1925 Lowell Lectures by proposing an alternative to it. "In this alternative scheme," that Whitehead unfolds in the lecture, "the notion of material, as fundamental, has been replaced by that of organic synthesis" (1925, p. 219). As noted earlier, Whitehead goes on to develop from this organic approach the doctrine of organism, which he champions as a replacement for traditional "scientific materialism" (1925, p. 53). Moreover, the organism is the fundamental unit for each of the sciences. "Biology is the study of the larger organisms;" argues Whitehead, "whereas physics is the study of the smaller organisms" (1925, p. 145). Finally, the organism for Whitehead is not a static thing but rather a dynamic process of events, what Tom Roberts calls "processual" events (2014, p. 968), in which agency is not external but inherent within the organism—which sets up examining new materialism.

What is at issue for materialism and also for physicalism is the notion of agency in terms of initiating change. Traditionally, matter or material is seen as inert and passive, and agency relegated to the efficient and external cause. But with Whitehead's doctrine of organism and its inherent agency, along with the advances in twentieth century physics, an avenue was opened up for a new type of materialism (Wolfe 2017). This new materialism locates agency within matter itself (Choat 2018, Dolphijn and Tuin 2020). Barad calls this agency "agential realism" in which "agency is a matter of intra-acting…doing/being in its intra-activity" (2007, p. 235). And intra-acting involves material entanglement that cuts across different scales from the quantal to the cosmic. In other words, agency is part of the material and not something conferred on it externally, such as in vitalism. In causal terms, materiality is not simply necessary but sufficient for processive change and development, whether in terms of autopoiesis (self-generating) or allopoiesis (other-generating) (Hongbao Ma 2005, Meincke 2019). Christopher Gamble and colleagues call Barnard's agential realism "performative" new materialism, and they base it on three entangled features of matter. The first is *pedesis* in that matter is in motion, and the next feature defines that motion in terms of iterative processes while the final feature states that "matter must be fully *relational* and immanently self-caused" (Gamble et al. 2019, p. 127).

Finally, the phenomenal is deeply material from a new materialism perspective—in contrast to an anti-phenomenological traditional materialism—in the sense that experience depends intimately on the material body itself qua self-creating agent (DeLanda 2021, Grosz 2017, McGregor 2020). As Kristidel McGregor claims,

> Any practice of phenomenology from a new materialist perspective must have a theory of experience that accounts for all that is entangled in the phenomena, including both the material, the discursive, the human, and the researchers themselves (2020, p. 511).

Phenomenology is materialistic in that experience begins with the lived body experience within a particular physical environmental context. Moreover, discursive practices of embodied agents engage and are also entangled within the environment that includes every agent—whether human and nonhuman. What is critical is the active and creative agency of the material body. Rather than an inert or a passive body, the phenomenal body vis-à-vis new materialism contains the necessary and sufficient agency for initiating and completing processual events.

Such phenomenological new materialism has important implications for systems medicine, especially P7 medicine, in contrast to the biomedical model based on traditional materialistic perspective (Marcum 2004, 2008a). From such a traditional perspective, the patient is composed of inert and passive material that requires external intervention in terms of either drugs or devices to treat the patient's disease. Outside of these interventions the biomedical model offers little else for treating the patient, which has had a major impact not only on the quality of care but also on the effectiveness of treatments for chronic diseases like diabetes, stroke, and heart disease. Moreover, the biomechanical model has had a profound impact on the patient–physician relationship. A patient's diseased body part often resembles an enigma or at worse an insoluble conundrum that concerns the physician or another healthcare practitioner as a technician or mechanic, to both diagnose and treat the disease. As a technician, the clinical gaze is generally myopic—often focused on a diseased body part and to the exclusion of the patient's overall illness experience and suffering.

For systems medicine from a phenomenal new materialism perspective, especially in terms of P7 medicine, the physico-biomolecular P (P1) is transformed from simply a traditional material component in which matter is inert and passive in terms of reductive mechanistic or machine perspective to an animated component, which exhibits a wholeness to account for the entangled intra-agency of the patient's material components. Not only is their entanglement within the P1 component itself but there is also entanglement of this component with the psycho-cognitive P (P2) such that the patient is now able to participate as a unique person in the clinical encounter and treatment options. Moreover, the P1 and P2 components are then entangled with the populational-public P (P3) such that the patient and other social and political factors allow the patient to participate from a wider perspective, whether in patient support groups or political advocacy. Finally, the P1-3 components are entangled to generate the personal P (P4), which permits the patient to engage fully and effectively in recovering from illness and restoring an operative or even optimal level of health.

5. Upward and Downward Causation

Causation is an important conceptual foundation for both biomedicine and systems medicine, especially in terms of the patient, whether as a machine that consists of mechanistic parts or as a whole organism that exhibits organic animation. It is at best a rather controversial and ambiguous concept, especially from a philosophical perspective (Beebee et al. 2009, Mumford and

Anjum 2013, Pearl 2009). Apart from this controversy, a working definition is proposed that captures especially the ontological and epistemological dimensions of causation. Specifically, the definition involves a relationship between two entities or events qua process such that one entity or event qua agent is required for the existence or emergence of the other qua product. For example, the synthesis of a chemical bond (process) involves the transfer of energy (agency) such that one atom is then connected or yoked to another atom (product). Importantly, this bonding can be caused ostensibly either through enzymes or not. But in a substantial sense, enzymes account not so much for the ontology of the causal relationship—that is accounted for through the energy transfer between the two atoms—but rather for its epistemology in that the enzymatic reaction explains why the bond formation occurs given specific conditions. Causation has been divided into various categories, such as direct or indirect causation, but for current purposes causation is divided into two related concepts: upward or bottom-up and downward or top-down causation (Ellis 2005a, Santos 2015).

5.1. Upward Causation

Upward causation is the concept that lower-level entities or events are responsible for higher-level complex entities or events (Coffman 2006, Martin 2008). In other words, it refers to the idea or notion that simple events are causally responsible for complex events. For the natural sciences, for example, material or physical entities account for the appearance of more complex entities like organisms and their behavior. Thus, to explain complex entities or events, particularly in terms of causality, requires a reduction of them into their constitutive or compositional parts. Importantly, lower-level or simple entities or events cause higher-level or complex entities or events and not vice versa. The causal chain is strictly one way, from the bottom to the top of a hierarchy. And the reduction of complex events to physical events, for example, is the basis for this causal relationship. "Particle physics," contests George Ellis, "is the foundational subject underlying—and so in some sense explaining—all the others" (2005b, p. 743). In other words, causation is related to or the result of a complex event's composition (Auyang 1999).

Upward or bottom-up causation, then, refers conceptually to "a certain causal process leading from the lower-level entities to the higher-level ones, so that the lower level can be seen as the cause and the higher level as the effect" (Emmeche et al. 2000, p. 18). Thus, to a significant extent, upper-level entities or events are simply epiphenomena and lack causal powers with respect to the lower-level phenomena that initially caused them. For example, the mind is simply an epiphenomenon of brain activity. The causal chain terminates then with lower-level physical entities, which permits biologists to predict a complex entity's behavior. Biological entities, for instance, are simply (special) arrangements or aggregates of physico-chemical components. In other words, a biological organism is the result of structuring macromolecules—like proteins and complex carbohydrates—in specific patterns. The organism's parts dictate its structural pattern. There is nothing ontologically distinct about the higher-level or complex entities or events vis-à-vis lower-level or simple entities or events in terms of causation.

Upward causation is predicated on the principle of causal closure and physicalism (Garcia 2014, Gibb 2015, Montero 2003, Papineau 2009, Tiehen 2015, Vicente 2006). According to David Papineau, for example, the principle states, "Every physical effect has an immediate sufficient physical cause, in so far as it has a sufficient [immediate] physical cause at all" (2009, p. 59). What is critical for the principle is that the physical cause must be both immediate and sufficient. In other words, the cause must be proximate and not distal to the effect such that there is not an intermediate nonphysical cause, and it must be adequate in toto to bring about the effect without reliance on an additional nonphysical cause. Also critical, according to Papineau, is

> that every physical effect has a sufficient immediate physical cause 'in so far as it has a sufficient immediate cause at all.' The reason for this latter qualification is to accommodate the indeterminism of modern quantum mechanics, which tells us that certain physical effects are random, without any sufficient determining cause (2009, p. 59).

And as he goes on to point out, this qualification is based on the fact that quantal indeterminacy is still based on physical and not nonphysical causes. Thus, upward or bottom-up causation is adequate to account for more complex entities or events without invoking nonphysical causation, which has important implications for the biomedical model. Finally, upward causation is possible because higher-level entities or events supervene on lower-level entities or events (Kim 1993, Welshon 2002). In other words, changes in higher-level entities or events require changes in lower-level entities or events.

The biomedical model relies almost exclusively on the belief that by reducing a disease to its physical cause the disease can be cured if not managed successfully (Ghaemi 2017, Marcum 2004, 2008a, Russell 2014, Valles 2020).

After all, the patient is a machine composed of aggregate parts and if a part fails then it simply needs to be fixed or replaced. And even a psychological or psychiatric disease, like depression, is reducible to a physical cause, such as a neurotransmitter (Bracken et al. 2012, Deacon 2013, Moncrieff 2008). This reliance on upward causation and its associated causal closure principle and physicalism has certainly supported the biomedical model, along with EBM, as the dominant means of providing healthcare throughout the world. But the model has come under criticism for failing to provide cures for many chronic diseases (Fuller 2017, Rocca and Anjum 2020). For example, substantial concerns are articulated over the translation of a molecular approach to cardiovascular biomedicine into effective therapy (MacRae et al. 2016). Systems medicine and its reliance on downward causation, however, can address the concerns over the biomedical model with its strict reliance on upward causation.

5.2. Downward Causation

Downward or top-down causation is possible because higher-level or emergent properties supervene on lower-level parts. In contrast to the strict causal closure or determinism of upward causation, it claims that higher-level entities or events determine or constrain causally the properties or behavior of lower-level entities or events (Auletta et al. 2008, Davies 2006, Heil 2017, Wagner 1999).[45] In other words, downward causation involves "a direct, 'downward' fashion, in contrast to the operation of a simple structural macro-property, whose causal influence occurs *via* the activity of the micro-properties that constitute it" (O'Connor 1994, pp. 97-98). Donald Campbell, who initially introduced the term into the literature, provides a well-known definition of downward causation: "all processes at the lower levels of a hierarchy are restrained by and act in conformity to the laws of the higher levels" (1974, p. 180). For example, the phenotypic behavior of a cell relies on the constraints that higher-order structures, such as the microenvironment or stroma, place on the individual parts or components making up the higher-order structure. As John Heil interprets Campbell mereologically, "wholes that depend on assemblages of parts causally constrain the parts' behavior" (2017,

---

[45] An important assumption underlying downward causation is the existence of various ontological levels, which serve to ground different types of downward causation (Emmeche et al. 2000). In this way, downward causation does not violate either physicalism or naturalism in terms of nonphysical or unnatural causes participating in any effect or event.

p. 43). In other words, downward causation refers to the ability of complex higher-level entities or events to cause or limit the behavior or properties of simpler lower-level entities or events that originally constituted them ontologically.

For many advocates of downward or top-down causation, especially for systems biologists, the upward causation associated with reductionism is insufficient to account fully or suitably for the causal powers that animate entities or events exhibit (Noble 2008, 2017, Farnsworth et al. 2017, Szentágothai 1984). For them, higher-level entities or events exhibit causal powers in controlling or bringing about lower-level entities or events that would not exist simply because of the causal powers of those simpler entities or events. The phenotypic behavior of a cell, for instance, relies on the constraints of higher-order structures, such as the microenvironment or extracellular matrix as part of the tissue level, places on the individual parts or components that make up the higher-order of cellular structure and behavior that is responsible for its microenvironment (Teufel 2011). A striking example of downward causation is the causal relationship between tumor cells and their extracellular matrices in terms of carcinogenesis (Pickup et al. 2014, Walker et al. 2018).

Just as the concept of upward causation relies on notions of causal closure, physicalism, and supervenience, so does downward causation to avoid overdetermination, especially in terms of nonphysical causes (Ellis 2020, Funkhouser 2002, Kroedel 2015, Schaffer 2003). Although for downward causation higher-level entities and events do supervene on lower-level entities and events, the supervenience is only partial such that properties of the higher-level entities and events are ontologically distinct such that these entities and events can shape lower-level entities and events. In other words, the supervenient properties can cause changes in subvenient properties without changes in their properties. However, the causal effect does not violate causal closure and its associated notion of physicalism in that the higher-level entities and events are sufficiently accounted for in terms of physical causation. Finally, what makes downward causation possible is the emergence of novel properties at higher levels such that these properties are not supervenient on properties of lower-level entities and events (Campbell and Bickhard 2011, Macdonald and Macdonald 2010, Prosser 2012). But further discussion of emergence is reserved for the next chapter.

Although downward causation has attracted numerous advocates, critics raise several problems with it (Paoletti and Orilia 2017). One important problem with downward causation, especially Campbell's version of it, is the relationship between the laws or principles at lower levels and those at higher levels. Specifically, the problem is whether higher-level laws or principles are real or genuine or are simply the appearance of causation in terms of lower-level entities or events (Hulswit 2006, Tabaczek 2013). Instead of a strong notion of downward causation that is open to this criticism, some advocates of downward causation propose weaker forms in which the causal action is indirect, i.e., a medium downward causation, or represents an organization principle, i.e., a weak downward causation (Flack 2017, Emmeche et al. 2000, Green 2018). However, such forms run the risk of reducing higher-level phenomena vis-à-vis causal efficacy to epiphenomena.

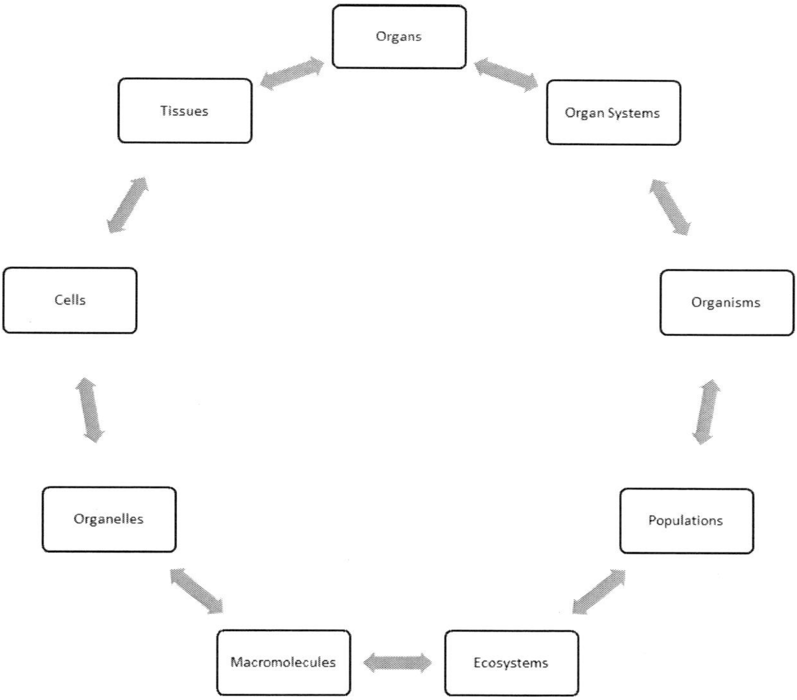

Figure 8. Circular causality (see text for details).

Although downward and upward causation are often contrasted with one another, several models are proposed that relationally combine the two (Craver and Bechtel 2007, Ellis 2005a, Santos 2015). For example, Noble and colleagues have proposed a circular causality model for living systems that integrates both downward and upward causation (Noble 2012, 2017, Noble et al. 2019). Their proposed model extends more traditional circular causality to include the principle of biological relativity in which no particular hierarchal level is privileged vis-à-vis another level. They provide an example of cardiac rhythm to illustrate the model. As Noble points out, "there is not a program for cardiac rhythm in the genome" (2012, p. 58). Rather, the rhythm reflects the constraints of higher-level structures such as the cell membrane has an impact on ion channel behavior. As depicted in Figure 8, causation runs in both directions in which macromolecules are causally responsible for higher-level entities such as the membrane which then serves to regulate the behavior of membrane components such as ion channels. Finally, Noble (2012, 2017) stresses that the circular causality relationship is not symmetrical in the sense that downward causation is not the reverse of upward causation but rather represents a feedback circuit.

Just as upward causation fuels contemporary biomedicine, so downward causation fuels systems medicine (Lourida and Louridas 2021, Tretter and Löffler-Stastka 2019, Vogt et al. 2014). Downward causation particularly provides the causal power for transforming the patient from a passive recipient of healthcare services to an active agent involved in participating enthusiastically and efficaciously in those services. However, systems medicine also incorporates upward causation with respect to representing the patient as a whole individual. In other words, feedback exists between the two types of causation as articulated by Noble and colleagues. In terms of P7 systems medicine, then, the personal P (P4) is the active agent that then impinges causally onto the P1-3 components. In other words, the patient qua P4 can reshape causally the biological (P1), mental (P2), and social (P3) components personally in order to treat illness. Importantly, the causal relationship is cyclical in terms of the changes that take place. Thus, as upward causation gives rise to the P4 component from the P1-3 components, downward causation from the P4 component onto the P1-3 components changes these components, which then gives rise to an altered P4 component until the illness is successfully treated. In sum, a trajectory is generated as the upward and downward causal powers shape the P1-4 components.

Conclusion

In sum, then, the main conceptual foundation for systems medicine is organicism and its associated concepts of wholism, new materialism, and downward causation. For P7 medicine, organicism, indeed, captures the organic vitality of the patient, especially as the P1-3 components entangle to give rise to the personal P (P4), which is both whole and expresses the necessary agency to participate actively in requisite treatment. In contrast, the biomedicine's concept of mechanism imprisons and dehumanizes the patient as a machine, which when broken is simply "fixed" by repairing the broken part or by replacing it. The patient's materiality or physicality is simply passive. Although the organismic and mechanistic approach to medicine is incommensurable with one another, yet both approaches can be integrated especially in terms of complementing and enriching each other in order to provide a comprehensive understanding of the patient. Also, the other associated concepts of systems medicine and biomedicine can be integrated with one another.

Even though wholism and reductionism are often contrasted with one another, advocates for systems approaches to the biomedical sciences argue for a paradigm that combines or integrates both concepts (Latterich 2005, Looijen 2000, O'Malley and Dupré 2005). According to Francisco Ayala, for example, the majority of these advocates "agree that the study of problems at a given level of complexity of the living world must proceed by exploring lower as well as higher levels of organization" (1974, p. ix). In other words, both wholism and reductionism are opposite poles on a continuum in which possible intermediate paradigms are available between "microscopic 'nothing but' statements" and "macroscopic 'all or nothing' statements" (Boogerd et al. 2007a, p. 12). Such intermediate paradigms provide a comprehensive picture of the natural world. "In order to understand Nature," claims Peter Schuster, "we can neither dispense from the reductionist's program and its results nor can we totally abolish the holistic view" (2007, p. 12). Rather both are integral to understanding nature.

For contemporary systems medicine both wholism and reductionism are critical for practicing clinical medicine (Berlin et al. 2017, Federoff and Gostin 2009). This approach is pluralistic and opportunistic in its nature and takes its cue from the problem at hand. "The consensus view," suggest Marc Van Regenmortel and David Hull, "leads to pluralism: both reductionist methods and a more holistic approach to biological complexity are required, depending on the questions being asked" (2002, p. 13). Such an approach has important implications for P7 systems medicine, especially in terms of new materialism. Specifically, the P1 component is still reducible to its material parts but there is no reason to invoke a causal force outside of its materiality. Rather the entanglement of P1's material components is the basis of its agency, especially in terms of efficient causation. Consequently, the personal P's materiality or physicality is not passive as for the mechanistic patient of biomedicine but rather dynamic.

Also, as noted earlier, both upward and downward causation can be integrated, such as Noble (2017) conjoining the upward causation of reductionist molecular biology with the downward causation of wholistic systems biology to generate circular causality. Whereas upward causation provides the formative and material components and processes that account for higher-level phenomena, those phenomena in turn causally impinge on lower-level components (Bruggeman and Westerhoff 2007, Westerhoff and Hofmeyr 2005). Thus, advocates of these intermediate paradigms connect both system properties and molecular properties in a reciprocal relationship such that changes in either one has causal consequences for the other. In other words, lower-levels events cause higher-level events, which in turn cause lower-level events. The implications for P7 systems medicine are important in terms of a wholistic causation that can reshape the personal P (P4) ontologically and thereby open up avenues for healing.

In conclusion, although systems medicine does rely on integrating its conceptual foundation of organicism with biomedicine's mechanistic approach, still its approach, especially for P7 systems medicine, is strictly organicistic in the sense that the patient ultimate is a whole qua personal P (P4) who has agency inherent within its embodied state that can exhibit downward causation in terms of participating in the healing process with respect to the P5-7 actions. Certainly, biomedicine's mechanistic approach, with its associated reductionism, materialism, and upward causation, are important for a robust systems medicine, particularly P7 medicine, but still, it is the concept of organicism that drives the conceptual framework for P7 systems medicine. The reason is that for the personal P (P4) novel properties emerge that are not properties of the P1-3 components. And so, the concept of emergence must be explored next.

Chapter 3

Resultant and Emergence

Abstract

In this chapter, the concept of the mechanistic resultant and its impact on the biomedical model is examined initially and is then contrasted to the concept of emergence and its impact on systems medicine, particularly P7 systems medicine. Next, systems medicine's conceptions of emergent synthesis and synergy, epigeneticism, and stochasticity are compared and contrasted to biomedicine's conceptions of synthesis, geneticism, and determinism. The chapter concludes with a discussion of a possible intermediate position or concept called emergent mechanism (Glauer 2012).

Keywords: determinism, emergence, epigeneticism, geneticism, resultant, stochasticity, synergy, synthesis

1. Introduction

Traditionally, the concept of emergence is contrasted often with mechanism, especially in terms of the latter's resultant output (Corning 2012, O'Connor 2020, Stephan 1992). "The concepts of mechanism and emergence," Fred Boogerd and collaborators insist, "have long been considered to be mutually exclusive" (Boogerd et al. 2007b, p. 329). The reason is that the concept of mechanism generally depends on a reductionist approach, as discussed in the preceding chapter, in which biomedical scientists analyze a system in terms of its mechanical parts and the resultant properties of those parts. These scientists then combine and synthesize aggregate parts and properties into an integrated system, which is then responsible for the system's resultant properties (Jones 2000, 2013). They utilize this method of analysis and synthesis of parts and properties to account for or to explain a system's mechanical state, especially in terms of disease etiology or even health. The success of twentieth century biomedicine, especially its molecular biology paradigm, depended on identifying the mechanisms underlying complex living phenomena (Allen 2018).

Emergence, on the other hand, involves the appearance of a system whose properties are unaccountable for or not explainable simply in terms of its constituent and aggregated parts or the properties of those parts (Bersini et al. 2012, Gillett 2016, Humphreys 2016, Kim 2006, O'Connor 2020, Vintiadis 2013). Rather, according to emergentists, a system—especially a complex adaptive system—and its properties arise or emerge from the synergistic interaction of the system's component parts. In contrast to mechanistic biomedical scientists, many, if not most, advocates of systems medicine claim that complex living phenomena exhibit emergent properties that are not reducible to or predictable precisely from a system's parts or its parts' properties (Hood and Flores 2012, Marcum 2020, Noble 2017, Wang et al. 2015, Wolkenhauer et al. 2013). In fact, the parts have limited, as discussed in the previous chapter, causal influence upon the emergence of a system and its properties. Rather, the organism reflects the emergence of a novel ontological entity, such as the personal P (P4) of P7 systems medicine.

2. Resultant and Emergence

In this section, the concepts of resultant and emergence are explored, especially as they relate to the biomedical model and systems medicine, respectively. The resultant, briefly, refers to an entity's properties that are reducible to its parts and represents a result or consequence of the parts' configuration. And the resultant is determinable or predictable from the combined or aggregate behavior of the parts without remainder or residue. According to emergence, in contrast, an entity is not simply reducible to the aggregate properties or behavior of its parts. Rather, an emergent property or behavior outstrips the simple combination or configuration of an entity's parts. In other words, the emergent entity represents the appearance of a new property or behavior that could not be predicted from the parts' aggregate properties or behavior.

2.1. Resultant

The concept of resultant has an extended history that parallels the history of mechanism, especially with Descartes' notion of the body as extended matter

(Baigrie 1996). In more contemporary terms, the concept involves the notion of an aggregation of parts that account for an entity or event (Jones 2000, 2013, Tu et al. 2021, Zhang et al. 2020). For example, the mass of a molecule is simply the aggregate mass of its individual atoms. Moreover, resultant properties are the outcome of the analysis of complex or higher-level entities or events into their component parts, with no reference to other parts or their properties. In other words, an entity and its properties can be accounted for in terms of its parts and their properties. As Dave Elder-Vass explains,

> The resultant properties of an entity are not dependent upon the relations between its parts, since they are already possessed by the parts themselves, and the resultant property of the higher-level entity is merely the result of the aggregation of the equivalent properties of its lower-level parts. It is therefore possible to explain the property purely in terms of the parts, neglecting any relations between them that are constitutive of the higher-level entity (2005, p. 322).

In other words, the entity can be explained simply and completely in aggregate terms, with no remainder or residue, i.e., it needs no further explanation than the configuration of its parts and their properties.

William Wimsatt identifies four conditions to account for a system's or an entity's resultant properties vis-à-vis what he calls aggregativity, i.e., "the system property must remain invariant or stable under modifications of the system in the specified way, a kind of independence of the property over changes in the mode of organization of the parts" (2000, p. 272). The first condition is "Inter Substitution" or the invariance of the system when "rearranging" its parts. The next condition is "Qualitative Similarity" of the system when adding or subtracting parts. The third condition, similar to the first, is "ReAggregation" or the invariance of the system when "reaggregating" its parts. The final condition is "Linearity" such that no cooperative or inhibitory interactions exist among the system's parts. In sum, a system exhibits resultant properties when it satisfies these conditions.

Richard Jones makes a similar argument for resultant properties. For Jones, such properties are

> strictly the product of the lower levels, or they are not new properties at all but only "resultant" properties (i.e., larger aggregates of the same lower-level properties) or a mechanical assembly (e.g., tables and radios) in which higher-level phenomena result solely from the structure of the

> lower-level realities and so are entirely explainable by the lower-level properties and hence are reducible. Resultant properties are simply the accumulations of lower-level properties, or at least no higher-level properties or structures are involved (2000, p. 19).

Consequently, the properties of a higher-level or complex entity or event are simply the straightforward combination of its parts. In other words, the assembly or compilation of an entity's parts accounts or is responsible for the resultant properties of the whole entity. Such a position denies, then, the need for anything extra—either ontologically or epistemically—to account for the properties of higher-level entities.

As discussed previously, mechanism is a founding concept of the biomedical model and evidence-based medicine (EBM). The reason is that the body and its properties, whether healthful or ill, are a resultant of the body's parts because causal flow is strictly and exclusively upward. Unfortunately, the impact of resultant mechanism, with its reductionistic approach, robs patients of their agency in clinical encounters and treatment regimes. And its impact also affects the biomedical sciences themselves in terms of their approach to investigating and developing therapeutic protocols and treatments. What drives that research is the notion of the "magic bullet" (Mann 1999, Rosen 2017). Paul Ehrlich introduced this notion in the early twentieth century and provided the first bullet, Salvarsan, to treat syphilis (Strebhardt and Ullrich 2008, Winau et al. 2004). Although the pharmaceutical industry strives to discover magic bullets for various diseases, especially chronic diseases, few if any drugs have been discovered or developed that are efficacious in curing the diseases plaguing contemporary industrialized society (Strasser 2008). Regrettably, many of the drugs have injurious side-effects that often cause more harm than good (Brandt 2020). For example, chemotherapy drugs developed to treat cancer are often fraught with debilitating side-effects (Velchiti and Punekar 2022). This situation has led to the reemergence of medical nihilism, according to Jacob Stegenga (2018), who proposes *la médicine douce*, or gentle medicine, in contrast to an aggressive medicine that is often promoted by the pharmaceutical industry.

2.2. Emergence

The concept of emergence has a prolonged history, with its roots in Aristotle's notion of entelechy (Clayton 2006, Corning 2012, Goldstein 1999, Stöckler

1991). For Aristotle, according to Philip Clayton, entelechy is "the internal principle of growth and perfection that directed the organism to actualize the qualities that it contained in a merely potential state" (2006, p. 5).[46] In other words, entelechy is a force or principle that realizes the organism's potential in terms of self-generation or development. In subsequent history, entelechy became associated with the notion of a vital force—a force that exists independently from the physical material upon which it acts (Allen 2018, De Klerk 1979, Sheldrake 1981a). For example, the German developmental biologist, Hans Driesch, defined entelechy not in terms of physico-chemical mechanisms. Rather, Driesch defined it as "something acting univocally with regard to the inorganic, as we know, and therefore there must be something in this relation that is comparable with the principle of reaction in a general logical sense though beyond inorganic causality" (1908, p. 228). In other words, entelechy transcends and at the same time controls or directs inorganic or physical entities vis-à-vis vital forces.

The contemporary roots of emergentism are in the late nineteenth and early twentieth centuries, especially in terms of the British Emergentist movement (Blitz 1992, McLaughlin 1992, 2019, O'Connor 2020).[47] British emergentists, who are the best-studied group of the emergentist movement, arose in response to the excesses attributable to both reductionism and vitalism.[48] "According to British Emergentism," claims Brian McLaughlin, "there is a hierarchy of levels of organizational complexity of material particles that includes, in ascending order, the strictly physical, the chemical, the biological, and the psychological level" (1992, p. 50). Each level contains various entities and processes specific to that level, and these entities and processes exhibit novel, emergent properties associated with a given level. For example, properties like consciousness and cognition emerge from the unique

[46] Aristotle defines entelechy in terms of the soul, as an actuality or a "substance *qua* form of a natural body which has life potentially" (1993, II, i, 412^{a}20).

[47] Stephan (1992) divides the history of contemporary emergentism into four periods, beginning with Mill and Lewes in the late nineteenth century. The next period covers the work of Alexander, Morgan, and Broad in the early twentieth century, while the third period starts in 1926 with the "Sixth International Congress in Philosophy" and includes the work of Driesch, Arthur Lovejoy, and others. The final period covers the second half of the twentieth century with the work of Sperry and Karl Popper, among others. Jeffrey Goldstein (1999), however, divides the history into two periods: proto-emergentism and neo-emergentism. The first refers to emergent theories prior to the 1930s, in which the mechanics of emergentism was unknown. The latter refers to theories after that date, in which commentators explicate emergentism in terms of complexity theory.

[48] The emergentist movement, however, did include a large number of scholars from various nations, such as the French philosopher Henri Bergson and the American philosopher Arthur Lovejoy.

and novel structure of neural circuitry. In addition, British emergentists aimed to provide a comprehensive view of the world in terms of evolutionary mechanisms.

Traditionally, John Stuart Mill is identified as the person responsible for initiating British Emergentism, although he did not use the word emergence. In *A System of Logic*, Mill (1865) argued that some physical or chemical properties are not reducible to their component parts and their properties or to the simple combination of these parts. For example, he claimed that water's property of wetness is not reducible to the individual properties of either hydrogen or oxygen.[49] In the late nineteenth century, the British psychologist, G.H. Lewes, argued that reductionism is incapable of capturing the completeness or wholeness of an entity or event and introduced the term "emergent" in contrast to the reductionist term "resultant" (McLaughlin 2019). According to Lewes, the "resultant…is clearly traceable in its components, because these are homogeneous and commensurable," while the "emergent is unlike its components insofar as these are incommensurable, and it cannot be reduced to their sum or their difference" (1875, p. 412). Lewes' intuition concerning the difference between emergent and resultant properties formed the conceptual basis for the development of British Emergentism.

Two figures that loomed large in the development of British Emergentism are Australian-born British philosopher, Samuel Alexander, and British zoologist and psychologist, C. Lloyd Morgan. Alexander developed his idea of emergence in his 1916-1918 Gifford lectures, later published as *Space, Time, and Deity*. According to Alexander (1920), the universe exhibits a layered ordering with higher-level entities constructed from lower-level ones. However, at the higher levels new properties or qualities emerge and can exhibit causal activity, even on lower-level entities. "Like the other British Emergentists," observes Carl Gillett, "Alexander holds that new 'emergent' properties come into being as microphysical individuals and their microphysical properties are aggregated in this manner" (2006, p. 264). Specifically, the aggregation is according to structured hierarchical levels, with high-level properties emerging from lower-level properties.

In 1922, Morgan also delivered the Gifford lectures, which were later published as his major opus—*Emergent Evolution*. For Morgan, as for

[49] "The chemical combination of two substances produces, as is well known," argues Mill, "a third substance with properties entirely different from those of either of the two substances separately, or both of them taken together. Not a trace of the properties of hydrogen or of oxygen," he proceeds to illustrate, "is observable in those of their compound, water" (1865, p. 408).

Alexander—who influenced Morgan—the world exhibits a layered ordering, with novel entities and events emerging from lower layers. He contrasted the emergent with the mechanical or mechanistic, which is discernable "in terms of resultant effects only, calculable in algebraic summation. It ignores the something more," Morgan went on to argue, "that must be accepted as emergent" (1927, p. 8). It was that "something more" that Morgan and other British emergentists strove to articulate; and, as the physicist P.W. Anderson argued later that this "more is different" in the sense that "the whole becomes not only more than but very different from the sum of its parts" (1972, p. 395).

The British philosopher, C.D. Broad, represents the pinnacle of British Emergentism, according to McLaughlin, "since the main doctrines of British Emergentism receive their most mature and careful formulation" with his work (1992, p. 52). His major tome was *The Mind and Its Place in Nature*, published in 1925. In it, Broad gave a straightforward definition of an emergent property or quality: "a quality which belongs to a complex as a whole and not to its parts" (1925, p. 23). In contrast to biological mechanism and substantive vitalism, Broad proposed an emergent vitalism, which he claimed depends not on entelechies, as did substantive vitalism. Rather, he grounded emergent vitalism on a conception of emergentism in which "the characteristic behaviour of the whole *could* not, even in theory, be deduced from the most complete knowledge of the behaviour of its components, taken separately or in other combinations, and of their proportions and arrangements in this whole" (Broad 1925, p. 59). In other words, a system's emergent properties outstrip the system's parts and their properties but not necessarily their arrangements or combinations.

British Emergentism was certainly not without its critics, which included Charles Baylis, Rudolph Carnap, William McDougall, Stephen Pepper, and Bertrand Russell, to name a few (Corning 2012, McLaughlin 1992, Symons 2018). For example, the American philosopher, Stephen Pepper (1926), raised a number of philosophical objections to the concept of emergence, especially in terms of the propositions used to defend the concept. For Pepper, emergentism is simply epiphenomenalism and lacks the necessary scientific rigor or empirical support to account for evolutionary change. Specifically, Pepper argued that "either the emergent laws they [emergent evolutionists] are arguing for are ineffectual and epiphenomenal, or they are effectual and capable of being absorbed into the physical system" (1926, p. 244). In other words, emergent laws, if any exist, are simply ineffectual or, if effectual, are reducible to physical laws.

Although there were a number of philosophical problems with the concept of emergentism, British Emergentism—as well as emergentism writ large—eventually failed not because of any one philosophical problem but because of the perceived empirical success of science that supported reductive mechanism, especially support from genetics and quantum physics (Corning 2012, McLaughlin 1992, Richardson and Stephan 2007b).[50] Although emergentism faded from the limelight, it did continue to find adherents throughout the twentieth century, especially in disciplines like ecology and systems science (Corning 2012, Stephan 1992). Its contemporary resurgence at the end of the twentieth century and the beginning of the twenty-first century is the result of developments in complexity and chaos theories, especially as illustrated by the Santa Fe Institute and its emphasis on complexity science (Corning 2012, Cunningham 2001, Goldstein 1999, Strogatz 2018, Waldrop 1992).

Although the goal of contemporary emergentists is comparable to the goal of earlier emergentists: "to find an approach that avoids both the Scylla of vitalism (or dualism) and the Charbdis of reductionism (or materialism)" (Boogerd et al. 2005, p. 145), they struggle with articulating a consensus definition for emergence.[51] Moreover, philosophers and scientists often emphasize different approaches to defining emergence (Bersini et al. 2012, Corradini and O'Connor 2010). Most scientists take a practical or pragmatic approach to defining emergence in terms of research discipline. According to evolutionary biologist Lynn Rothschild (2006), for example, pragmatic emergence represents a research strategy for investigating natural entities or events. For Rothschild, where reductionist approaches to investigating complex biological entities or events may be too time consuming or expensive, "a higher-level approach, which acts *as if the characteristic were emergent*, may lead more quickly to results" (2006, p. 163). In other words, pragmatic emergence is a methodological approach for understanding emergence in which an investigator pretends that a complex biological phenomenon exhibits emergent properties in order to expedite scientific investigation and analysis. She claims that this approach is particularly suited for biological research,

[50] Broad admitted that he could not provide a "conclusive example" of emergence, but he still defended emergence as "logically possible" (1925, p. 59).

[51] No consensus or precise definition of emergence is currently available because of an inherent paradox (Bedau 1997, Deguet et al. 2006). On the one hand, the emergent depends on lower-level parts and yet, on the other hand, it transcends them.

especially problems concerning origin of life, eukaryotic cells, multicellularity, and self-replication—to name just a few.[52]

The pragmatic approach of scientists to the conception of emergence vis-à-vis specific disciplinary research leads to a plethora of definitions. For example, computer scientist Aleš Kubĵk defines emergence in terms of "a property of the system that can be produced by interactions of its agents (components) with each other and with the environment and cannot be produced by summing behaviors of individual agents in the environment" (2003, p. 47). "Emergence"' as evolutionary biologist Robert Reid defines it, "is the spontaneous appearance of novel qualities through the interactions and constraints of generative conditions, consisting of the dynamic structure of the original, and properties of its environment" (2007, p. 290). Neuroanthropologist Terrence Deacon defines it as the "unprecedented global regularity generated within a composite system by virtue of the higher-order consequences of the interactions of composite parts" (2006, p. 122). Based on modeling flock behavior, physicists Manuel Berrondo and Mario Sandoval define emergence as a global effect that arises "from local interactions producing a collective coherent behavior" (2015, p. 69). Finally, according to computer scientist Sophia Kivelson and quantum physicist Steven Kivelson, "An emergent behavior of a physical system is a qualitative property that can only occur in the limit that the number of microscopic constituents tends to infinity" (2016, p. 1).

For many contemporary emergentists, as the above definitions attest, the concept of emergence refers commonly to processes by which emergents appear or manifest themselves at higher levels of complexity and organization (Agazzi and Montecucco 2002, Fernández et la. 2014, Gregersen 2006, Holland 1998).[53] For example, complexity scientist Jeffrey Goldstein defines emergence as "the arising of novel and coherent structures, patterns, and properties during the process of self-organization in complex systems" (1999, p. 49). Noble (2006) provides an apt illustration of emergence from physiology. The heart—composed of various cells and tissues—functions to pump blood throughout the body. Both the structure of the heart qua pump and its function qua pumping represent emergents, which are not reducible in toto to its component cells and tissues or to the properties of those components. In

---

[52] Although pragmatic emergence appears feeble, as Rothschild admits, its real power is in providing a means by which to evaluate whether reductionism is sufficient to investigate and explain complex biological entities.

[53] Emergents can refer to a variety of things, including agency, behaviors, effects, entities, events, laws, phenomena, properties, and even reality, to name a few (Ellis 2006, Stephan 1992).

other words, the heart is a novel entity and its ability to pump blood is a unique property vis-à-vis its component parts and their properties. Thus, while ascending a hierarchical scale from elementary components, such as macromolecules and cells, to higher-level entities, such as organ systems and organisms, both novel entities and their unique properties at higher levels emerge. In general, then, a higher-level property of a complex entity (E_1) is emergent if a different complex entity (E_2) lacks E_1's emergent property even though E_2 is composed of the same parts as E_1 but those parts resemble a different structure from E_1 (Marcum 2008a).

Based on different definitions for emergence, contemporary emergentists identify and explicate a variety of characteristics for emergence and emergent properties (Clayton 2006, Goldstein 1999, Humphreys 2016, Richardson and Stephan 2007b, Stephan 1992). The most common characteristic is naturalism, i.e., "only natural factors play a role in the various phenomena of life and mind" (Richardson and Stephan 2007b, p. 92). In other words, supernatural or unnatural entities and processes are unnecessary to account for emergents. This key feature distinguishes emergentism from vitalism. The next characteristic, related to the first, is novelty. According to Goldstein, novel "emergents have features that are not previously observed in the complex system under observation…[and] are not able to be anticipated in their full richness before they actually show themselves" (1999, p. 50). This characteristic relates to and depends upon another characteristic, hierarchical organization. Hierarchical organization refers to the segmentation of natural phenomena into higher (macro) and lower (micro) levels of organization. Emergents appear, in terms of being ostensive, during the scaling or ascending of the hierarchy from lower to higher levels. One of the historically relevant characteristics of emergence is its nonadditivity. According to this characteristic, the emergent is not the result of an algebraic sum or difference of the causes but rather a nonlinear geometric result.[54]

An emergent property is systemic, which is irreducible, nondeducible, unpredictable, and dynamic (Kim 1999, O'Connor 2020, Stephan 1999). "A property is a systemic property," argues Achim Stephan, "if and only if a

[54] Joris Deguet and colleagues analyzed several definitions of emergence present in the literature; and from their analysis, they identified several key elements of emergence (Deguet et al. 2006). Besides dynamics, they also identified the construction of a new language to articulate the novel phenomenon and its properties. Another element pertains to criteria needed to identify an emergent phenomenon or property as such. They list a variety of criteria for this last element found in the literature, including downward causation and simulation optimality. Deguet and collaborators suggest that these elements may help to guide future efforts to define precisely the nature of emergence.

system possesses it but no part of the system possesses it" (1999, p. 50). The first characteristic of a systemic property is that it is irreducible to its component parts. As Robert Richardson and Achim Stephan articulate it,

> the properties of higher-level entities do not appear to be a result of the properties of the components, even if the properties of the system are inevitable given the components together with their organization: the organization might not be a consequence of the properties of the constituents (2007b, p. 92).

Nondeducibility is the next characteristic of a system property and refers to the inability to deduce organizational principles from underlying physical laws. Because of both irreducibility and nondeducibility, a systemic property is unpredictable—even from first principles. Finally, a systematic property is dynamic in that it develops or evolves over time.

Rather than a practical or pragmatic approach to emergence, many contemporary emergentists, especially philosophers, take an ontological and/or epistemological approach (Humphreys 2016, O'Connor 2020, Rothschild 2006, Silberstein 2002, Van Gulick 2001, Wilson 2021, Yates 2013). Ontological emergence refers to the appearance of novel, substantive entities and properties at higher levels that are irreducible to fundamental components at lower levels. According to philosopher Paul Humphreys, for example,

> Ontological emergence asserts that some emergent features or objects are real features of the world and their status as emergent does not depend either on the state of knowledge of cognitive agents or on the degree of sophistication of the representational apparatus employed by such agents (2016, p. 56).

Epistemological emergence refers to the emergence of novel laws and principles at higher levels of organization, which are unpredictable or nondeducible from lower-level laws. According to Srdjan Kesić, for example, "*Epistemological emergence* occurs in situations when we do not have satisfactory explanation of the higher-level phenomena by those that exist at a lower level" (2016, p. 589).

Although emergentists classify the concept of emergence in terms of various taxonomic categories, they generally divide the concept into two main categories: strong and weak (Bedau 1997, Chalmers 2006, Clayton 2006, Emmeche et al. 2000, O'Connor 2020, Paoletti 2018, Rothschild 2006, Stephan 1999, 2006, Vintiadis 2013, Wilson 2021). David Chambers, for example, defines strong emergence "with respect to a low-level domain when the high-level phenomenon arises (in some sense) from the low-level domain, but truths concerning that phenomenon are not deducible even in principle from truths in the low level domain" (2006, p. 244). Although Chambers considers nondeducibility of strong emergents too radical, he is confident in pointing to one example in the natural sciences—human consciousness. All other examples of emergence he believes are examples of weak emergence. "A weakly emergent property of a system," according to Chalmers, "is an interesting property that is unexpected, given the underlying principles governing the system" (2006, p. 253). He admits, however, that a weakly emergent property is ambiguous in that such a property may be unexpected in terms of principles at lower levels but less so at higher levels. As he illustrates, an organism's behavior may be unexpected with respect to genetic principles but not with respect to organismal principles.

Chalmers acknowledges that his analysis of the categories of emergence is a "first approximation" and might need further elaboration. Stephan (1999, 2006) provides such elaboration. He identifies two subcategories of strong emergence, which depend on the notions of irreducibility and of unpredictability, respectively. The basis of the first subcategory, which he calls synchronic emergence, is irreducibility. By irreducibility, Stephan argues that the systemic or emergent property "cannot be deduced from the arrangement of its system's parts and the properties they have 'isolated' or in other (more simple) systems" (1999, p. 51). He goes on to identify two types of irreducibility. The first pertains to the behavior of a system's components that is not deducible from the components in isolation or in a simple arrangement. This type of irreducibility implies downward causation from the system's overall organization onto its parts. The second type pertains to unanalyzable properties of a system's micro or macro structures. These properties are not causal in a mechanistic sense but rather epiphenomenal.

Stephan predicates the second subcategory of strong emergence on the notion of the unpredictability of systemic properties. He calls this subcategory, diachronic emergence. For this subcategory, emergent properties "could not have been predicted in principle before their first instantiation" (Stephan 1999, p. 49). As such, these properties are novel. Importantly, the notion of unpredictability may reflect the variability or indeterminacy in the overall structures or configurations generating the novel properties. Stephan calls such variability or indeterminacy the "unpredictability of structure." This structural unpredictability gives rise to novel properties, especially when "laws of deterministic chaos" are responsible for their creation. An alternative reason for unpredictability is that, even if the structures are predictable, their properties are irreducible. And since novel properties are irreducible, they are then by definition unpredictable in terms of their first occurrence.

As with many other emergentists (Bedau 2013, O'Connor 2020), Stephan (1999, 2006) postulates only one category of weak emergence, and he identifies the following characteristics for this category of emergence. The first, which is common to the strong categories of emergence, is that weakly emergent properties are systemic properties. Also, in conformity with the irreducible categories of strong emergence, the weak category denies a strong sense of reductionism. The next two characteristics of the weak category, however, differ from the strong categories. The weak category exhibits a physical monism in that all systems are composed of material parts. Moreover, this category exhibits synchronic determination in that the systemic property depends on the system's structure or arrangement of its parts.[55] Consequently, the weak category is compatible with property reductionism because a systemic property depends on a system's structure. For some emergents, weak emergence is not especially useful (Boogerd et al. 2005), but certainly not for all (Bedau 2010, 2013).

Finally, a controversial philosophical issue with emergence is the interaction between emergent higher-order entities and their lower-order parts, in terms of downward causation (Bedau 2002, El-Hani and Emmeche 2000, Ellis and Kopel 2019, Emmeche et al. 2000, Macdonald and Macdonald 2010, Stephan 2002). As detailed in the previous chapter, downward causation represents the regulatory control over lower-level parts by higher-level entities. The American neuropsychologist, Roger Sperry, provides the classic example of downward causation in terms of emergent mental or conscious phenomena. According to Sperry, emergent mental phenomena exert "an active control role as causal determination in shaping the flow patterns of cerebral excitation" (1980, p. 201). However, a number of problems face emergentists who advocate downward causation through emergent entities or

[55] Stephan provides the following definition of synchronic determinism: "A system's intrinsic properties and dispositions depend nomologically on its micro-structure, that is to say, on its parts' properties and their arrangement" (2002, p. 80).

agencies.[56] The chief problem with downward causation vis-à-vis emergence, especially with Sperry's example, is that it is unclear how to connect or combine higher-level entities with their lower-level parts in a causal manner (Stephan 1992). How can emergent higher-level entities qua agents cause physically or materially new or different patterns of lower-level parts? In other words, the problem of downward causation is that it fails to account for or to demonstrate the causal powers of emergent entities or properties in terms or conditions that satisfy the mechanistic criteria for upward causation.[57]

While traditional biomedicine relies on a resultant mechanistic conceptual foundation, systems medicine relies on a conceptual foundation of emergence (Green 2017, Kaminsky et al. 2011, Louridas and Lourida 2017, Yan 2017). As Guillaume Noell and colleagues stress, "Human health and disease are emergent properties of a complex, nonlinear, dynamic multilevel biological system: the human body" (Noell et al. 2018, p. 1). And they go on to advocate for a P4 systems medicine approach to healthcare. The human body and its physiology and pathology certainly represent an emergent entity and its properties. However, P7 systems medicine incorporates not just the biological and biochemical in terms of the physico-biomolecular P (P1) but also the psychological and populational/public of patients and healthcare practitioners and society in terms of the psycho-cognitive P (P2) and population-public P (P3), respectively. Furthermore, the personal P component (P4) is also an emergent agent with emergent properties, which arise from the interactions among and entanglement of the P1-3 components. But to understand fully the emergence of P4 requires several supporting concepts, including emergent synthesis, epigeneticism, and stochasticity (Table 1), which are discussed in the next three sections.

[56] For example, is the emergent property or agent new or distinct ontologically from the properties or agents that compose it? For an emergent property, this seems to be the case since the emergent property is not similar to the properties of the parts composing it. The problem is with the emergent agent (Humphreys 2016). Is such an agent simply describable as an aggregation or even a fusion of the component parts? Emergentists claim, and some reductionists agree, that emergent agents are simply more than an aggregation of component parts but rather the structuring or patterning of those parts are what make emergent agents unique ontologically and permit them to exhibit downward causal powers.

[57] As noted earlier, some philosophers hold that higher-order phenomena supervene on lower-order phenomena in a causal manner, while other philosophers acknowledge that higher-order phenomena supervene on lower-order phenomena but without any direct causal interaction between them (Kim 1993, Mendonça 2002). According to Jones, however, the notion of supervenience does not address the causal question concerning emergent realities, "since the question merely becomes: why is there a process of some realities supervening on others?" (2000, p. 335).

3. Synthesis and Emergent Synthesis

The concept of synthesis is the foundation of biomedicine and EBM in which the patient represents the aggregate combination of mechanical parts. Disease and health then are simply the proper synthetic function of those parts, and synthesis guarantees the ability to then predict possible dysfunction, especially in terms of a reductive precision medicine. In contrast, the concept of emergent synthesis states that the patient's pathophysiological condition is an emergent product or property of the synergy among the mechanical parts. Disease and health then are not reducible to the simple aggregation of a system's parts but the emergent property of the system itself. Inherent in this conception is a paradox of uncertainty in that on the one hand diagnosis and therapy might be efficacious for one patient but on the other hand not for another similar patient, and the current biomedical model struggles to explain the difference between them.

3.1. Synthesis

For mechanists, as noted earlier, an entity like a machine is composed of parts and the method for investigating it is through analysis and synthesis, which has a long history in both science and philosophy (Beaney 2014, Hall 1995, Jones 2000, 2013, Ritchey 1991). For example, Newton's method of scientific investigation was grounded on both analysis and synthesis of natural phenomena (Ducheyne 2011, Guicciardini 2009).[58] In the *Opticks*, Newton characterized analysis accordingly, "we may proceed from Compounds to Ingredients, and from Motions to the Forces producing them; and in general, from Effects to their Causes, and from particular Causes to more general ones" (1730, p. 404). For synthesis, he claimed it "consists in assuming the Causes discover'd, and establish'd as Principles, and by them explaining the Phænomena proceeding from them, and proving the Explanations" (1730, p. 405). As Giorgio Tonelli sums up Newton's method, "the analysis should always precede the synthesis, because it allows us to proceed from the compounds to the composing parts, and in general from the effects to the causes, until we reach the most general causes" (1976, p. 180).

[58] Besides Newton, other prominent natural philosophers promoted the scientific method of analysis and synthesis such as Francis Bacon (Jardine 1974).

As the analysis-synthesis method developed in the natural sciences during the last several centuries, especially within the chemical and biological sciences, analysis was reductive in nature while synthesis was combinative of the analytic parts as a resultant entity (Hall 1997, Poli 2011). Importantly, the entity is simply the result of a synthetic aggregation of its parts and their properties. This synthesis does not depend on an additional ontic property or component, but it does depend epistemically on the structure of the parts vis-à-vis the intact entity. In other words, the structural interaction of the component parts is important and sufficient for explaining the resultant or mechanistic properties of the synthetic entity.

Synthesis, then, refers to the recombining or reassembling of components obtained through reductive analysis. And it is an important methodological strategy for understanding entities or events, especially biological ones. The notion of biological life, for instance, is intelligible in terms of structuring an organism's component parts. "Life, like a machine," claim Anthony Forster and George Church, "cannot be understood simply by studying it and its parts; it must also be put together from its parts" (2006, p. 1). Synthesis represents the ability to structure a biological entity through stepwise addition of parts or subsystems of parts. For example, Craig Ventor and colleagues recently synthesized a minimal cell called JCVI-Syn3.0, which has a genome of a little over 500,000 nucleotide base pairs and only 438 protein-coding genes and 35 RNA-coding genes (Hutchison et al. 2016).

For biomedicine and EBM, the patient represents a synthesis of analyzed clinical and laboratory data from which a diagnosis is made, and therapy is then recommended derived from metanalyses or systematic reviews (Catillon 2017, Marcum 2004, 2008a, Tucker et al. 2020, Valles 2020). And based on this diagnosis, the general approach to treatment is "one size fits all" in terms of either drugs or devices, especially for chronic diseases like cancer—although there is a push towards precision or personalized medicine (Friedman 2015, Yau 2019). Unfortunately, the recent COVID-19 pandemic illustrates this approach in which patients were disempowered from engaging in treatment options and treated homogenously with a "one size fits all" approach (Santos 2020). Moreover, this approach often results in more harm than benefit. For example, the treatment of patients suffering from mental illness and suicide ideation from a "one size fits all" approach in terms of inpatient care and medication-only treatment has failed to treat these patients effectively and has only exacerbated their suffering (Cohen et al. 2019, Jobes and Chalker 2019). In the end, patients often become digital entities that have lost their dignity as human persons (Floridi 2016, Rubeis 2021).

3.2. Emergent Synthesis

Whereas mechanists utilize the concept of synthesis based on reductive analysis to account for the interactions among component parts and to explain a system's features, emergentists use emergent synthesis and its associated concept of synergy (Bruton and O'Dwyer 2018, Bushev 1994, Roell et al. 2017, Ueda 2001).[59] Emergent synthesis refers to "a system synthesis methodology by which system behavior emerges as a global structure that is built up through bottom-up and top-down dynamic processes" (Ueda et al. 2007, p. 463). In other words, during the synthesis of a system or an entity through structuring its parts from the bottom-up, a system or an entity emerges that is the result of top-down agency. According to Jones, for example, "in a system the higher-level properties are not located in the parts, their sum, or their spatial relation with each other—the patterns are caused by something other than the forces at work in the parts" (2000, p. 29). Rather, emergent synthesis involves cooperative interaction or entanglement among its parts that give rise not simply to novel entities but to entities that also exhibit causal effect or agency on its constituent parts.

Closely associated with emergent synthesis is the concept of synergy, which is critical for understanding the emergence of novel entities and their properties (Corning 2012, Floyd and Carson 1993, Haken 2020, Rothman 1974). Peter Corning provides a comprehensive definition of synergy, which has important implications for the concept of emergence: "the *combined or cooperative effects produced by the relationships among various forces, particles, elements, parts or individuals in a given context—effects that are not otherwise attainable*" (2012, p. 303). Inherent in this definition are several types of synergy. The first involves what Corning calls "functional complementarities" and pertains to the enhancement of an entity's effect in combination with other entities, such as the emergent property of crystallinity for NaCl crystals. Importantly, the appearance of the novel property is not reducible to the properties of the individual components. Another type is what he calls "synergy of scale" and involves the aggregation of similar parts such that a novel entity or effect emerges, such as sand dune, which is related to another type of synergy called "threshold effects" resulting in an avalanche. Finally, Corning applies the concept of synergy to emergence and proposes a definition of emergent phenomena "as a 'subset' of the vast (and still

[59] "New" synthesis represents another approach to capturing the complexity of interacting subsystems, especially in explaining consciousness (Feinberg and Mallatt 2016) and moral psychology (Haidt 2007).

expanding) universe of cooperative interactions that produce synergistic effects of various kinds, both in nature and in human societies" (2012, pp. 304-305).

In sum, just as the concept of mechanism helps to explain biological entities or events in terms of the synthetic interactions among their component parts, so the concept of emergent synthesis serves a similar explanatory function with respect to synergistic interactions and the emergence of causal agency, especially in terms of top-down causation, irreducible to its constituent parts (Baas and Emmeche 1997, Humphreys 2016, Kim 1997, Markič 2004). Emergent synthesis is a strong form of emergence, and it can account for the complexity of biological entities and their behavior. For as Richardson and Stephan attest, "the system is the explanatory unit" (2007a, p. 141). In other words, the system as a unit is the basis for explaining it. Emergent explanations, then, are an alternative to traditional scientific explanations, such as deductive-nomological explanations.

However, emergent explanations are prone to a stinging paradox (Goldstein 1999). That paradox rests on epistemological features of emergence such as unpredictability, irreducibility, or nondeducibility. Emergent explanations cannot provide an explanation in terms of definitive causal factors in that the emergent cannot be determined or predicted with certainty prior to its appearance, as with the resultant. In other words, emergent explanations account for higher-level entities or events, which cannot be predicted from lower-level principles. For example, the emergent properties of living cells are the result of the synergistic interactions of molecular components and of a unique cellular structure. The synergistic interactions are responsible for the higher-order structures that exhibit downward causation. For strong emergentists, downward—and not upward—causation provides an accurate account of complex entities or events in that a downward cause explains the activity of lower-order entities or events and not vice versa.

Systems medicine represents a paradigmatic shift from the biomedical synthetic view of "one size fits all" treatment to an emergent synthetic view of "one size fits one" treatment in which synergy plays a critical role in enhancing treatment efficacy (Bland 2017, Megahed et al. 2020). In terms of P7 systems medicine, emergent synthesis and synergy operate at two levels, especially in terms of health or wellbeing and disease or illness. The first is with respect to the emergent synthesis of entities and processes that constitute P1, such as biomacromolecules, cellular elements and cells, tissues, organs, and organ systems; P2, such as psychological and behavioral factors; and P3, such as population, public, social, political, and environmental factors.

Synergy among the P1-3 components is critical for maintaining the functional integrity for each of the Ps.

The second level concerns the synergy among the P1-3 components that is then responsible for the emergent synthesis of the personal P (P4). Together with the entanglement of new materialism, synergy contributes to the functional agency of the patient qua P4, which has important implications for empowering the patient for responsible agency and participation. Moreover, rather than a digital patient constructed from synthesizing clinical and laboratory data, the personal P can be represented through construction of an avatar or a virtual patient that can be used in the classroom for pedagogical purposes (Isaza-Restrepo et al. 2018, Kononowicz et al 2019) and eventually in the clinic for making diagnoses and for exploring treatment options (Chase et al. 2018, Niederer et al. 2020, Viceconti and Hunter 2016).

Finally, several examples aptly illustrate the role and impact of emergent synthesis and synergy in systems medicine. Although emergent synthesis and synergy are operable in most clinical specialties, oncology is probably the best and most prolific example to date. Genetically modified mammary epithelial cells, for instance, that overexpress the genes encoding for both cyclin D1 and c-MYC concomitantly develop more aggressive and invasive tumors in SCID mice, than mammary cells that overexpress the genes encoding for either cyclin D1 or C-MYC separately (Wang et al. 2007). Besides at the genomic level, emergent synthesis and synergy are also operative at the epigenomic level, especially in terms of therapy. For example, experimental studies demonstrate a significant synergistic effect of microRNA on small interfering RNA in silencing the ovarian oncogene *Epha2* and thereby reducing tumor growth (Nishimura et al. 2013). Moreover, mathematical models can be used to demonstrate a strong synergistic effect between cancer immunotherapy and radiotherapy (Serre et al. 2016). Recently, a Deep Learning computational approach called DeepSynergy was developed to produce optimal synergistic combinations of chemotherapeutic drugs (Preuer et al. 2018).

4. Geneticism and Epigeneticism

In this section, the two concepts of geneticism and epigeneticism are examined with respect to their historical origins and then to their impact on both biomedicine and systems medicine, respectively. Conceptually, geneticism or genetic determinism refers to the information contained within an organism's genome, i.e., its genotype, which is responsible for its development with respect to both morphology and physiology, i.e., its phenotype. Epigeneticism, on the other hand, includes the roles environmental or external factors play in the expression of the genome such that these factors introduce variability or plasticity into the final outcome of the organism's structure and function. To that end, geneticism and biomedicine are discussed first, followed by epigeneticism and P7 systems medicine.

4.1. Geneticism

The concept of geneticism was introduced in the early twentieth century to describe James Baldwin's genetic method towards historicism in psychology (Bawden 1904). For Baldwin, the genetic method referred to "the explanation of things, for purpose of instruction, according to their genesis or manner of coming into being" (Fletcher 1921, p. 422). In other words, explanation or meaning arises from a serial relationship of entities that depends upon their antecedent factors, i.e., akin to genetic or transmissible factors. And inherent within that transmission is the information responsible for the appearance of the contemporary from the historical. In other words, there is a flow of information from the past that is responsible for the present and thereby dictates or determines the future.

In the latter half of the twentieth century, the biologist Peter Medawar championed the concept of geneticism or genetic determinism to account for biological phenomena. "Geneticism," according to Medawar, "is the doctrine of the primacy of the genetic make-up in determining every aspect of the human mind, constitution and social behaviour" (1984, p. 255). Later, Abby Lippman introduced the term "geneticization" to substitute for Medawar's geneticism and defined it as "an ongoing process by which differences between individuals are reduced to their DNA codes, with most disorders, behaviors, and physiological variations defined, at least in part, as genetic in origin" (1991, p. 19). In other words, biological determinism claims that biology is destiny (Allen 1984, Lewontin 1983, Peggs 2012).

Consequently, the concept of geneticism could be summed up in the phrase, "genotype dictates phenotype" (Taylor and Lewontin 2021). In other words, an organism's structural and functional characteristics are completely explainable in terms of its genes, which are responsible for specifying the proteins and other biomolecules responsible for its characteristics. Indeed, the idea that genes are fundamental factors that determine or dictate an organism's phenotypic morphology and behavior was not simply the predominant idea during the latter half of the twentieth century but has also survived into the twenty-first century (Plomin 2018). Historically, besides genetic determinism geneticism has taken a variety of other conceptual forms, including genetic essentialism, genetic reductionism, and genetic fatalism.

Genetic determinism is defined straightforwardly "as the view that genes (genotypes) cause traits (phenotypes)" (Resnik and Vorhaus 2006, p. 3). And it "refers to a belief system that locates the cause of all biological development in an organism's gene" (Keller 1994, p. 115). It is usually divided into two forms based on the strength of the determinism, i.e., either into strong or weak form (Resnik and Vorhaus 2006, Zwart 2014). For strong genetic determinism, genotype "always" dictates phenotype. Organisms and their behavior are just expressions of genes. For weak genetic determinism, genotype "sometimes" dictates phenotype. Often determinists articulate this form of genetic determinism in terms of potentials or predisposition, which the genes confer upon the organism but are then actualized environmentally (Moore 2003, Zwart 2014). Finally, a moderate genetic determinism occupies an intermediate position between strong and weak genetic determinism (Dawkins 1976, Resnik and Vorhaus 2006).

There are other forms of genetic determinism. For example, Sebastian Schuol (2017) divides genetic determinism into simple and covert. The former claims that "only genes characterize the phenotype" (p. 46), and it is comparable to the strong form of genetic determinism. The latter is covert in the sense that the information stored in the nucleotide sequence, which is still of primary importance causally, is regulated in terms of environmental cues. Moreover, Ted Peters (2003) divides genetic determinism into puppet determinism, in which the genes function as puppeteers, promethean determinism, in which scientists manipulate the genes, and playing-god determinism, in which scientists create the genes.

Besides genetic determinism, geneticism also includes genetic essentialism, reductionism, and fatalism (Kampourakis 2017, Wachbroit 2002). Although these forms of geneticism are sometimes used interchangeably within the professional literature, significant differences exist among them (Wachbroit 2002). Genetic essentialism refers to "the belief that our identity and personal traits are 'hard wired' by our genomes and that they are intrinsically defined and can be predicted by our genetic makeup" (Sabatello and Juengst 2019, p. S11). In other words, genes are "essential" rather than "accidental" units of heredity. Since genes are essential for the phenotypic traits, "if even one gene in the organism changes…the result is a different organism" (Wachbroit 2002, p. 355). Since "genes underlie a person's identity—they ultimately contribute to make the person who they [sic] are" (Heine et al. 2019, p. S20). Finally, Dorothy Nelkin and Susan Lindee insist the "idea of genetic essentialism has been readily adopted in popular forums where DNA—the invisible, eternal, and fundamental basis of human identity—has acquired many of the powers once granted to the immortal soul" (2004, p. 57).

Genetic reductionism refers to the belief that "genes provide the ultimate explanation for characters, and so the best approach to explain these is by studying the phenomena at the level of genes" (Kampourakis 2017, p. 6).[60] In other words, nongenetic explanations, such as environmental or social explanations, are epistemically inconsequential and thereby negligeable. Ontologically, genetic reductionism states that phenotypic traits are "nothing but" the expression of the genotype since the phenotype is reducible to its genotype (Sarkar 1998). Moreover, it has important implications methodologically in that "investigations that focus on the genetic aspects of biological phenomena are more likely to come up with important and interesting results. The patterns that emerge are more likely to reflect fundamental principles of biology than accidental or derivative correlations" (Wachbroit 2002, pp. 354-355).

Finally, genetic fatalism pertains to the conviction that if a phenotypic trait is genetic in its origin, then it is "fixed and unchangeable" (Alper and Beckwith 1993, p. 511). In other words, such a trait is the fate or providence of its genotype and is thereby unalterable. Probably the best illustration of this position is by James Watson, who is quoted as saying, "We used to think our future was in the stars. Now we know it is in our genes" (Sabatello and Juengst 2019, p. S15). For example, when patients are told they have "a gene for heart disease" they often become fatalistic about their future health (Bates et al. 2003). In sum, then, for genetic determinism, genes determine traits; for genetic essentialism, genes are essential entities responsible for traits; for genetic reductionism, traits are reduced to genes; and for genetic fatalism, traits are the fate of genes.

Geneticism and its various forms are the foundation of the biomedical model of healthcare (Sabatello and Juengst 2019, Zwart 2009). Specifically, biomedical scientists presume that diseases have strictly a genetic basis, i.e., genetic defects or mutations are responsible for disease etiology. For example, Huntington disease represents a fully penetrant autosomal dominant

[60] Genetic explanations of behavior based on strident reductionism is at best problematic in terms of providing a simplistic view of complex behaviors (Krimsky 2012).

neurodegenerative disorder (Testa and Jankovic 2019). But most diseases are not Mendelian monogenic but rather polygenic in origin (Kumar 2008). For example, many cardiovascular disorders are not only polygenic but also pleiotropic in that a single gene can contribute to multiple disorders (Cerrone et al. 2019).

The major fear among critics of biomedicine's geneticism is that the patient is simply reduced to the genome with little regard for lifestyle and social factors that can have a major impact on health and illness (Arribas-Ayllon 2016, Brenner 2004, Strohman 2003, Weiner et al. 2017). "The widespread use of genetic information to identify individuals or groups at risk for disease, or to guide provision of any social benefits and services or classify people, may," warns Melodie Slabbert, "change or challenge the way we think about what it means to be human" (2006, p. 251). In other words, patients are viewed simply as their genes and not as people.

The best example of geneticism's impact on biomedicine is the Human Genome Project (Gannet 2008, Zwart 2014). In discussing the Project, Jacquelyn Kegley (1999) identified three important assumptions undergirding its foundation of geneticism. The first is that genotype or the genetic makeup of an organism shapes its phenotype. The next assumption is that the genotype determines an organism's capacities and the boundaries of those capacities, which are invariant. The final assumption is that the genotype defines an organism's tendencies, especially physiological and behavioral. Although the Project has been highly successful in terms of identifying the biomolecular basis for living and pathological processes, it—along with geneticism in general—has its limitations and critics (Revel 2005, Strohman 2003).

In sum, as one critic, Richard Strohman, opines given numerous problems voiced against geneticism within the professional literature,

> But if genes don't determine us, if our disease causality cannot be located in genetic agents alone, if develop mental processes characterized by high fidelity adherence to species form cannot be reduced to genetic programs, if the source of evolutionary change is not traced solely to random genetic mutation, then what does determine us? (2003, p. 170).

And Strohman goes on to give a "short" answer, "that the program is in no one place; it is *distributed* at many levels of the organism, and all levels are open to environmental signals" (2003, p. 170). And he then turns to epigenesis, and its cognate epigeneticism, to unpack the answer.

4.2. Epigeneticism

Conceptually, epigeneticism has a long history (Goy 2018, Maienschein 2005, Nicoglou and Wolfe 2018), dating as far back as to Aristotle's concept of epigenesis in which an embryo develops from amorphous material through accretion of parts (Zagris 2022). In 1651, William Harvey articulates the concept precisely in the *Anatomical Exercises on the Generation of Animals* (Goldberg 2017, Harvey 1989). According to Harvey, the embryological development of "animals commences from some one part as its nucleus and origin, by the instrumentality of which the rest of the limbs are joined on, and this we say takes place by the method of epigenesis, namely, by degrees, part after part" (1989, p. 334). Thus, epigenesis refers to the step-by-step process by which an organism develops embryologically in contrast to preformation in which the organism was already fully developed, such as the homunculus, and simply grows in mass and size (Maienschein 2005). The concept of epigenesis was to play a key role in the history of embryology through the ensuing centuries, as biologists struggled to investigate and understand the mechanistic process of differentiation during embryological development (Horder et al. 1986, Needham and Hughes 1959).

After the genetic revolution in the early twentieth century, the role of the gene began to factor majorly in embryological development (Horder 2010, Morgan 1934). But the issue facing biologists was how to explain embryological development in terms of the organism's genetics. Or, as Woodger (1930) articulated it, how are genes responsible for the differentiation of smooth muscle cells and glandular cells, for example, from undifferentiated cells. In other words, how could the gap between genotype and phenotype be bridged? This question was to occupy the efforts of mid-twentieth century biologists, especially Waddington (Burian 2005, Deichmann 2016, Nicoglou and Merlin 2017).

In his 1939 book on modern genetics, Waddington (2016) introduced the concept of epigenotype to bridge the gap between genotype and phenotype. In a subsequent 1942 article on the epigenotype, Waddington (2012) coined the term epigenetics to account for the "causal mechanisms" that control developmental processes. And he went on to define the epigenotype in terms "of concatenations of processes linked together in a network, so that a disturbance at an early stage may gradually cause more and more far-reaching abnormalities in many different organs and tissues" (2012, p. 10). In other words, a change in the genotype would lead to changes within the organism's ontogeny and he gave the example of the grey-lethal gene in mice to support his theory. The network of concatenations would later become Waddington's epigenetic landscape (2014). Although epigenetics was present within the first half of the twentieth century literature, it was to become more prevalent within its second half (Holliday 2006, Streelman and Karl 1997).

A second genetic revolution, which was associated with the molecular biology revolution, took place during the second half of the twentieth century and led to the discovery of the molecular mechanisms responsible for epigenetics (Deichmann 2016, Birnstiel 1996, Morange 2020, Watson et al. 2017). One of the first major discoveries was the silencing or inactivation of the mouse X-chromosome and the proposal that the effect was the result of DNA methylation (Holliday and Pugh 1975, Riggs 1975). Subsequent research demonstrated that CpG sites or islands were the primary target for methylation (Bird 1986). Another major discovery was the role of histone modification in regulating gene activity. As early as mid-twentieth century, histones were implicated in regulating gene activation (Stedman and Stedman 1950). With the subsequent discovery of the nucleosome, the basic unit of chromatin structure comprised of chromatin wrapped around histones, acetylation or methylation of histones was associated with gene regulation (Li and Reinberg 2011, Quina et al. 2006). In short, epigenetic changes can have a significant impact on the course of both development or ontogeny of the individual organism and evolution or phylogeny of the species (Kiefer 2007, Laland et al. 2015, Noble 2006, Van De Vijver et al. 2002).

Contemporary epigenetics, as it developed during the latter half of the twentieth century, refers to the ability of nongenetic or environmental factors to determine phenotypic behavior (Feil 2008, Holliday 2006, Moore 2015). In contrast to geneticism, epigeneticism involves control of morphological development due to changes other than alteration of the DNA nucleotide sequence.[61] Moreover, a variety of definitions were proposed for the concept of contemporary epigenetics, although none of them adequately captures the various nuances for epigenetic control of biological entities or events (Baedke 2018, Lederberg 2001, Meloni and Testa 2014, Wu and Morris 2001). Arthur Riggs and colleagues, for example, proposed a useful definition of epigenetics as the "*mitotically and/or meiotically heritable changes in gene function that cannot be explained by changes in DNA sequence*" (Riggs et al. 1996, p. 1). Part of the problem with defining epigenetics is that a variety of mechanisms

---

[61] While some contrast genetic and epigenetic controls (Newman 1999), others integrate them to provide a comprehensive regulation of complex entities or events, which may involve "the reciprocal relationships between genes, organisms and their environment" (Van Regenmortel 2004, p. 1018).

exists to account for nongenetic control of biological events, from DNA methylation to chromosome imprinting. Adrian Bird also proposed the following definition of epigenetics, "the structural adaptation of chromosomal regions so as to register, signal or perpetuate altered activity states" (2007, p. 398). But research in the early part of the twenty-first century has expanded and advanced the understanding of epigenetics and its mechanisms.

The Human Genome Project has spawned the current third genetic revolution (Choudhuri 2011, Felsenfeld 2014, Kumar et al. 2017). One of the major epigenetic mechanisms discovered during this revolution is noncoding RNA (ncRNA) (Liu and Pan 2015, Wei et al. 2017). ncRNA is transcribed from DNA but is not translated into proteins. And ncRNA is distinct from messenger, ribosomal, and transfer RNAs. In general, ncRNA ranges in epigenetic functions from DNA methylation and gene inactivation to chromatin remodeling. And ncRNA is divided into two major groups: short ncRNA, which is <30 nucleotides in length, and long ncRNA, which is >200 nucleotides in length (Hombach and Kretz 2016). Short ncRNA is divided into several types: microRNA, which binds messenger RNA and prevents its translation, short-interfering RNA, which shares a similar function to microRNA and also induces heterochromatin formation, PIWI-interacting RNA, which binds the PIWI proteins and suppresses transposon activity, and small nucleolar RNA (this ncRNA is intermediate in size compared to short and long ncRNAs), which is involved in regulating translation through ribosomal activity (Ozata et al. 2019). Long ncRNA is the largest group of ncRNAs and is involved in chromatin remodeling and other molecular mechanisms (Kazimierczyk and Wrzesinski 2021). Two important types of long ncRNA are enhancer RNA and circular RNA, which are involved in transcriptional regulation.

The third genetic revolution has had a considerable impact on how epigenetics is currently defined, even though there has been little consensus on how to define it.[62] Although not meant to be a consensus definition, Carrie Deans and Keith Maggert proposed a rather comprehensive definition of epigenetics: "the study of phenomena and mechanisms that cause chromosome-bound, heritable changes to gene expression that are not

[62] Shelley Berger and colleagues, in an effort to achieve consensus within the scientific community, offer the following "operational" definition: "An epigenetic trait is a stably heritable phenotype resulting from changes in a chromosome without alterations in the DNA sequence" (Berger et al. 2009, p. 781). And they go on to parse the definition in terms of the ensuing steps: an epigenator that serves as a signal to trigger the epigenetic mechanism, an epigenetic initiator that translates the signal into an epigenetic chromatin state, and an epigenetic maintainer that sustains the chromatin state.

dependent on changes to DNA sequence" (2015, p. 892). Their definition connects the changes in gene expression to chromosomes that are independent of their DNA sequence or composition, and it acknowledges that these changes are heritable. The term "phenomena" is broad enough to include not only developmental or embryological processes but also other biological and pathological processes. Moreover, the term "mechanisms" can refer to both the molecular, including ncRNAs, and morphological dimensions of epigenetics. Finally, much of the conceptual evolution of epigenetics parallels that for genetics, especially with respect to terminology that emerged from the Human Genome Project. For example, terms like epigenome and epigenetic code mimic terms like genome and genetic code. Epigeneticism, then, represents a promise for control of biological entities or events unfulfilled by geneticism, especially its form of genetic determinism (Silverman 2004).

Epigenetics is important in implementing systems medicine, with respect to both the clinic and the laboratory (Auffray et al. 2009). It is certainly considered an essential element in establishing personalized lifestyle medicine.

> What makes each individual different is not just due to genetic variations. Environmental factors, epigenetics, gene-environmental interactions, and many others together modify our nutritional requirement, metabolism, and predisposition to disease, as well as our response to drug or lifestyle intervention. Integrating these pieces of information will allow healthcare professionals to provide personalized nutrition and lifestyle recommendations that minimize side effect and optimize efficacy (Band et al. 2017, p. 2).

An important role for epigenetics vis-à-vis systems medicine is longevity in that it can play a significant role in treating chronic diseases, such as cardiovascular diseases, type-2 diabetes, Alzheimer's disease as well as other neurological degenerative disorders, and cancers (Roukos 2012). For example, Hood and colleagues incorporate epigenetic techniques for diagnosing and treating patients suffering from various cardiovascular diseases (Trachana et al. 2018).

Epigenetics has also had a major impact on investigating and understanding disease mechanisms, especially carcinogenesis (Cazaly et al. 2015, Feinberg et al. 2016, Marcum 2019, Rodenhiser and Mann 2006, Strohman 1995, Waggoner 2007). As the epigenome consists of the normal architecture of chromosomal structure for the transmission of epigenetic information, the cancer epigenome consists of an abnormal chromosomal architecture that results in a distortion of epigenetic information (Dawson 2017). The cancer epigenome "harbors myriad abnormalities that are based on somatically heritable alterations that are not due to primary DNA sequence changes" (Baylin and Jones 2011, p. 726). Besides DNA methylation, histone modifications, and ncRNAs, one of the chief hallmarks of the cancer epigenome is chromosomal instability, which is the result of genomic instability—especially with mutation of DNA repair genes and other mitotic regulatory elements, such as chromatin remodeler complexes (Bakhoum and Landau 2017). Moreover, chromosome territories are also involved in tumorigenesis through their rearrangement so genes that are often insulated from one another intermingle (Umlauf and Mourad 2018). Finally, epigenetics plays a significant role in cancer therapies (Bates 2020, Häfner and Lund 2016, Nebbioso et al. 2018). For example, azacytidine and decitabine—two epidrugs that regulate DNA methylation—have been used to treat acute myeloid leukemia and significantly extend patient overall response rate to treatment (Pan et al. 2020).

As for systems medicine, epigenetics also plays an important role in P7 systems medicine's implementation into clinical practice. It functions for each of the first three P components, especially the physico-biomolecular P (P1). Along with genomics, transcriptomics, proteomics, metabolomics, and nutrigenomics (Table 2), epigenomics is essential for the development, growth, and health of the patient's P1 component. And just as it functions in terms of P1, so too for the psycho-cognitive P (P2). Epigenetics knits these two P components together so that the personal P (P4) can emerge through epigenetic interactions with the population-public P (P3). Indeed, it is the epigenetic interactions between the P1-2 and P3 components that account for P4's development as a unique individual person that then makes possible personalized and precision medicine. Finally, Strohman (2003) in his criticism of biomedicine's genetic determinism chastised it for ignoring the patient's experiential world, claiming that through epigenetics "the organism integrates its world of experience into a phenotype of health and well-being" (2003, p. 173). P7 systems medicine ensures that P4's phenotype includes that world of experience through acknowledging the importance of epigenetic mechanisms.

5. Determinism and Stochasticity

The concept of determinism has already been introduced when discussing the concept of genetic determinism. But the context for that discussion was the contrast between geneticism and epigeneticism, even though there is a certain amount of stochasticity or indeterminism and randomness associated with the concept. Stochasticity in general refers to an inability to predict or to determine precisely a system's future state given its present state. In contrast to determinism, stochasticity depends mathematically on probability theory and includes a variety of stochastic processes. In this section, the concepts of determinism and stochasticity are explored in greater detail and compared with one another, especially as they relate to biomedicine and systems medicine.

5.1. Determinism

The concept of determinism certainly has a long history, reaching back to the ancient Greeks. According to Presocratic philosopher Leucippus, "Nothing occurs at random, but everything for a reason and by necessity" (Guthrie 1965, p. 415). And through the subsequent centuries, the concept continued to have an impact on Western thinking, especially within the natural sciences. No person best represents determinism than Newton and his mechanistic world. For Newton, knowing the initial conditions and the laws of motion are sufficient to determine subsequent movement of a given body, which eventually led to Laplace's concept of determinism and to his demon (Janiak 2008, Weinert 2016).

Although the concept of determinism entered professional academic literature within the mid-nineteenth century, the concept itself was controversial (Bunge 2017, Earman 1986, Hacking 1983). For example, the nineteenth-century logician Henry Mansel in his discussion on determinism defined it as "the uniform sequence of phenomenon B from A" (1851, p. 303). In other words, a necessary relationship holds between A and B in that A is the cause of B. This definition depends on the two important notions: necessitarianism and causation or causality. Necessitarianism is the metaphysical notion that "anything possible is necessary" (Mandelkern and Rothschild 2021, p 89). Related to necessitarianism is the notion of predeterminism, which Jaclyn McKewan defines as, "All future actions and events are already decided or known (by God, fate, or some other force)" (2009, p. 1034). Based on these notions, Roy Weatherford provides the following general definition of determinism, "all events without exception are effects—events necessitated by earlier events. Hence any event of any kind is an effect of a prior series of effects, a causal chain with every link solid" (1995, p. 194). Although his definition exhibits reasonable simplicity, still the concept is terribly problematic; and philosophers and scientists continue to debate determinism conceptually.

One of the chief problems concerning determinism is the notion of causation or causality, which contributes significantly to the former's ambiguity (Anscombe 2001, Bunge 2017, Earman 1986, Pereboom 1995). In other words, is causation adequately and sufficiently precise to stich events together such that the determinate history of those events weaves a seamless garment? In partial response to this problem, determinism is categorized into distinct types, based on particular ideologies and disciplines, which include adequate determinism, anthropological determinism, causal determinism, ethical determinism, historical determinism, linguistic determinism, logical determinism, nomological determinism, structural determinism, and theological determinism—to name just a few (Hoefer 2003, Honderich 1988, Lucas 1970, Taylor 2006). The chief type of determinism traditionally is scientific in nature (Deese 1985, Maar 2019, O'Connor 1971). According to Robert Ackermann, scientific determinism "involves predictability in that it claims that human scientists can predict the future and will one day be able to predict all interesting facts about the future on the basis of current information" (1976, p. 130). The four common types of scientific determinism include physical determinism, biological determinism, psychological determinism, and ecological determinism, along with environmental and social determinism.

Physical determinism is the most prevalent type of scientific determinism both historically and contemporarily, which is commonly associated within the physical sciences, particularly classical Newtonianism—although this is a simplistic view (Earman 1986, Lucas 1970, Swinburne 2019). David Hodgson defines it succinctly as "*earlier circumstances and the [physical] laws of nature uniquely determine later circumstances*" (2012, p. 114). Physical determinism is often yoked with chemistry to form a physico-chemical determinism, which pertains to the reduction of chemical reactions to physical forces (Lightman 2005). Although physico-chemical determinism pertains to the inanimate world, it is also ascribed to the animate world in terms of biological determinism, which includes the concept of genetic determinism (Alper 1977, Lewontin 1983). Genetic determinism, as noted earlier, is the belief that phenotype is simply the expression of the genotype. Next, behavioral determinism, at least a radical and metaphysical type, claims that "Nothing but the behavior that did occur could have occurred, given the antecedent causal circumstances" (Slife et al. 1999, p. 77). And finally ecological determinism claims that "whatever the historical changes in distribution (dispersal or vicariance) [of species], present-day ecological factors are the major determinant of distributions" (Endler 1982, p. 349).

These various types of determinism can also be applied to humanity and its communities. For example, biological determinism holds that "the roots of human social behavior and personality lie in the biology of individuals and groups (racial or ethnic) and thus determine fundamental aspects of social life" (Allen 1984, p. 141). Behavioral or psychological determinism, on the other hand, refers to the belief that "there are certain psychological laws…enabling us to predict, usually on the basis of his experiences in early infancy, how a man will respond to different situations throughout his later life" (Lucas 1970, pp. 65-66). Environmental determinism, as David Livingstone briefly defines it, is the concept that "human activities are controlled by the environment" (Livingstone 2011, p. 368). In other words, the environment shapes the general and regional features of and differences between human cultures and societies, especially with respect to life worlds, cultural beliefs, and wellbeing. Finally, social determinism refers to the belief that "a person's essential character is shaped by social factors" (Rangel and Keller 2011, p. 1056). In sum, scientific determinism pertains to forecasting events, from the physical to the environmental to the social, that depend on both prior events and the laws governing those events—whether human or not.

Determinism is certainly at the heart of biomedicine and its associated EBM (Daschner 2019, Downie 1975, Timmermans and Kolker 2004).[63] Without a clear and consistent relationship between the etiological factors and the requisite disease, biomedical scientists and clinicians are powerless to treat the patient effectively. As Rudy Rijke acknowledges, "The principle aim of medical research is to determine which factor (or factors) causes a particular disease" (1993, p. 58). But not only physical and biological determinism are at the heart of contemporary biomedicine and EBM, although they are the chief types of determinism operative in biomedicine, but so are psychological-behavioral, environmental-ecological, and social-cultural determinism. The patient is simply a product of these deterministic factors so that knowing the conditions from the physical to the social, the patient's illness is just a matter

[63] Although EBM can accommodate uncertainly in terms of probabilistic diagnosis and treatment (Soltani and Moayyeri 2007), still the accommodation is statistical in nature rather than indeterminant.

of identifying the factors causally responsible for the disease and then simply intervening in those factors, with the expectation that a cure is guaranteed.

Unfortunately, the biomedical deterministic approach to treating patients successfully, especially of chronic illness, has been at best problematic (Stegenga 2018, Strohman 2003). Moreover, as Alvaro Daschner claims about the biomedicine's deterministic approach, "The doctor's dilemma in the face of scientific determinism is the difficulty to decide extrapolation of clinical studies results to the individual patient" (2019, p. 67). In other words, for the individual patient indeterminacy is a compounding or confounding factor for successful personalized treatment. To address that indeterminacy, as well as the patient's uniqueness, systems science and medicine depend on the concept of stochasticity or randomness in examining and understanding natural and biomedical phenomena (Buiatti and Longo 2013, Calude and Longo 2016, Heams 2014, Nikolova 2020, Van Kampen 1992).

5.2. Stochasticity

The concept of stochasticity, as previously noted, pertains to an inability to predict precisely a system's future state given its present state. The concept includes a variety of stochastic processes, such as Bernoulli process, Branching process, Brownian motion, Markov chain, Martingales, Poisson process, and Wiener process—to name but a handful (Brémaud 2020, Olofsson and Andersson 2012). According to Joseph Doob, a stochastic process represents "simply a probability process; that is, any process in nature whose evolution we can analyze successfully in terms of probability" (1942, p. 648). In more technical parlance, it is "a collection of random variables that take values in a set S, the state space…[and that] collection is indexed by another set T, the index set" (Olofsson and Andersson 2012, p. 444). The state space refers to either continuous or discrete random field variables, while the indexed set to either continuous or discrete time variables. A stochastic process, then, has various possible outcomes and a given outcome is referred to as a sample path or realized state.[64] In sum, it represents "the most

[64] According to Nico Van Kampen, "a stochastic process is simply a function of two variables, one of which is time t, and the other a stochastic variable X…On inserting for X one of its possible values x, and ordinary function of t obtains: $Y_x(t) = f(x, t)$, called a *sample function* or *realization* of the process. In physical parlance one regards the stochastic process as an 'ensemble' of these sample functions" (1992, p. 52).

prominent possibility to combine dynamical phenomena and randomness resulting from incomplete information" (Schuster 2016, p. 199).

Stochastic processes involved in biological and biomedical phenomena range from gene expression and cell growth to community ecology and species evolution, as well as from disease etiology to treatment (Andrews et al. 2009, Mode et al. 2013, Nikolova 2020). Importantly, gene expression is basically a stochastic process in which intrinsic randomness or noise associated with transcription and translation results in varying levels of mRNAs and proteins, which then influences phenotype even for genetically identical cells (Kærn et al. 2005, Raj and Van Oudenaarden 2008). Besides intrinsic randomness, extrinsic randomness in terms of external cell constituents—such cell cycle stage, RNA polymerase concentration, mRNA degradation machinery, and general cellular environment—also plays a significant role in the stochasticity of gene expression (Swain et al. 2002). Closely associated with gene expression is cellular metabolism, growth, and division, which also involve a variety of stochastic processes (Kiviet et al. 2014, Thomas et al. 2018). Besides cell growth, stochasticity is also involved in cell fate and pluripotency (Losick and Desplan 2008, MacArthur et al. 2008, Wennekamp and Hiiragi 2012).

Psychological phenomena, both neurobiological and behavioral, are also subject to stochasticity and stochastic processes (Townsend and Ashby 1983, Tuckwell 1989, Ueltzhöfferet al. 2015). Various psychological, including neurobiological and behavioral, phenomena range from synaptic transmission to cognitive faculties to personality traits. For example, release of neurotransmitter from the presynaptic membrane exhibits stochasticity as the transmitter diffuses across the synaptic cleft to bind to the postsynaptic membrane, which then has an impact on neuroplasticity (Choquet and Triller 2013, Ribrault et al. 2011). As for cognitive faculties, Dean Simonton proposes that even "scientific creativity constitutes a form of constrained stochastic behavior" (2003, p. 474). What Simonton means is that such creativity is an outcome of the stochastic processes that have an impact upon the integration between the scientist and the scientific process and product. Finally, Kyle Honegger and Benjamin de Bivort introduce the notion of stochastic individuality, which they claim is the result of "non-heritable, inter-organism behavioral variation, observable as contrasts between pairs of individuals, or, at the level of populations, as variance in a measure of behavior" (2018, p. R9). Such stochastic individuality has important consequences for a person's personality and a population's composition.

Stochasticity also plays a major role in an organism's environmental and ecological conditions, as well as in its evolution (Lande et al. 2003, Ovaskainen et al. 2016). "Environmental stochasticity," according to Masami Fujiwara and Takenori Takada, "refers to unpredictable spatiotemporal fluctuation in environmental conditions, affecting biological processes" (2017, p. 1). Stochastic environmental conditions depend on abiotic factors, such as geological architecture, nutrient accessibility, precipitation, and temperature, and on biotic factors, such as competitors, cooperators, food resources, and predators. Stochastic fluctuations of these factors have a significant impact on population size and structure, especially on a community's ecology (Shoemaker et al. 2020). Environmental and ecological stochasticity also has an impact on the life history of not only individuals and populations but also species (Engen et al. 2020). Stochasticity in evolution involves the fluctuations in genotypes, particularly in terms of genetic mutations and drift, and in environmental and ecological conditions, with respect to the adaptation and selection of novel phenotypes (Lenormand et al. 2009, Rice et al. 2011). For example, stochastic branching processes have been used to model the establishment of a beneficial mutation under fluctuating environmental conditions (Uecker and Hermisson 2011).

Finally, stochasticity also has an impact on cultural and social evolution (Buskell et al. 2019, Cantor et al. 2021, Zhukov et al. 2020). Cultural and social evolution refers to the evolutionary changes in cultural and social traits ranging from beliefs, myths, and material artefacts to social structures such as cultural norms and social institutions and technologies. Historically, models constructed to investigate and explain cultural and social evolution mimicked models of population genetics. "Cultural patterns of transmission, innovation, random fluctuations, and selection," according to Oren Kolodny, "are conceptually analogous to genetic processes of transmission, mutation, drift, and selection, and many of the mathematical techniques used to study genetics can be useful in the study of culture" (Creanza et al. 2017, p. 7782). Although such a genetic approach has yielded much insight into cultural and social evolution, evolutionary change within cultures and societies often involves stochastic processes and architectures exclusively associated with them. For example, according to Sylvain Billiard and Alexandra Alvergne,

> there are several other potential sources of stochasticity that might impact patterns of cultural diversity: cognitive processes at the individual level, random copy errors during the expression of traits, interactions between

> individuals in social networks, and random sampling at the population level (2018, p. 17).

Lastly, just as species become extinct so can cultures and societies, especially artifacts associated with them such as language, which can also be influenced by stochastic processes (Zhang and Mace 2021).

Before turning to the role of stochasticity in both systems medicine and P7 medicine, the relationship between determinism and stochasticity is an important question that must be addressed. That question is whether the two concepts, even though mostly if not completely incommensurable, are still concurrently operative but simply in different domains. In other words, are deterministic or stochastic processes the appropriate approach for modeling a particular biological phenomenon? Although many developmental processes appear to generate a deterministic product, major variation in that product is possible, which requires different modeling strategies (Lecca et al. 2013). To some extent, the distinction between determinism and stochasticity is a false dilemma (Zernicka-Goetz and Huang 2010). For example, in terms of cell fate decisions during development, variation is certainly observable but still the final product is predictable and so the appropriate analogy is not the randomness of a coin-flip but of a weighted coin-flip (Zechner et al. 2020). Rather than a strict dichotomy, developmental processes like most biological processes result in a range of possible but constrained outcomes. Even epigenetic influence on gene expression is to some extent deterministic (Waggoner and Uller 2015). In sum, both determinism and stochasticity play an important role conceptually in understanding biological phenomena and require careful consideration both in terms of etiology and treatment of disease.

As noted earlier, stochasticity is very important conceptually in systems medicine. It has been incorporated into the investigation of the etiology of a number of diseases, including macular degeneration, metabolic diseases, and children's diseases such as measles and whooping cough, as well as the spread of diseases including COVID-19 (Hjelmeland 2011, Kim et al. 2019, Maltsev and Stern 2021, Panzeri and Pospisilik 2018, Rohani et al. 2002). However, it plays a particularly key role in investigating and understanding cancer (Feinberg 2014, Foo et al. 2011, Sabino et al. 2018, Teschendorff et al. 2016). One study in particular commanded quite a bit of attention not only from the scientific community but also from the public. Christian Tomasetti and Bert Vogelstein (2015) conducted the study and what they discovered by analyzing the relationship between stem cell divisions and carcinogenesis was a direct correlation between the number of stem cell divisions and the incidence of cancer. Tomasetti and Vogelstein concluded that a significant number of cancers are "due to 'bad luck,' that is, random mutations arising during DNA replication in normal, noncancerous stem cells" (2015, p. 78). Although their study initiated considerable debate, Barry Meisenberg, a practicing oncologist, lamented that "It is perfectly fine for cancer in the abstract to be stochastic; but cancer in the individual should not be deprived of meaning" (2015, p. 576). Meisenberg's perceptive insight belies that although stochasticity is important in systems medicine, it is often relegated to the biological level and fails to engage the patient at the personal level.

P7 systems medicine provides a larger perspective to include not simply the impact of stochasticity with the physico-biomolecular P (P1) but also with the psycho-cognitive P (P2) and population-public P (P3), especially in terms of forming the unique personal P (P4). Briefly, stochasticity provides the source for variation that makes each patient qua P4 not simply personal but also individually unique. Given this uniqueness, implementation of P7 medicine requires that healthcare practitioners integrate as best as possible each of the first three P-components, especially in terms of the P-actions. In other words, the practitioner must integrate both the P5-predictive and the P6-participatory actions in order to prevent the illness or to treat it efficaciously if manifested. By considering the impact stochasticity can have on either preventing the illness or treating it, the P7 practitioner strives to incorporate random variation into the clinical consult to provide the best healthcare possible.

Conclusion

Whereas the biomedical model depends on the concept of mechanistic resultant for providing clinical care, systems medicine, and P7 systems medicine in particular, depends on the concept of emergence. The biomedical mechanistic resultant includes the concepts of synthesis, geneticism, and determinism, while P7 systems medicine includes the concepts of emergent synthesis, epigeneticism, and stochasticity. Synthesis is an important concept in terms of integrating the various component parts that comprise a biomedical entity, such as the patient, but it fails to acknowledge that some of its properties do not reduce to the properties of its parts, whereas emergent synthesis does acknowledge this and uses it to provide a more comprehensive analysis and understanding of the whole system that includes the patient as unique. Both geneticism and determinism supplement the biomedical mechanistic resultant in that the patient is simply determinable in terms of the genome, e.g., genetical determinism. In terms of the personal P (P4) of P7 systems medicine, the emergent, in its fully vigorous form, takes into consideration both epigeneticism and stochasticity for understanding the patient as a unique individual.

Although the mechanistic resultant and the emergent appear to be mutually exclusive or incommensurable concepts, several intermediate paradigms that combine both have been proposed within the literature (Boogerd et al. 2005, Boogerd et al. 2007b, Ellis 2006, Glauer 2012, Orsucci 2003, Richardson and Stephan 2007a, Schouten and De Jong 2006). Richardson and Stephan, for example, argue that complex biological entities can exhibit "emergent phenomena that are mechanistically explainable" (2007a, p. 126). The distinction is not so much between emergent and resultant as it is between emergent mechanism and reductive mechanism. Briefly, the emergent mechanism is not eliminative as is reductive mechanism; rather than eliminating or bracketing the context at higher levels, it takes into consideration that context in which a higher-level phenomenon occurs or emerges. According to Richardson and Stephan (2007a), an emergent mechanistic approach to biological entities or events is two-dimensional, including not only the vertical relationships among levels of organization—which is reductive in nature—but also the horizontal relationships among grades of resolution—which is emergent in nature. This two-dimensional approach allows biomedical scientists to explain the behavior of a complex biomedical phenomenon through redescription of the phenomenon at different grades of resolution rather than simply through reduction to a lower level of organization.

Ramiro Glauer (2012) also proposes the notion of emergent mechanism to bridge the gap between emergence and mechanism. Glauer postulates a continuum between a strong form of emergence and a weak form. On the weak end of the continuum, emergent properties can be accounted for mechanistically, or in his words, "systems that are characterized by [differential] equations that can be solved analytically and whose quantitative and qualitative system behavior can be determined quite easily" (2012, p. 120). On the strong end, emergent properties cannot be solved using differential equations quantitatively and are unexplainable qualitatively in terms of mechanism. He gives the example of strange attractors within a chaotic system. In between the two ends of the continuum is an emergent mechanism, which, although a complex dynamic system cannot be solved in terms of differential equations, can be explained in terms of qualitative mechanisms. "Emergent mechanisms," concludes Glauer, "were introduced in order to distinguish systems that somehow escape our naïve mechanistic thinking but are explained in terms of an organized collection of components nonetheless" (2012, pp. 127-128). Importantly, then, emergence is not a simple concept but requires attention to the context under which a phenomenon develops, which has important implications for systems medicine and its practice.

In conclusion, although biological and biomedical processes appear on average to be deterministic the practitioner of P7 systems medicine realizes that uncertainty or indeterminacy is always a possibility during the patient's illness experience and in treating the illness. Indeed, as Atul Gawande writes,

> The core predicament of medicine—the thing that makes being a patient so wrenching, being a doctor so difficult, and being a part of society that pays the bills they run up so vexing—is uncertainty. With all that we know nowadays about people and diseases and how to diagnose and treat them, it can be hard to see this, hard to grasp how deeply uncertainty runs. As a doctor, you come to find, however, that the struggle in caring for people is more often with what you do not know than what you do. Medicine's ground state is uncertainty. And wisdom—for both the patients and doctors—is defined by how one copes with it (2002, p. 229).

P7 systems medicine equips and empowers both the clinical practitioner and patient not only to appreciate the uncertainty of the illness experience but also to incorporate it into the clinical encounter to provide the best possible care and clinical outcome, which raises the final conceptual foundation for achieving that end—robustness.

Chapter 4

Homeostasis and Robustness

Abstract

In this chapter, the concept of homeostasis is initially examined by reconstructing its history and then exploring its various definitions, followed a discussion of homeostatic regulatory mechanisms, along with the different processes for maintaining a system's internal state. Besides homeostasis, the associated concepts of linear dynamics and stasis or stability, along with the concepts of homeodynamics, heterostasis, and allostasis, are introduced and discussed. Next, the concept of robustness, in terms of its history and definitions, are examined, along with the architecture of robust systems in terms of its bow-tie or hour-glass structure. Finally, nonlinear dynamics as well as evolvability and fragility—concepts closely associated with robustness—are introduced and discussed.

Keywords: dynamics, evolvability, fragility, homeostasis, robustness

1. Introduction

One of the chief or core concepts of the biomedical paradigm is homeostasis (Billman 2020, Michael et al. 2017). According to Cecie Starr and colleagues, homeostasis "is one of the defining features of life" (2019, p. 7).[65] Fundamentally, the concept of homeostasis including its homeostatic regulatory mechanisms, refers to the capacity or capability of an organism to maintain a stable internal environment in a changing external world, i.e., maintenance of a system's state around a particular pre-set value or set point. For example, a sudden and dramatic change in the external temperature causes but a momentary and modest change of the internal temperature of a warm-blooded or homeothermic organism. Such an organism relies on homeostatic regulatory mechanisms, such as shivering and peripheral vasoconstriction, to

[65] For further discussion, see also Agutter and Wheatley (2007), Chiras (2015), Epstein (2003), Fowler et al. (2017), Gánti (2003), and Thomas (1996).

maintain its internal temperature in the face of cold temperatures. Besides thermoregulation, other examples of homeostasis include regulation of blood glucose and calcium levels.

In general, homeostatic regulatory mechanisms are involved in restoring an organism's internal stability or stasis when confronted with an external perturbation or challenge and as such plays a pivotal role in defining health and disease (Billman 2013, Chiras 2015, Patton and Thibodeau 2014, Ventriglia and Murgia 2011). These mechanisms usually involve the concept of linear dynamics or oscillations constituted by negative and positive feedback and feedforward loops. The internal environment's constancy entails only a spatiotemporal slice of a natural phenomenon and relies on the concept of stasis or stability. From such a slice, biologists and biomedical scientists identify and investigate the parts that constitute the homeostatic mechanism in a static or stable fashion. Finally, the concept of stasis or stability involves the capacity of a system to maintain its structural and functional pre-set steady state with respect to its physical or chemical equilibrium. However, this equilibrium is invariable in nature given the fixed value of a pre-set steady state value or condition that is preserved within a limited range.

Robustness is one of the chief features of systems biology and medicine, especially with respect to systems complexity (Bertolaso et al. 2018, Carlson and Doyle 2002, Marcum 2009, Nijhout et al. 2019, Whitacre 2012). "Robustness," observes Hiroaki Kitano, "is one of the fundamental characteristics of biological systems" (2007a, p. 1). It denotes a system's capacity to accommodate or endure a variety of perturbations that might compromise not only its structural but also its functional integrity. Importantly, accommodation conceptually refers to a "stationary state, a regulatory scheme (e.g., topological features of a regulatory network), or a function of a living system, or a developmental pathway (that is, the sequence of 'choices' or 'decisions' made at each step in the making of an organism)" (Lesne 2008, p. 511). In addition, perturbations may exhibit a wide range of characteristics, including magnitude, i.e., strong or weak; scale, i.e., large or small; spatiality, i.e., system or environment; and temporality, i.e., transient or sustained. In contrast to the linear dynamics of homeostasis, robustness depends on nonlinear dynamics (Ahn et al. 2006, Strogatz 2018).

Systems scientists distinguish robustness from homeostasis in that the former depends on strategies for maintaining functionality, even if those strategies forfeit stasis or stability, while the latter does not (Bizzarri et al. 2013, Stelling et al. 2004). "Although robustness will often entail maintaining the system within a narrow range of parameters," as Peter Hammerstein and coworkers explain, "it will also often entail strategically shifting the system into dramatically different mode of operation" (Hammerstein et al. 2006, pp. 90-91). That shifting of the system involves the notion of evolvability, which pertains to the notion of the system's plasticity but also includes its fragility (Kitano 2007a, Wagner 2005). Finally, robustness exhibits bow-tie or hour-glass architecture, composed of highly conserved core processes that are responsible for reacting to perturbations (Alon 2019, Kitano 2004a, 2007a).

2. Homeostasis and Robustness

As noted above, homeostasis is the maintenance of a constant or stable physiological state or condition in which the organism can function optimally, especially when confronted with external perturbations or challenges to that stability or stasis. To that end, several homeostatic mechanisms are responsible for maintaining an organism's internal stability when confronted with an external perturbation, including the linear dynamics of negative or positive feedback or feedforward loops. Homeostasis is the fundamental concept for the biomedical paradigm, especially in terms of health and disease. Robustness can also involve the maintenance of a constant or stable physiological condition, but that stability need not represent a permanent pre-set value but one that can be redefined to establish a new value. It is not limited to static or even linear dynamic control but rather to a nonlinear dynamic control. And robustness is the foundational concept for systems medicine, particularly P7 systems medicine.

2.1. Homeostasis

Although Walter Cannon (1929, 1939) acknowledged the role of the Greek physician, Hippocrates, and the notion of *vis medicatrix naturae* (natural healing powers) in his historical reconstruction of homeostasis conceptually, the historical origin of homeostasis is recent (Billman 2020, Cooper 2008, Eskov et al. 2017, Pennazio 2009). Cannon identified several nineteenth century physiologists who contributed to or presaged the concept of homeostasis. The first is the German physiologist, Eduard Pflüger. Cannon claimed that Pflüger's 1877 "dictum" advocated the presence of "natural adjustments which lead toward the maintenance of a steady state of organisms" (1939, p. 21).[66] Next is the Belgium physiologist, Léon Fredericq, whom Cannon quotes approvingly,

> The living being is an agency of such sort that each disturbing influence induces by itself the calling forth of compensatory activity to neutralize or repair the disturbance... [This activity] tend[s] to free the organism completely from the unfavorable influences and changes occurring in the environment (1939, p. 21).

Finally, Cannon cited at length the French physiologist, Charles Richet:

> The living being is stable...It must be so in order not to be destroyed, dissolved or disintegrated by the colossal forces, often adverse, which surround it. By an apparent contradiction it maintains its stability only if it is excitable and capable of modifying itself according to external stimuli and adjusting its response to the stimulation. In a sense it is stable because it is modifiable—the slight instability is the necessary condition for the true stability of the organism (1939, p. 21).

But Cannon credited particularly one of Bichat's compatriots as the important predecessor to the conceptualization of homeostasis—Claude Bernard (1957).

In a chapter on the body qua fluid matrix, Cannon (1939) acknowledged Bernard's experimental work and specifically his notion of *milieu interieur*. For example, Cannon claimed that "Claude Bernard...first suggested that a highly important factor in the establishment and maintenance of steady states in the body is the internal environment" (1939, p. 37). Cannon pointed out that Bernard enlarged the notion of the *milieu interieur* to include not only the blood and then lymph, but also the whole of bodily fluids. Cannon then quoted Bernard on the importance of a fixed internal environment vis-à-vis a varying external environment:

> It is the fixity of the '*milieu interieur*' which is the condition of free and independent life...all the vital mechanisms, however varied they may be, have only one object, that of preserving constant the conditions of life in the internal environment" (1939, p. 38).

---

[66] Cannon had earlier identified Pflüger's 1877 "dictum" as, "The cause of every need of a living being is also the cause of the satisfaction of the need" (1929, p. 399).

Cannon then extended Bernard's notion by invoking the automatic or homeostatic mechanisms involved in maintaining the internal milieu's constancy.[67]

Cannon also acknowledged the impact of Ernest Starling on the formulation of homeostasis, particularly as it relates to medicine. "Only by understanding the wisdom of the body…," wrote Cannon sympathetically of Starling, "shall we attain that 'mastery of disease and pain which will enable us to relieve the burden of mankind'" (1939, p. xv).[68] In the 1923 Harverian Lecture, "The Wisdom of the Body," Starling discussed his research on the heart, which led to Starling's law of the heart, and on hormones, a term he coined, and on how the body adapts to changes in its environment. Starling concluded from his research on the heart's response to challenging stimuli: "the heart has a marvelous power of adapting its work and its performance in accordance with the needs of the body as a whole" (1923, p. 686). For example, according to Starling's law of the heart an increase venous return stretches cardiac fibers or cells so that the heart contracts more forcefully to meet the demand of the body's metabolizing tissues. Cannon found these innate properties of the heart suggestive of automatic mechanisms by which the body maintains an internal stability in an unstable world, i.e., the body's "wisdom" to know how to act when threatened by harmful or challenging stimuli.

Obviously, Cannon's own research work was instrumental in the formulation of the concept of homeostasis. As Donald Fleming observes,

> The main source of the new concept lay in Cannon's own topics of research broadening out from digestion to adrenaline and thence to the sympathetic system and finally to the autonomic system in general. The whole thrust of his career had been pointing him toward a heightened

---

[67] Importantly, Bernard subscribed to a reductive strategy for experimental research in medicine, as evident from this following claim: "a living organism is nothing but a wonderful machine endowed with the most marvelous properties and set going by means of the most complex and delicate mechanism" (1957, p. 63).

[68] Cannon's quote represents the last line of Starling's published lecture. Interestingly, Starling embedded this charge for the relief of pain and suffering in the secularized religious language of sin: "when as physicians we stand on the other side of good and evil, we know that the sin for which man is continuously paying the penalty is not necessarily failure to comply with someone or other of the rough tribal adjustments to the environment, which we call morality, but is always and in every case ignorance and disregard of the immutable working of the forces of Nature which is being continually revealed to us by scientific investigation" (1923, p. 690).

awareness of self-regulatory processes in physiology (1984, pp. 622-623).[69]

And, although Cannon's discovery of the role of adrenaline in the release of sugar from the liver was necessary for the elucidation of the concept of homeostasis, the discovery of insulin in the early 1920s provided the crucial exemplar for developing the concept (Bliss 1982). Now Cannon had an antagonistic agent that could counter the effects of adrenaline (Cannon 1994, Fleming 1984). In other words, insulin causes the liver to take up and store sugar while adrenaline causes it to release the carbohydrate when the body needs it. Cannon directly saw his way clear to articulating the concept of homeostasis, which he first introduced in a mid-1920s article published in a Jubilee volume honoring Charles Richet (Cannon 1926). He further elaborated the concept in a review article (Cannon 1929) and ultimately in a book (Cannon 1939).

From the historical analysis and from his experimental work, Cannon concluded, "Organisms, composed of material which is characterized by the utmost inconstancy and unsteadiness, have somehow learned the methods of maintaining constancy and keeping steady in the presence of conditions which might reasonably be expected to prove profoundly disturbing" (1939, pp. 21-22). From this conclusion, he provided a precise definition for homeostasis, which he coined from two Latin words: *homeo*, which means the same or similar, and *stasis*, which means standing or state. For Cannon, homeostasis is "the steady states in the body…a condition which may vary, but which is relatively constant" (1939, p. 24). Cannon made a distinction between equilibrium and homeostasis, in that the former reflects the "relatively simple physic-chemical states, in closed systems, where known forces are balanced" (1939, p. 24). The latter, however, refers to the state of living organisms that represent open systems able to respond to varying environmental conditions. Homeostasis is the "normal state" of the organism that when perturbed by outside stimuli returns to normalcy.

Contemporary literature contains a plethora of definitions for homeostasis. For example, one commentator defines it accordingly: "a specialized form of regulation that precisely maintains the function of a system at a set point level of activity" (Davis 2006, p. 307). Another defines it as "a self-regulating process by which an organism can maintain internal stability

---

[69] Besides Fleming, see also Saul Benison et al. (1987), Bradford Cannon (1994), and Elin Wolfe et al. (2000), for summaries of Cannon's research.

while adjusting to changing external conditions" (Billman 2020, p. 1). While another defines it as the "stability, balance, or equilibrium within a cell or the body" (Palaparthi 2017, p. 1). Finally, other definitions refer to homeostasis as "the maintenance of a constant internal environment within the body" (Givens and Reiss 2002, p. 56), as the "maintenance of static or constant conditions in the internal environment" (Guyton and Hall 2005, p. 3), or as the "the maintenance of a constant internal environment by active functioning of cells, tissues, and organs organized into a negative feedback system" (Michael et al. 2017, p. 45).

Although the above definitions suffice for capturing the basic conceptual meaning of homeostasis, Cannon made an important distinction between homeostasis *per se* and homeostatic reactions or mechanisms for maintaining a stable inner environment. Whereas homeostasis *per se* represents an organism's constant condition or normal state, homeostatic mechanisms refer to the "coördinated physiological processes which maintain most of the steady states in the organism" (Cannon 1939, p. 24). These processes, then, are essential for "preserving" an organism's steady state. Cannon also distinguished homeostatic conditions, which refer to the "details of the stability," from homeostasis *per se* (1926, p. 91). He identified two classes of homeostatic conditions (Cannon 1929). The first involves the material provisions for cellular functions, such as energy sources, water, and electrolytes, while the second class consists of environmental factors, such as temperature and osmotic pressure.

Cannon (1926, 1929) listed a half-dozen "postulates" or "tentative propositions" concerning the concept of homeostasis, which he felt provided heuristic explication and guidance for development and application of the concept and for further research. The first and most important postulate is,

> In an open system, such as our bodies represent, composed of unstable structure and subjected continually to disturbance, constancy is in itself evidence that agencies are acting or are already to act to maintain this constancy (Cannon 1926, p. 91).

These agencies, according to Cannon, are often antagonistic to each other in terms of their actions, such that the agencies counter each other's activities to maintain overall stability. Another important postulate is that homeostatic mechanisms are composed of various cooperating systems, either successively or contemporaneously. Finally, homeostatic mechanisms involve involuntarily regulation. "When a factor is known which can shift a homeostatic state in one direction," observed Cannon, "it is reasonable to look for automatic control of that factor or for a factor or factors having an opposite effect" (1926, p. 93).

The chief processes or mechanisms for maintaining homeostasis include regulatory systems composed of negative and positive feedback and feedforward loops (Hagen 2021, Kim et al. 2006, Modell et al. 2015, Palaparthi 2017). The basis of feedback mechanism is the simple principle that an output derived from a particular process has an effect, i.e., feedback, on the input of that process and either inhibits (negative) or stimulates (positive) it (Figure 9). Importantly, examples of negative, as opposed to positive feedback mechanisms, abound in nature. Feedforward mechanisms involve the inhibition (negative) or stimulation (positive) of a latter step (C, Figure 10) in a pathway by an earlier step (A, Figure 10). Finally, coupling of these homeostatic mechanisms, whether feedback or feedforward loops, with one another provides the necessary regulation to maintain homeostasis.

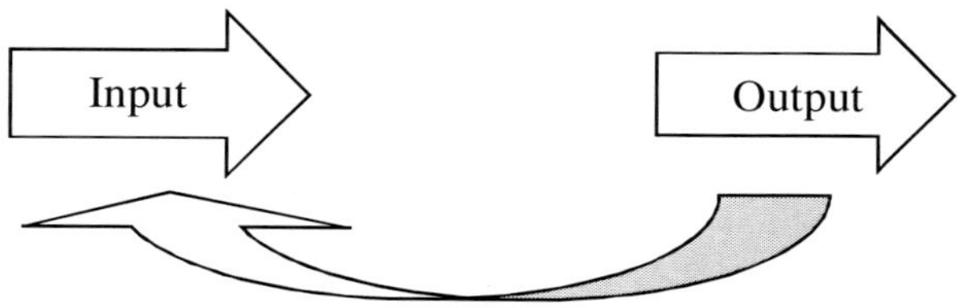

Figure 9. Feedback mechanism or loop.

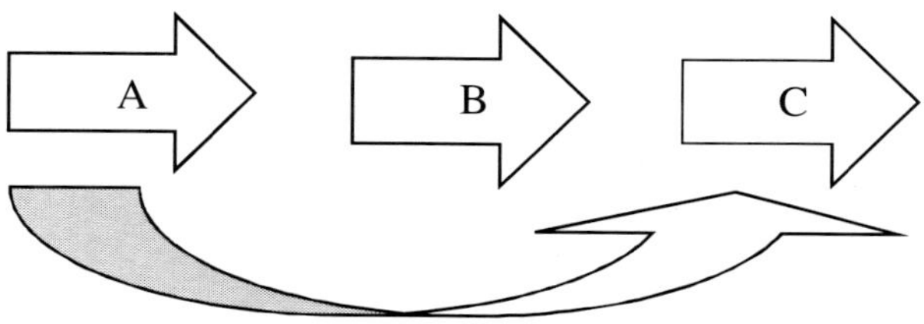

Figure 10. Feedforward mechanism or loop.

The schema for a regulatory system involving feedback and feedforward mechanisms consists of several basic or common components, including a regulated substance or activity with its set-point value, a measurement or sensor system, a control or an integrator system with its response mechanisms, and an effector system. A regulated substance is the entity of a system that is under control or regulation, such as blood sugar or body temperature. It falls within a rather narrow range of values, i.e., a set-point value. Significant change in the substance's value results in action taken by a homeostatic mechanism to return it to the set-point value. The sensor or measurement system involves the detection of any changes in the regulated substance. The control or integrator system compares the current value of the regulated substance with a set-point value. If a significant difference exists between the two values, then response mechanisms associated with the control system engage an effector system. The effector participates in returning the regulated substance's value to its set-point value.

Finally, homeostatic mechanisms are quantifiable or calculable, although considerable uncertainty or disagreement exists over how best to accomplish this (Dyson 1999, p. 82). One of the more notable examples of quantifying homeostasis is metabolic control analysis (MCA) (Cornish-Bowden 1995, Fell 2005, Joy et al. 2012, Meireles and Simões 2014, Wildermuth 2000). MCA involves the analysis of a metabolic system and its fluctuations with respect to its component parts. According to MCA, a cell's metabolism and its regulation can be accounted for with the notion of a rate-limiting reaction or step. The flux of the metabolic system is the result of the system's sensitivity to the activities of all the enzymes composing the system, and the measurement of that sensitivity is in terms of a control coefficient (C), which is the percentage change effected in the system by variations in an enzyme's activity. In addition, the enzyme kinetics can change in response to variations in metabolite concentrations, such as the enzyme's substrate. This latter parameter is measured in terms of an elasticity coefficient (ε). Daniel Kahn and Hans Westerhoff (1993) utilize both C and ε to provide a precise formulation for homeostatic strength (H):

$$H = -C \times \varepsilon$$

This formula reveals that the closer H is to 1 the more stable is the system's homeostasis, while the closer H is to 0 the less stable is its homeostasis.

Although homeostasis consists of various mechanisms for maintaining an organism's internal milieu, as noted above, negative feedback is unquestionably the predominant mechanism. According to Stephen Woods and Douglas Ramsay (20007), the physiologist Curt Richter, who utilized Cannon's notion of homeostasis to investigate various regulatory physiological processes, was partly responsible for limiting homeostatic mechanisms to negative feedback loops. As Woods and Ramsay conclude, "homeostasis became operationally defined as a series of inter-related negative feedback loops" (2007, p. 391). However, as biomedical physiologists continued to explore the role of homeostasis in maintaining bodily equilibrium, various types of homeostasis were introduced, including "predictive homeostasis, reactive homeostasis, homeorheusis, homeorhesis, homeokinetics, rheostasis, homeodynamic regulation, heterodynamic regulation, heterostasis, allostasis, and allodynamic regulation" (Woods and Ramsay 2007, p. 395). The three most common types are homeodynamics, heterostasis, and allostasis.[70]

Homeodynamics was developed to account for the body's equilibrium and its regulation in dynamic rather than static terms (Ahn et al. 2006, Berntson and Cacioppo 2007, Buchman 2002, Lloyd et al. 2001). Rather than linear stasis or statics, in contrast to homeostasis, it accounts for bodily equilibrium in terms of dynamic stability in which the "regulatory mechanisms are multiple and complex" (Berntson and Cacioppo 2007, p. 436). Homeodynamics is dynamically interactive and not static in that a system reaches balance with respect to integrated regulatory mechanisms (Emerson 1954, Irizarry et al. 2001). For example, David Lloyd and colleagues define homeodynamics as "the continuous transformation of one dynamical system into another through instabilities at bifurcation points" (Lloyd et al. 2001, p. 136). A dynamic system represents an open system's self-organization in which it cannot only maintain a stable state but can also switch among stable states. A chief feature of a homeodynamic system is its spatiotemporal coherence, which refers to "the synchronisation in space and time of molecules, or the architecture or supermolecular or supercellular structures, through self-organisation, in an apparent, 'purposeful,' functional way" (Lloyd et al. 2001, p. 136). Besides bottom-up mechanisms, homeodynamics also includes top-down mechanisms to account for a system's complex behavior. Although it includes bifurcation points for explaining system behavior, it still relies on linear mechanisms.

In 1973, Hans Selye championed the notion of heterostasis to account for external or exogenous stimuli or signals that can alter the regulatory set-point value or range of values, in contrast to homeostasis in which the set-point varies only slightly within a constrained range. According to Selye,

[70] One important variant of homeostasis, since the appearance of Woods and Ramsay's article, is adaptive homeostasis to account for transient adaptations to mild changes in bodily conditions (Davies 2016).

homeostasis "maintains the normal steady state [for a given set-point] by physiological reactions," whereas heterostasis involves resetting the set-point so that the body can defend itself against an exogenous pathological entity (1973, p. 443). The classic example is fever, which is an increase in bodily temperature caused by a foreign pathogen. "The elevation in temperature associated with a fever," as Gary Berntson and John Cacioppo note, "may be of benefit in mobilizing energy resources to combat infections or other adaptive challenges" (2007, p. 436). Indeed, experiments with injection of an antipyretic drug into infected rabbits resulted in decreased blood leukocyte counts and increased bacterial count, which accounts for increased mortality of antipyretic-treated rabbits compared to controls (Vaughn et al. 1980).

In 1988, Peter Sterling and Joseph Eyer introduced the concept of allostasis to account for variation within set-points not only daily but also throughout a person's lifetime, especially in response to environmental and even sociological factors. For example, the set-point for blood pressure can vary during the day, whether a person is awake or asleep. According to Berntson and Cacioppo,

> These alterations in set-point are not consonant with simple homeostatic or homeodynamic models. Nor do they necessarily involve the exogenous agents or pathological conditions of Selye's model. Rather, they are seen as reflecting the natural adaptive readjustment of regulatory levels in view of changing physiological demands (436).

Moreover, allostasis also expands the extent of homeostatic control of a single physiological process to include a variety of, if not all, physiological processes. "To maintain stability," insisted Sterling and Eyer, "an organism must vary all the parameters of its internal milieu and match them appropriately to environmental demands" (1988, p. 636). The biomedical community has certainly embraced the concept of allostasis to describe and understand health and disease (McEwen and Wingfield 2003, Ramsay and Woods 2014, Schulkin 2003, Sterling 2020).

Homeostasis, along with its variations, is the cornerstone concept of the biomolecular and biomedical paradigm, especially in terms of accounting for health and disease (McEwen and Wingfield 2003, Rattan 2020, Ventriglia and Murgia 2011). It represents the system's property that depends on the regulation of linear interactions of a system's components (Nijhout et al. 2019). It is reductionistic in two important ways (Ahn et al., 2006). First, a single factor, such as the set-point for blood glucose, is often the focus of attention, especially with respect to restoring or correcting a divergent factor or set-point to its normal value, within a well-defined range. Second, interaction of the system's parts is linear and static with respect to a wide range of pre-set values. Although variants of homeostasis, such as homeodynamics or allostasis, include variation of set-points given daily or developmental conditions, still divergent set-points not limited to these conditions are outside its regulatory control—even though they are evolutionary diachronic (Torday 2015). Homeostasis and stability, especially static linear stability, are utilized to account for the interactions among a system's parts—even if it includes all the system's regulatory mechanisms as in allostasis. These interactions are sufficient to explain system behavior as an organism attempts to remain within a limited range of values for a given parameter. The patient vis-à-vis biomedical homeostasis and its variants is a static system that when set-point values drift outside a prescribed range are treated to restore the normal value otherwise biomedicine has failed. The patient's illness story then defines the patient qua person.

2.2. Robustness

In the last several decades, the concept of robustness, although not a new concept in the biomedical sciences, has taken on greater significance for describing and understanding complex biological and biomedical systems (Bertolaso et al. 2018, Crespi et al. 2021, Kitano 2007a, Masel and Siegal 2009, Nijhout et al. 2017, Whitacre 2012).[71] In the late 1960s and the early 1970s, Michael Savageau (1969a,b, 1970) introduced the concept of robustness as an important design principle in the analysis of metabolic and genetic circuits (Alon 2019, Savageau 1976, 1991, Voit 2013). Savageau initially called the principle "Biochemical Systems Analysis," which later became known as "Biochemical Systems Theory" (BST). BST is a mathematical analysis of a system based on power laws that describe a system's overall nonlinear behavior. In other words, a metabolic system is analyzed using the simple addition or subtraction of the power law

[71] Erica Crespi and colleagues distinguish between robustness and resilience. Briefy, robustness refers to a system's stability when faced with a perturbation, while resilience to its ability to regain stability (Crespi et al. 2021). They proceed to model both robustness and resilience with respect to network theory. Frederik Nijhout and colleagues also make a distinction between robustness and plasticity, claiming that "the overall system may show stability or robustness in the face of perturbation, even while the underlying components are showing plasticity" (Nijhout et al. 2017, p. 181).

approximations for various metabolic reactions. From such an analysis, Savageau demonstrated that unbranched metabolic systems with feedback loops are more robust vis-à-vis fluctuations in metabolite concentrations than systems without such loops. Importantly, these robust systems are more stable and selectable with respect to evolutionary development.

Robustness, then, is an important concept for understanding the behavior of complex biological and biomedical systems not only in terms of maintaining structural and functional integrity but also for developmental and evolutionary change (Alon 2019, Kischner and Gerhart 2005, Klipp et al. 2016, Lenski et al. 2006, Masel and Trotter 2010, Wagner 2005). Robustness is an important design concept for analyzing fluctuations within biological systems—but systems that are still able to maintain themselves in terms of their structural and functional integrity. According to Uri Alon, robustness reflects the "biological systems special robust designs that make their essential function work precisely despite naturally occurring noise" (2019, p. 117). In addition, fluctuations in certain biological parameters are critical for species evolution or evolvability, especially in terms of mapping phenotype onto genotype (Kaneko 2012, Krakauer 2006, Nijhout et al. 2017). Finally, an important notion for understanding robustness is the fragility—the obverse of robustness—of biologically complex systems (Klipp et al. 2016). Often robust systems develop a particular fragility that can be important for development of therapeutic modalities, especially against diseases like cancer (Kitano 2004b, Tian et al. 2011).

Although no consensus exists in the literature for defining the concept of robustness, many of the definitions share a common thread with respect to a system's capability or property to maintain not only its structural but also its functional integrity or performance (Crespi et al. 2021, Kitano 2004a, Krakauer 2006, Lesne 2008, Nikolov et al. 2007, Stelling et al. 2004). For example, Jonna Masel and Mark Siegal succinctly define robustness as the capacity "of a system to produce relatively invariant output in the presence of a perturbation" (2009, p. 395).[72] Jose Fernandez-Leon provides a rather helpful working definition: "robustness is the capacity that allows an agent (artificial or biological) to continue functioning *via* tolerance or adaptation to

[72] Masel and Siegal call attention to the similarity between robustness and canalization, in that for the latter a "system need not return to its pre-perturbation state, but instead returns to the same developmental trajectory" (2009, p. 395). Indeed canalization—a concept introduced by Waddington (1942)—plays an important role conceptually in understanding the evolution of complex traits, as well as disease etiology (Flatt 2005, Gibson and Lacek 2020).

internal and external perturbations, where this capacity is partially determined by an agent–environment history of interactions" (2014, p. 561). In other words, robustness maintains a system's integrity even in response to either internal or external perturbations or disturbances, which could compromise its integrity or performance. It is a relative or relational concept in that various systems can be insensitive or sensitive to exact pre-set values and parameters (Alon 2019, Barkai and Leibler 1997, Fernandez-Leon 2014).

According to Kitano (2004a, 2007a), robustness generally manifests itself in complex biological or biomedical systems in two different ways. The first is the ability of a system to adapt to a perturbation by returning to its steady state value, which is often denoted as an attractor. An example is bacterial chemotaxis in which a bacterium adapts to changes in chemical signals within its environment (Hansen et al. 2008). The attractor can be either static, which represents a fixed value, or oscillatory, which cycles in terms of its value under varying conditions. The second type of robustness represents a transition from one attractor to another. In this sense, robustness is heterodynamic in that regulatory mechanisms are highly complex and exhibit acute fluidity such that while homeostasis represents "wisdom of the body" robustness represents "wisdom of the heterodynamic body" (Goldberger 2001, p. 1290). An example is the G1/S phase transition, which represents a robust function during the cell cycle (Swat et al. 2004). Stochastic or random processes are at times instrumental in the transition from one attractor to another (Vasconcelos et al. 2017). Besides this transition to a new attractor, the system can simply become unstable or chaotic (Abarbanel 1996).

One of the key challenges for understanding robustness and for discovering its underlying principles responsible for the development and evolution of complex biological systems is their analytic formalization. Kitano (2007a, p. 3) proposed a mathematical formula (Figure 11) to define system robustness and to calculate the robustness (R) of a system (S) in terms of a function (a) and a perturbation set (P). The term $\psi(p)$ represents the probability of perturbation (p), while D(p) represents an evaluation function given p. When D(p) = 1, a system maintains its functional integrity; however, under this condition the system is too inflexible and therefore unable to adapt or respond to a treacherous perturbation. When D(p) = 0, the system fails since it degrades too quickly upon perturbation. Obviously, D(p) ranges between 0 and 1 for many biological systems, thus avoiding either scenario. One of the more important challenges for this formulization, as Kitano acknowledges, is its application to concrete thermodynamic constraints and situations involved in biological events such as evolution and development.[73]

$$R^{s}_{a,P} = \int_{P} \psi(p) D^{s}_{a}(p) dp$$

Figure 11. Mathematical formula to define and calculate a system's robustness (see text for details).

Several principles or mechanisms responsible for robustness in biological and biomedical systems have been articulated within the literature (Kitano 2004a, Krakauer 2006, Stelling et al. 2004, Whitacre 2012). One of the most important principles pertains to fail-safe mechanisms, such as redundancy and diversity or distributed robustness (Crespi et al. 2021, Félix and Barkoulas 2015). Redundancy involves the presence of several identical or similar parts so that when one part fails another takes its place.[74] These parts, then, have "overlapping functions...up to a certain point" (Crespi et al. 2021, p. 5). In other words, they are not strictly identical but comparable enough to perform the same function, more or less, so the system continues to function, more or less. Diversity or distributed robustness refers to heterogeneous parts such that their function is "robust because the flow of information is distributed among several alternative components and flow paths, with no two parts performing the same function" (Fernandez-Leon 2014, p. 559). What distinguishes diversity from redundancy, then, is that the former involves "variations in responses to heterogeneous challenges that can enable the system to function under different conditions" while the latter does not (Crespi et al. 2021, p. 6).

Several other principles are important to understanding the concept of robustness, including antiredundancy, modularity, decoupling, and systems control, especially in terms of feedback/forward loops. Antiredundancy, according to David Krakauer and Joshua Plotkin, involves "mechanisms that sensitize cells or individuals to genetic damage and thereby eliminate them preemptively from a population" (2002, p. 1405). And they contend that such

[73] Another challenge is quantifying robustness and developing simulation models of it for investigating complex biological and physiological systems (Kamapantula et al. 2017, Kitano 2010, Lee et al. 2014, Walsh et al. 2013).

[74] Paul Mason distinguishes between redundancy, which pertains to "structural duplication," and degeneracy, which refers to "structural variation" (2014, p. 12). And Mason goes on to claim that degeneracy plays an important role in complexity, robustness, and self-organization.

antiredundancy is responsible for robustness in terms of redundancy. In other words, it is the principle that a biological system purges itself of defective components, in order to maintain its integrity (Wagner 2005). Another principle relies on modularity or compartmentalization in which physical, functional, spatial, temporal, or even logical modules, subsystems, or compartments are arranged hierarchically and can maintain a system's robustness (Holme 2011, Wagner et al. 2007). Decoupling is an additional principle in which variation is isolated or decoupled from important functional states of the biological system, thus protecting the system from dangerous perturbations (Bich et al. 2016). The final principle is systems control, which involves negative or positive feedback or feed-forward loops (Cosentino and Bates 2012, Dethier et al. 2015, Freeman 2000). Negative feedback is instrumental in returning a system to its pre-set value upon perturbation, while positive feedback often consists of a transition to another attractor through amplification. Interestingly, besides normal developmental processes, robust systems also incorporate both positive and negative feedback mechanisms in terms of disease mechanisms (Hannezo and Heisenberg 2019).

The standard framework or structure of robustness is the bow-tie or hourglass architecture (Csete and Doyle 2004, Ghosh Roy et al. 2021, Kitano 2004a, Zhao et al. 2007, Whitacre 2021). This architecture is composed of various modules that interact with one another according to protocol rules to generate system robustness. The key or central module to the architecture is a core module—the bow-tie's knot or the hour glass's constriction—composed of highly conserved processes or mechanisms. This module's function is to respond to perturbations received through input-process modules and to correct system fluctuations through output-process modules. In addition to the core module, there are several weak linkages closely associated with the core module, which also participate in responding to perturbations and correcting fluctuations. The weak linkages can also involve "the addition of new processes to the existing core process using common versatile mechanisms that operate on diverse inputs and outputs" (Kitano 2004a, p. 832). This process of responding to perturbations and correcting fluctuations is referred to as buffering. Finally, robustness architecture can occur at any hierarchical level and individual bow-ties can be nested into higher levels to generate an integrated whole.

Metabolism provides one of the best known and studied examples of nested bow-tie architecture (Csete and Doyle 2004, Hao et al. 2012, Ma et al. 2007, Zhao et al. 2007). Marie Csete and John Doyle (2004) deconstruct the overarching or global bow-tie architecture for metabolism into three separate—but interacting—bow-tie architectures. Two of the architectures are associated with the central core or knot of the bow-tie, which represent central processes in metabolism. Although both core processes of these two bow-ties share the same input processes associated with catabolism, which in turn is fed by a nutrient stream—along with its perturbations and fluctuations—the two core processes respond differently to the inputs. The knot associated with carriers generates energy-rich molecules like ATP and NADP, while the knot associated with precursors generates metabolic antecedents such as amino acids and nucleotides for the anabolic or trans bow-tie associated with the output processes of the global bow-tie. These carriers and precursors are important components for the anabolic pathways of the output processes associated with protein synthesis. The trans bow-tie knot includes the conserved processes of transcription and translation.

The importance of the bow-tie architecture is associated with the robustness of various regulatory processes (Friedlander et al. 2015, Krauss et al. 2012, Nielsen and Keasling 2016). This robustness allows the cells to respond to perturbations or fluctuations in the extracellular and intracellular environments. In other words, the robustness of this architecture "facilitates control, accommodating perturbations and fluctuations on many timescales and spatial scales" (Csete and Doyle 2004, p. 447). At rapid timescales, for example, the core processes consist of allosteric and competitive inhibition that average out the requirements placed upon a system through input and output processes. In addition, proximity to the central core processes has an influence on the conservation of regulatory processes so that core enzymes are generally more specialized than enzymes found at input or output process modules. Thus, reactions that are upstream or downstream from the bow-tie knot need not be as robust as those within the knot itself. This regulatory architecture has important implications for biological processes, such as evolution.

Interestingly, the concepts of homeostasis and robustness are often used interchangeably within the literature (Nijhout et al. 2019). For example, Zhe Tang and David McMillan, when discussing the regulatory mechanisms for maintaining stability, denote them as "robustly homeostatic" (2016, p. 276). And Gerard Eberl (2018) equates the two concepts in that homeostasis provides biological organisms their robustness. However, for present purposes the two concepts are not interchangeable but significantly different, especially in terms of medical practice. Robustness is not concerned directly with a system's steady state but with the dynamic processes or behavior responsible for the integrity of its function or performance, versus the static processes or simple structural integrity of homeostasis (Stelling et al. 2004). Thus, a robust system may shift between various steady states to maintain its functional integrity (Kitano 2007a). In addition, robustness differs from homeostasis in terms of maintaining a system's functional rather than simply its structural integrity. In other words, a system's robustness refers to its behavior rather than simply to its state (Ahn et al. 2006). A system's nonlinear dynamism ensures its proper functioning. Moreover, a system may gain robustness through instability in one of its subsystems. For example, chromosomal instability enhances tumor robustness towards chemotherapy, because it increases the tumor cell's genotype and phenotype heterogeneity (Kitano 2004b). In the end, although a close similarity exists between the two concepts, they play different roles in medicine.

Finally, just as the concept of homeostasis was the foundation of the biomedical model, the concept of robustness is P7 systems medicine's foundational concept. The personal P (P4) represents an entanglement of the P1-3 components, which accounts for the patient robust state with respect to the biomolecular, psychological, and social dimensions. And each of the P1-3 components are composed of elements that can combine to operate at a value different from the original pre-set value and not outside that value as required by homeostatic mechanisms. For the physico-biomolecular P (P1), robustness is an important concept for understanding the etiology of diseases, such as cancer and cardio-vascular diseases, and for developing effective therapies (Kraushaar et al. 2018, Tian et al. 2011). Also for the psycho-cognitive P (P2), robustness is a significant concept for explaining the origins of psychological and psychiatric diseases, like Alzheimer's and Parkinson's diseases (Kalampokis et al. 2003), especially the genetics of such diseases (Gershon and Goldin 1986, Robert and Plantikow 2005). Lastly, robustness is key to understanding the impact of environmental and social factors comprising the P3 component (Duijndam and Denollet 2019), especially in terms of aging (Kraushaar and Bauer 2021, Kriete 2013).

In sum, robustness of the personal P (P4) is a key element for the patient's capacity not only to survive an illness but also to forge a new life even if a biomedical cure is not possible or available. In contrast to biomedicine's homeostasis, which is constrained in terms of a cure, i.e., returning the patient to a pre-set value or pre-disease state, P7 systems medicine's robustness allows the patient to heal in the sense of constructing a post-set value or post-disease state, which is born out with respect to the P-actions. For treating a disease, the participatory P (P6) empowers the patient to engage in the therapeutic plan to choose what is best or robust in terms of the patient's values and preferences. But more importantly, the P-actions can be used not simply reactively with respect to treating the disease but proactively in terms of preventing it. The robust patient qua the personal P (P4) is empowered to choose a lifestyle that optimizes the patient's health and decreases the probability of disease onset due to poor lifestyle choices. Robustness in P7 systems medicine then represents entanglement of both the four P-components and the three P-actions, so that the patient can prevent predicted potential healthcare risks.

3. Linear and Nonlinear Dynamics

Homeostasis depends upon linear systems, while robustness upon nonlinear systems (Hespanha 2018, Sastry 1999, Thyagarajan and Kalpana 2021). Linear systems are composed of nonbranching sequential events often with a well-defined single equilibrium, while nonlinear systems are composed of branching events that are not necessarily sequential and can exhibit multiple equilibria. Both type of systems involve feedback and feedforward processes and mechanisms that are responsible for system control and dynamics. Linear dynamics are often straightforward in their operations and are generally easily modelled or simulated to provide outcomes that are determinate in terms of both predictability and certainty. Nonlinear dynamics, however, are complex and often more difficult to model or simulate, and they generally exhibit chaotic outcomes that are problematic in terms of predictability and certainty. The biomedical model of healthcare depends on linear dynamics, while systems medicine upon nonlinear dynamics.

3.1. Linear Dynamics

The processes and mechanisms associated with homeostasis are linear in terms of their dynamics, as well as with respect to feedback and feedforward regulation and control (Brin and Stuck 2002, Grigoriu 2021, Layek 2015, Luenberger 1979, Thieffry 2007). The concept of linear dynamics refers to the rectilinear or nonbranching structure or temporal sequence or interaction of a mechanism's or system's components. For example, as detailed earlier, a linear mechanism exhibits the following sequential structure.

$$A \rightarrow B \rightarrow C$$

In this linear mechanism or system, A gives rise to B and then B to C in that particular successive and undeviating order or pattern. In a simple enzymatic reaction, for example, A may represent a substrate that an enzyme converts into the product B, which in turn B serves as a substrate for another enzyme that converts it into the product C. Given the linearity of enzymatic reaction, the reaction's output is deterministic, predictable, and certain.

Systems or mechanisms that exhibit linearity or linear dynamics display two important features or properties (Brin and Stuck 2002, Grigoriu 2021, Luenberger 1979). The first is proportionality, i.e., for a system composed of several components the output of that system is proportional to the initial input into the system. In other words, the relationship between input and output is strictly linear. The linearity of a system can be expressed mathematically as

$$O = \alpha I + \beta$$

where O is the system's output and is a dependent variable that is contingent on the input I, which is the independent variable, while α and β are the constants defining the system's linear proportionality. The second property is independence of the system's components such that the system's output is the algebraic sum of the system's inputs and can be expressed as

$$O = \alpha I_1 + \alpha I_2$$

and the system's output is scalar in terms of representing the summation of the various independent inputs.

Feedback or feedforward mechanisms are a critical feature for regulating or controlling linear dynamical systems (Åström and Murray 2021, Hu et al. 2014, Thieffry 2007, Thomas and D'Ari 1990).[75] Importantly, the impact or effect of the regulatory mechanism can be either positive in which the output is either increased, or negative in which the output is decreased. Although feedback or feedforward regulatory mechanisms appear to introduce branching into the overall mechanism, as illustrated accordingly:

[75] Besides being deterministic, dynamical systems can also be stochastic (Kaplan and Glass 1995, Layek 2015, Luenberger 1979).

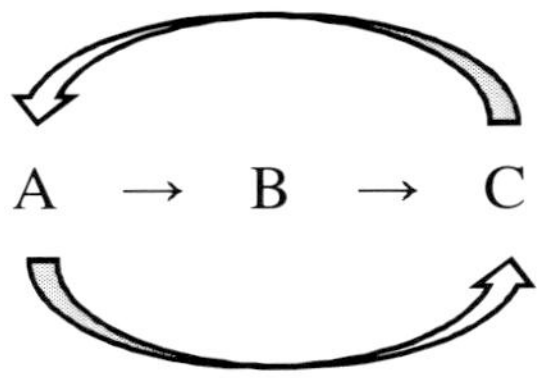

still the regulatory mechanism does not change the overall linear relationships of the mechanism's components or the proportionality of the system's input or A and output or C. In other words, whether the feedback (C to A) or feedforward (A to C) mechanism decreases or increases the system's output, the output or C is still linearly proportional to the input or A.

At its core, a system's linearity or linear dynamics includes both the structure or sequence of its mechanism and its function, especially in terms of its outcome vis-à-vis its input. For many, if not most, linear homeostatic mechanisms, the outcome is proportional to or depends directly on preceding events, and a simple mathematical relationship or formula predicts and determines the outcome. In other words, the linear relationship is with respect to the interaction of the system's component parts, in that it can respond directly to perturbations in the external environment or internal milieu and thereby maintain the conditions required for both the system's structure and function. Given the system's linear dynamics, its function is deterministic, predictable, and certain, which has important implications for the biomedical model of healthcare.

Linearity and linear dynamics comprise the critical conceptual foundation for biomedicine and EBM, as well as their clinical practice (Higgins 2002, Klonowski 2007). Indeed disease is viewed as a disruption in the linear mechanisms and dynamics constituting a particular physiological function. For example, carcinogenesis under the standard somatic mutation theory results from the mutation of specific genes involved in the regulation of cell growth (Davis et al 2017, Fearon and Vogelstein 1990, Hanahan and Weinberg 2000, Vaux 2011). Therapy, then, is based on targeting the mutated genes and their products that constitute the linear mechanism. Such linearity provides the biomedical scientist with the theoretical foundation for identifying pathological mechanisms and correcting the disruption caused in the normal mechanistic order. The outcome is often a drug or device that can restore the patient's normal functioning. The importance of such linearity is that the clinician can precisely pinpoint the pathological problem and potentially correct it.

3.2. Nonlinear Dynamics

Nonlinearity changes the rules and principals of the system that often define or determine the system's behavior. Assuming determinism always guarantees the same result, while non-determinism does not because of chaos. A confounding factor for systems biology and for understanding the complexity of biological systems is that many, if not most, biologically complex systems exhibit nonlinear dynamics or nonlinearity (Janson 2012, Scott 2007, Socolar 2006). "Nonlinearity in a system," according to Neil Rasband, "simply means that the measured values of the properties of a system in a later state depend in a complicated way on the measured values in an earlier state" (2015, p. 2). In other words, nonlinearity or nonlinear dynamics refers to a system and its properties that are not directly relational or proportional to the summation of its parts and their properties. Rather, nonlinear systems are complex in which the outcome of the system's function is not additive in a straightforward manner (Tranquillo 2019).

Consequently, systems scientists express nonlinear dynamics mathematically as an outcome of complex interactions that do not equal the sum of the parts. According to Joshua Socolar, for example,

> the equations of motion include at least one term that contains the square or higher power, a product of system variables (or more complicated functions of them), or some sort of threshold function, so that the addition of two solutions does *not* yield a valid new solution, no matter how the system variables are defined (2006, pp. 121-122).

In other words, the system's output is a nonlinear function of the interaction of its components. In contrast to linear systems, then, nonlinear systems are often unpredictable and nondeterministic such that the system's outcome is highly uncertain given initial starting conditions.

Nonlinear dynamics also involve branching structures, in which the mechanistic interactions of complex processes yield bifurcations, as illustrated in the following scheme:

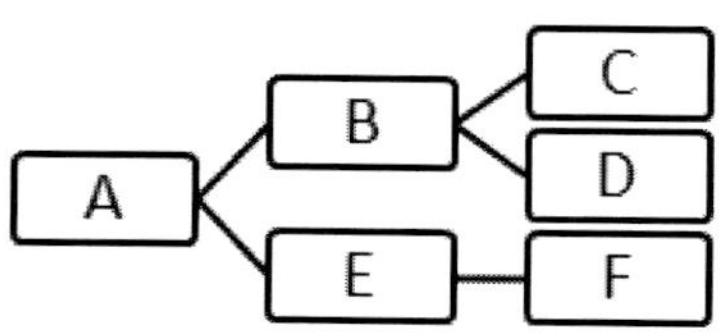

In the above scheme, A represents a bifurcation point that can follow either the B pathway, which also serves as another bifurcation point, or the E pathway. In addition to branching, feedback and feedforward mechanisms add to the complexity of nonlinear dynamic systems. For example, in the above scheme F could feedback on B in a negative fashion to reduce the level of C. An important consequence of nonlinear dynamics is the appearance of a new type of attractor coupled with chaotic events (Socolar 2006). And, according to Steven Andrews and colleagues, "essentially any system that is governed by nonlinear dynamics…rapidly becomes chaotic as the system size is increased beyond a few molecules, and thus becomes effectively unpredictable" (2009, p. 8732).

Chaos and nonlinearity or nonlinear dynamics are intimately related to one another, especially in terms of modeling or simulating complex systems (Aguirre and Letellier 2009, Klonowski 2006, Knüpfer and Beckstein, 2013). "Whenever dynamical chaos is found," observes Rasband, "it is accompanied by *nonlinearity*" (2015, p. 2). Although nonlinear systems can exhibit chaotic dynamics, the outcomes of such systems are not necessarily random in terms of no causal relationship among events, like flipping a coin, rather they are causally related to initial conditions even though the outcome cannot be predicted with certainty—only approximately. Although the outcome is dependent on the initial conditions, small perturbations in those conditions, which occur constantly given the system's dynamic nature, result in unpredictable outcomes. In essence, chaos is one of the chief features of the system's complexity, especially for living organisms (Bizzarri et al. 2020, Coffey 1998, Eskov et al. 2013, Rickles et al. 2007). Finally, control or regulation for a complex, chaotic system involves an adaptability of the system to perturbations detrimental to it (Iglesias and Ingalls 2010, Sastry and Bodson 2011).

Whereas linearity and linear dynamics are the conceptual foundation of the biomedical model, nonlinearity and nonlinear dynamics, along with the associated notions of complexity and chaos, undergird conceptually systems medicine (Chamberlain and Bütz 2013, Higgins 2002, Klonowski 2007, West 2013). Although the biomedical model has made progress on treating diseases, it has yet to provide cures for many of them, especially chronic diseases. Part of the problem involves defining disease in terms of homeostasis (Varela et al. 2010). As Ary Goldberger contends,

> findings from non-linear dynamics have also challenged conventional mechanisms of physiological control based on classic homoeostasis,

> which indicates that healthy systems seek to attain a constant steady state. By contrast, non-linear systems with fractal dynamics (such as the neuroautonomic mechanisms regulating heart-rate variability) behave as if they were driven far from equilibrium under basal conditions. This kind of complex variability, rather than a single homoeostatic steady state, seems to define the free running function of many biological systems (1996, p. 1314).

And so disease represents more than simply disruption of homeostatic linear dynamics. Carcinogenesis is an excellent example of how the biomedical model has struggled to account for tumorigenesis, especially in terms of the somatic mutation theory (Brücher and Jamall 2016, Soto and Sonnenschein 2014). Nonlinear dynamics and complexity are providing productive avenues or approaches for explaining and treating cancer (Dinicola et al. 2011, Gatenby and Brown 2018). Finally, nonlinearity and linear dynamics have important implications for clinical practice (Buchman 2004, Goldberger 1996, Tuffin 2016).

Nonlinearity and nonlinear dynamics, along with complexity and chaos, are particularly critical for P7 systems medicine and its clinical practice. Specifically, nonlinear systems account for not just the physical dimension or even for the psychological dimension but also for the social dimension of the patient (Woehle 2007). For P7 medicine, nonlinear dynamics are important for shaping the behavior of the patient in terms of the physico-biomolecular P (P1), as well as the psycho-cognitive P (P2). The complexity of the interactions among the biomes comprising the various P components provide the network, and in some cases fractal patterns, in which novel behavioral features can emerge given well-defined initial conditions, including the environmental and social factors associated with the population-public P (P3). For example, analysis of omics data based on nonlinear dynamical modeling has provided insights into carcinogenesis with potential therapeutic benefits (Chen 2019, Knox 2010). In the end, nonlinear dynamics are responsible for the unique individuality of the patient qua personal P (P4), especially as defined in terms of the physiome, pathome, and personome (Table 2), and how that patient not only experiences a specific illness but also how that patient responds to treatment.

4. Stasis and Evolvability

Two important concepts related both to homeostasis and linear dynamics and to robustness and nonlinear dynamics are stasis and evolvability, respectively. The two concepts are often portrayed as antithetical to one another, and in evolutionary biology stasis presents a problem or paradox for species evolution (Lidgard and Hopkins 2015). Specifically, the paradox is that stasis or morphological constancy is commonly observed over geological time scales even though the potential for rapid evolutionary change exists because of drastic alterations in environmental conditions. In other words, the paradox centers on the diverse variability within species; but species often exhibit a stasis over evolutionary and geological eras. In this section, the concept of stasis as it relates to homeostasis is initially discussed, which sets the stage for examining the concept of evolvability and associated concepts of plasticity and fragility and how these concepts relate to robustness, especially in terms of how a patient responds to an illness.

4.1. Stasis

The concept of stasis or stability is a fundamental concept for the biomedical model, especially in terms of homeostasis and allostasis (McEwen and Wingfield 2003). The concept within medicine has an interesting history. Generally, it is associated with disease mechanisms. For example, stasis or stagnation of the four humors was thought, according to proponents of humoral pathology, to be the etiology of certain diseases, especially those diseases associated with the blood circulatory system and the circulation of other fluids (Arikha 2007, Long 1965). With Cannon's introduction of homeostasis, stasis takes on a new meaning—one pertaining to a constant or unchanging equilibrium, which defines the optimal functioning of a system. And the stasis Cannon introduces represents a system state that is not stagnant but rather dynamic. "Stasis," according to Colleen Clements, "is a process situation or controlled state, not a steady state with implications of immutability and eternality" (1976, p. 139). In other words, the concept pertains to a system state that maintains an intact structure through regulatory mechanisms in order to function consistently and properly.

Besides stasis, Cannon also relied on the related concept of stability. Although he distinguishes the concept of homeostasis from the notion of equilibrium, he utilizes the concept of stability to define homeostasis. In fact,

Cannon's earliest definition of homeostasis is in terms of the "stability of the organism" (1926, p. 91). Consequently, over the years, stability became intimately associated with the concept of homeostasis. Homeostasis, then, represents "the stability of physiological systems that maintain life" (McEwen and Wingfield 2003, p. 3). Generally, homeostatic mechanisms are critical for maintaining a stable internal environment in which the organism can function normally, when either the internal or the external environment is changing. For example, developmental pathways for a given organism yield expected species morphology or phenotype vis-à-vis variations in the internal and/or external environment because of genetic homeostatic adjustments. Developmental or genetic homeostasis represents "a mechanism for promoting the stability of phenotypic expression of a genotype when grown over a wide range of environments" (Miglani 2006, p. 297). Thus, homeostasis qua stability involves an organism's structural integrity vis-à-vis a pre-set value or range of values.[76] However, this stability is static in that it represents fixed values of pre-set values maintained within predetermined ranges (Ahn et al. 2006, Nikolov et al. 2007).

4.2. Evolvability

A notion closely related to the concept of robustness is evolvability (Kirschner and Gerhart 1998, 2005, Nehaniv 2003, Sniegowski and Murphy 2006, Wagner 2005, 2008). Loosely defined, evolvability refers to the ability of biological organisms and systems to evolve, which makes it a rather trivial and very "slippery concept with a variety of meanings and implications" (Sniegowski and Murphy 2006, p. R831). Although biologists propose various definitions for evolvability, these definitions generally fall into two categories: genotype-oriented and phenotype-oriented definitions (Wagner 2005, 2008).[77] Genotype-oriented definitions focus on the capacity of an organism's nucleotide sequence or genetic capacity to respond to selection pressures. For example, Günter Wagner and Lee Altenberg define genotype-oriented evolvability as "the genome's ability to produce adaptive variants when acted upon by the genetic system" (1996, p. 970). Evolvability is the adaptive capacity of organisms to respond successfully to environmental changes *via* genetic mutations and mechanisms. It assumes fundamentally a rigid mapping

---

[76] Tibor Gánti, however, argues that homeostasis is the result of "inherent" stability, which is "a special organizational state of the system's internal processes" (2003, p. 77).

[77] For another classification of evolvability definitions, see McBride et al. (2008).

of phenotype onto genotype, with little flexibility (Krakauer 2006, Nehaniv 2003).[78] As such, the advantage of genotype-oriented evolvability is the emergence of a better adapted organism genetically to its environment vis-à-vis competitors. However, a disadvantage is the possible over-adaptation that may lead to extinction of the species under extreme selection pressures or environmental changes. Evolvability then results in genetic robustness, in which genetic mutations of a highly adapted, robust organism leads paradoxically to reduced evolvability for a species over time.

The above paradox is the consequence of a general interpretation of robustness as system stability and of evolvability as system change. Although at first glance robustness and evolvability appear antagonistic or incompatible with one another, they exhibit an interconnection to one another such that the paradox is more illusory than real. For example, Andreas Wagner (2008) divides robustness and evolvability into two categories: (1) genotype (sequence) robustness and evolvability and (2) phenotype (structure) robustness and evolvability. Utilizing studies with RNA secondary structure, Wagner concludes that high genotype (sequence) robustness results in low genotype (sequence) evolvability. The basis of the antagonistic relationship between genotype (sequence) robustness and evolvability is the fact that "genotypic robustness and evolvability are properties of one specific genotype" (Wagner 2008, p. 99). However, these studies also support the conclusion that high phenotype (structure) robustness leads to high phenotype (structural) evolvability. The reason, claims Wagner, is that "phenotypic robustness and evolvability are properties of all genotypes with the same phenotype" (2008, p. 99). He argues that the paradox vanishes when taking a phenotype-oriented approach to examining the relationship between robustness and evolvability, which leads to the second type of definition for evolvability.

For the second type of definition, evolvability focuses on phenotype. For example, Marc Kirschner and John Gerhart define phenotype-oriented evolvability as "an organism's capacity to generate heritable phenotype variation" (1998, p. 8420). Wagner (2005, 2008) also defines evolvability in terms of heritable phenotypic variants. For him, these variants are the result of mutations, especially neutral mutations, within a biological organism. These mutations provide a population of organisms the opportunities to capitalize on evolutionary novelty or innovations. This type of evolvability represents the

[78] For example, James Sethna and collaborators propose a notion of sloppiness to account for evolvability's flexibility but at the same time maintaining inflexible parameters to ensure robustness (Daniels et al. 2008).

ability of organisms to utilize a single heritable mutation in the production of a different functional modular system, which then has the capacity to adapt more efficiently and effectively to a new environment or selection pressure and to out-compete those organisms that do not have the mutation. For example, a neutral mutation to an enzyme within a metabolic pathway might initially be silent, but it might permit the pathway to regulate itself more effectively under different environmental conditions in the presence or absence of certain substrates and thus confer a selectable advantage over competitors that do not have the mutation. Importantly, the neutral mutation is not detrimental to the organism's survival and reproduction. However, even non-neutral mutations in this example might be harmless in that the other enzymes in the pathway are able to incorporate the mutated enzyme because of plasticity in their functional capacities. Thus, mutations—including even neutral mutations—that potentially lead to phenotypic variations are responsible for driving evolutionary novelty or innovation over time.

Biologists can approach the apparent paradox between robustness and evolvability from another phenotype perspective—the bow-tie architecture of robustness. Based on this architecture, evolvability and robustness share common purposes. "On long-time horizons," explain Marie Csete and John Doyle, "evolvability can be considered as the robustness of lineages to potentially large (environmental and/or internal) changes" (2004, p. 448). Bow-tie architecture provides the necessary structure such that evolvability resembles a robust response to changes over long periods. With respect to a geological timeframe, biologists envision evolvability as species robustness to major environmental perturbations or changes.

According to Jörg Stelling and collaborators, "robustness may in fact not impose barriers to evolution but instead enhance 'evolvability' because robustness enables genotypic variability without immediate functional consequences, [thereby] shortening the path to favorable phenotypes" (Stelling et al. 2004, p. 677). What is required for phylogeny, then, is a balance between evolvability and robustness (Lenski et al. 2006). In other words, if robustness is too strict, then systems cannot respond adequately to changes. However, if evolvability is too permissive, then systems respond too readily to changes and do not maintain their identity or integrity. The bow-tie architecture provides a mechanism for balancing robustness and evolvability, with core processes that maintain stability in response to perturbations but with peripheral processes that can shift operations to accommodate those perturbations.

Besides evolvability, another important concept closely associated with robustness is fragility (Doyle et al. 2005, Kitano 2004a, Kitano and Oda 2006, Lehár et al. 2008, Luan et al. 2007 Stelling et al. 2004). The concept of fragility, according to Csete and Doyle, refers to "large and deleterious changes in particular system properties, attributable to possibly small but specific variations in the environment or in components" (2002, p. 1669). In other words, fragility represents an increased sensitivity to perturbations. Biologists often view fragility as the inverse of robustness, i.e., as robustness or insensitivity of a system to changes increases, fragility or sensitivity decreases.

Importantly, fragility is the function of a system's complexity (Kitano 2004a, Stelling et al. 2004). Simple systems that are highly robust are often very fragile. In other words, a single perturbation that blocks an upstream node can attenuate or extinguish the system's output. However, if the system is complex and contains redundant nodes then a functional node can substitute for a blocked or dysfunctional node to maintain the system's output. Joseph Lehár and colleagues have taken advantage of system fragility to identify nodes of fragility in complex systems (Lehár et al. 2008). By removing nodes sequentially from a complex system, they determined the "combination order of fragility" in which downstream redundant nodes no longer compensate a blocked upstream node. Such analysis has important implications for therapeutic drug development (Kitano 2007b).

Although robustness and fragility appear antagonistic or incompatible, from a systems biology or medicine perspective, they are considered two sides of the same coin. As robustness in one part of a system increases through evolvability, for example, fragility in another part of the system may also increase. According to Kitano, "systems that are evolved to be robust against certain perturbations are extremely fragile to unexpected perturbations" (2004a, p. 835). This represents a tradeoff between robustness and fragility, often called the "robust yet fragile" (RYF) phenomenon (Doyle et al. 2005, Stelling et al. 2004). RYF has important consequences not only for evolution but also for disease explanation and therapeutic development (Kitano 2007a, b). In other words, as a disease exhibits robustness to certain perturbations or therapies it will also become more sensitive to other perturbations or therapies. For example, the current rise in type 2 diabetes can be explained in terms of adaptations to starvation in which food, especially high-energy food, is stored as fat (Csete and Doyle 2004). By approaching this type of diabetes as a systems disease, identification of possible nodes of fragility may lead to novel therapeutic approaches (Kitano et al. 2004).

Jeffrey Varner and colleagues provide a case study of blood coagulation that illustrates the notion of fragility and the issues surrounding it vis-à-vis robustness, i.e., RYF, especially for targeting nodes of fragility for drug discovery and evaluation (Luan et al. 2007). They tested the hypothesis that "computationally derived points of fragility of human relevant cascades could be used as a rational basis for target selection despite model uncertainty" (Luan et al. 2007, p. 1347). To that end, they examined the extrinsic blood clotting cascade using mathematical modeling and Monte Carlo sensitivity analysis. They found that thrombin and factor X/Xa are more sensitive, and thereby represent nodes of fragility, when compared to factor IX/IXa and factor VIII/VIIIa, which are more robust. Importantly, they found fragility spread across both initiation of blood clotting factor activation and amplification. Although their results predict the fragility and robustness for the clotting cascade network, application of the results to the clinic requires more translational research. "Perhaps embedding the network into a pharmacokinetic or physiologically based pharmacokinetic (PBPK) model and then exploring the sensitivity profile of the augmented system," conclude Varner and colleagues, "could give insight into factors such as bioavailability and therapeutic window" (Luan et al. 2007, p. 1356).

Just as stasis or stability is a fundamental concept for the biomedical model, so is evolvability, and its related concept of fragility, for systems medicine—as illustrated above (Alon 2023, Price et al. 2010, Wolkenhauer and Green 2013). Specifically, genotype-oriented and phenotype-oriented evolvability are critical concepts for understanding the genetic and/or other molecular, including cellular and organ, foundations of disease etiology and how best to treat a disease in a personal and precise manner. Both types of evolvability are particularly relevant for P7 systems medicine and its notion of the personal P or P4 component. P7 medicine takes into consideration the evolvability of the physico-biomolecular P or P1 component, the psycho-cognitive P or P2 component, and the populational-public P or P3 component, especially in terms of their entanglement with the appearance of the personal P. Finally, systems medicine provides the basis for investigating and explaining the evolutionary appearance of disease mechanisms (Berlin et al 2018, Cardinal-Fernández et al. 2014).

Conclusion

Biomedical scientists explain a system's response to external perturbations in terms of homeostasis, which relies on linear statics or stasis. Other biomedical scientists, however, account for a system's response in terms of homeodynamics, which depends on linear dynamics or dynamic stability. According to these latter scientists, homeodynamics incorporates homeostasis: "we regard homeodynamics as a more general, all-embracing concept from which homeostasis becomes a special case" (Lloyd et al. 2001, p. 136). Nonlinear stasis or statics is another feasible alternative for explaining the preservation of complex biomedical systems. For example, A.I. Kostyukov (1987) utilized nonlinear statics to account for the hysteretic response involved in the motor control of muscle contraction. However, many biomedical scientists do not adopt nonlinear statics as a way of explaining a system's robustness (Champneys 2006). Part of the reason for this is that nonlinear statics accounts for only a limited fragment of a complex biomedical system, especially when investigating a system's evolvability. Nonlinear statics is unable to account for the radical transition from one state to another.

The majority of advocates for systems medicine, including P7 systems medicine, explain a biomedical system's response to external changes in terms of robustness, which relies on nonlinear dynamics. According to some of these advocates, robustness incorporates both homeostasis and stability (Kitano 2007a, Stelling et al. 2004). For example, Timothy Buchman challenges these advocates to "embed homeostatic mechanisms into larger networks that themselves confer robustness to perturbation and thereby protect the community of the self" (2002, p. 251). Finally, these larger networks must also include homeodynamics and its linear dynamics or dynamic stability, as well as nonlinear stasis or statics, to account for a system's response to the considerable number of external perturbations challenging a system.

Chapter 5

Challenges Facing Systems Medicine

Abstract

In this chapter, four major categories of challenges, including methodological, conceptual and theoretical, social and political, and ethical challenges, are discussed. To that end, the methodological, including technological and computational, challenges are examined first, followed by an exploration of the conceptual and theoretical, social and political, and ethical challenges, especially in terms of P7 systems medicine. Moreover, the COVID-19 pandemic has exposed the problems associated with biomedicine and EBM and the potential of systems medicine to resolve the problems, which is analyzed briefly in a separate section. The chapter concludes with a discussion of systems medicine's future, especially as applied to the clinic. If systems medicine cannot successfully tackle these challenges, then its future may not be as bright as originally promised.

Keywords: COVID-19 pandemic, ethics, methodology, politics, systems medicine

1. Introduction

According to most advocates of systems medicine, systems medicine offers tremendous promise and potential for addressing the problems beleaguering biomedicine and its related evidence-based medicine (EBM) and for explaining pathological and clinical phenomena (Apweiler et al. 2018, Capobianco 2012). For example, Alan Aderem articulates that promise for therapeutic medicine accordingly, "Knowledge of disease-perturbed networks will facilitate drug discovery, and pharmaceutical intervention will focus on preventing disease-mediated transitions" (2005, p. 513). However, as Aderem and other advocates of systems medicine acknowledge, to fulfill that promise or to realize its potential systems medicine must first tackle several significant challenges and barriers facing it, many of which are similar to those facing systems biologists (Doyle 2008, Marcum 2009). For example, one of the major challenges facing systems medicine is the overwhelming complexity associated with even the simplest physiological or pathological processes and phenomena. For systems medicine to realize its potential for reshaping medicine in the twenty-first century, however, its advocates must address a number of specific challenges (Adams and Petersen 2016, Blobel and Ruotsalainen 2019, Duffy 2016).

2. Methodological Challenges

Probably the greatest challenge facing both systems medicine, including systems biology, is methodological (Bai and Hur 2022, Balling 2007, Carusi 2014, Wolkenhauer et al. 2013). This challenge is fundamentally methodological in nature because it includes technological and computational challenges and barriers (Ayers and Day 2015, Srivastava and Varner 2007, Wang et al. 2015, Westerhoff and Kell 2007). Advocates of systems medicine divide the technological challenges into instrumental and experimental challenges. Instrumental challenges pertain to the need for rapid, accurate, and inexpensive technology to measure and quantify variations in concentrations of macromolecules within patients. At the forefront of meeting these challenges are the development of nano and microfluidic technologies. The experimental challenges pertain to experimental design, from hypotheses formation to microarray assays. Another significant challenge is the collection and storage of experimental data. Finally, advocates of systems medicine divide the computational challenges into model building, especially dynamic simulation models, computer languages and software, and hardware challenges such as supercomputers (Mardinoglu and Nielsen 2012, Wolkenhauer et al. 2014). The significance of these computational challenges cannot be overemphasized since conceptual advancement depends on computational advancement. In the remainder of this section, the technological challenges are examined first, followed by a discussion of the various computational challenges facing twenty-first century systems medicine—particularly in terms of P7 systems medicine.

2.1. Technological Challenges

The technological challenges facing systems medicine and biology can be divided into instrumental and experimental challenges, which are related to each other. The instrumental challenges include the development of small-scale technologies such as nanotechnology and microfluidics, along with sensor and actuator devices (Freire and Wheeler 2006, Helmke and Minerick 2006, Roco 2003, Wikswo 2004, Wikswo et al. 2006). Advocates of both systems biology and medicine are aware of the need for technologies to determine the concentration of macromolecular components at very small concentrations and to determine the rates of very fast reactions among them. Nanotechnology permits analysis at a molecular scale ranging from ~1 to 100 nm, which represents biological structures from a single ion channel to a cellular organelle (Emerich and Thanos 2003, Nagamune 2017).

Microfluidic technology allows analysis of sample volumes ranging from microliters to picoliters (Hartgerink et al. 2001, Segaliny et al. 2018, Thibault et al. 2019, Whitesides 2006). For example, bioactive nanofiber scaffolding was recently developed to promote recovery from spinal cord injury within a mouse model (Álvarez et al. 2021). One of the major challenges facing small-scale technologies is the combination of nano, micro, and macro materials (Agarwal et al. 2010, Golubewa et al. 2020). Also, microarray-based assays have been combined with microfluidics, for instance, to analyze large parallel samples of nucleic acids and proteins samples (Situma et al. 2006). However, several challenges still face such combinations, particularly with respect to nonspecific adsorption and optical readout technology (Ewis et al. 2005, Müller and Nicolau 2005, Yang et al. 2020).

The experimental challenges facing both systems medicine and biology involve the type, quality, and quantity of data generated from high throughput assays, particularly omics assays (Ahrens et al. 2007, Auffray et al. 2009, Loscalzo and Barabasi 2011, Silvestri et al. 2011, Waters et al. 2006). Paradoxically, systems medicine and biology are both data-rich and data–poor disciplines. One the one hand, both are data-rich disciplines in that they generate enormous amounts of data, especially over the last several decades, with respect to high throughput omics assays. Unfortunately, standardization and quality control do not exist to evaluate these data, as well as their databases. In addition, robust hypotheses and computational algorithms (see next section) need to be developed not only to curate and search large databases but also to analyze and interpret the data contained in them.

On the other hand, systems medicine and biology are data-poor disciplines in that the data are often only partially analyzed or that only particular segments of the various cellular pathways are analyzed thereby leaving many other segments unanalyzed (Capobianco 2012, O'Shea 2012, Wong 2016). Moreover, physiological and pathological processes need to be determined or measured in real time to identify the molecular components of those processes, particularly in terms of the dynamic interactions of the components. Finally, many experimental protocols involving physiological and pathological mechanisms depend on physical disruption or destruction of cells, tissues, organs, and even organ systems. A major challenge for systems medicine is the development of measurement techniques that maintain the patient's integrity and minimize the damage to it.

Moreover, the technology of imagining a single cell provides opportunities for quantifying cellular dynamics, which has direct applications to systems medicine (Hood et al. 2004, Saliba et al. 2014). But significant challenges face these imaging technologies (Coskun and Ozcan 2014, Du et al. 2006, Eils and Athale 2003, Kherlopian, *et al.*, 2008, Megason and Fraser 2007). The advantages of such technologies consist of observing the dynamics of cellular circuits over time, within a single cell of an organism. According to Mikael Benson and colleagues, imaging technologies provide the potential to transform systems medicine into an informational discipline to understand pathological processes in terms of encoded, genomic information (Gustafsson et al., 2014). For example, quantum dots are fluorescent semiconductor nanoparticles developed to image and measure cellular activities (Gao et al. 2005, Jaiswal et al. 2004, Kargozar et al. 2020). One of the major advantages these dots provide over organic dyes is that they do not photobleach as quickly and thereby are brighter longer. Moreover, given their unique optical and electrical properties, they can be excited simultaneously to multiple colors. Unfortunately, the challenges plaguing quantum dot technology include nonspecific binding and cytotoxicity. Another major challenge is to merge these imaging technologies with omics assays, in order to yield a comprehensive and precise picture of the cellular economy.

In terms of P7 systems medicine, the major challenge is to develop the necessary technology to measure the dynamics of biomolecular interactions not simply at the cellular level but also at the organismal level. Thus, for the physico-biomolecular P the standard omics assays, e.g., genomics, transcriptomics, and metabolomics, provide the essential data for determining the patient's human interactome. Moreover, recent phenome-wide association studies in which single-nucleotide variants are mapped onto a range of phenotypes have provided specific genetic variations across various disease phenotypes (Bastarache et al. 2022). In addition, technologies need to be developed for integrating and analyzing data from the physico-biomolecular P with data from connectomics and cognomics of the psycho-cognitive P (Anthony 2001, Paus 2013, Siddiqi et al. 2023) and from exposomics and enviromics/environomics of population-public P (Guchet 2022, Yadav et al. 2013, Teixeira et al. 2011). Finally, technological challenges to forging a robust personal P for delivering quality healthcare include measuring the physiome, pathome, and personome (Ranea et al. 2022).

2.2. Computational Challenges

The computational challenges facing both systems medicine and biology are associated with collecting, curating, analyzing, and interpreting vast amounts of data generated especially through high throughput omics assays (Burrage et al. 2006, Cary et al. 2005, Dhar et al. 2004, Krohs and Callebaut 2007, Schaffner 2007, Wong 2016). And many of these computational challenges are concerned with analyzing data through the development of mathematical and computer models and the integration of these models. For example, Charles Auffray and colleagues identify three specific challenges for systems medicine: "disease subtype discovery using integrated datasets, obtaining a mechanistic understanding of disease, and the development of an informatics platform for the mining, analysis, and visualization of data emerging from translational medicine studies" (Saqi et al. 2016, p. 43). One of the major challenges for computational models is the sheer complexity of physiological and pathological mechanisms, along with data sets obtained from investigating them. As Peter Coveney and Philip Fowler admit, "models operating at different length-scales need to be integrated into a whole that can, for example, correlate a disease symptom with genetic mutations" (2005, p. 268). And computational challenges are divided into model building (software and mathematics development) and high-speed computers (hardware development) (Finkelstein et al. 2004, Kitano 2002a).

One of the chief aims of systems medicine and biology is the development of models to explain and predict system behavior for a variety of biological, physiological, and pathological mechanisms and phenomena (Kahlem and Birney 2006, Mazein et al. 2018, Tuena et al. 2020, Wolkenhauer et al. 2014, You 2004). Moreover, this aim forms the basis for the definition of model itself. Coveney and Fowler, for instance, define a model as "an abstraction of reality with which we can make predictions that may be tested by experiment" (2005, p. 269). The goal of most medical models, then, is to interpret data and thereby to predict behavior of a patient's illness based on the interpreted data. However, these models must be tested experimentally to determine how well they represent physiological and pathological phenomena. Obviously, a crucial characteristic of a model is its fidelity to the observed data and the reality it represents. "The *fidelity* of a model," according to Mark Ragan and collaborators, "is the degree to which it captures the processes or mechanisms, the entities and their relationships that we believe occur in the real system" (Burrage et al. 2006, p. 391). In other words, fidelity should reflect a given level of complexity such that a model simulates actual system behavior.

Systems medicine and biology models are generally divided into two types (Kahlem and Birney 2006, You 2004, Zhang and Hua 2016). The first are qualitative models, which include diagrams and maps, and Boolean models are the best representatives (Hemedan et al. 2022, Mayer et al. 2016). Diagrams and maps, for example, are used to predict the behavior of disease mechanisms as illustrated by the Disease Maps Project (https://disease-maps.org/) (Mazein et al. 2018). Also, Boolean models permit the elucidation of a disease's dynamics with respect to on/off states of its various components, subsystems, or nodes and to presage behavior—although the predictions may not be exactly precise. The second type of modeling is quantitative, which allows for better predictions about the behavior of physiological and pathological systems (Wang et al. 2015, Wolkenhauer 2020). This type takes into consideration the stoichiometry of the mechanisms involved in physiological and pathological behavior. To predict temporal behavior, for example, may require including kinetic parameters into the modeling protocols. Including these parameters often involve both ordinary and partial differential equations to define reaction rates and variations among them.

The most informative models for both systems medicine and biology are those that simulate a system's behavior (Burrage et al. 2006, Daskalaki 2009, Hofmeyr 2007, Kahlem and Birney 2006, Olivier et al. 2016, You 2004). The distinction between a model and a simulation is that a model represents "a set of algorithms that represent some biological process that is reproduced mathematically, whereas a simulation is built on top of a model with additional functionality, e.g., animation" (Patel and Nagl 2006, p. 60). And there are a variety of models available for simulating biological and pathological processes, from enzymatic pathways to disease mechanisms such as cancer (Deville et al. 2003, Harel 2003, Karimi et al. 2022, Takahashi et al. 2002, Tomita, 2001). For example, cell-based models are being developed to simulate cancer cell biology (Metzcar et al. 2019). Virtual Cell or VCell is one of the better-known models for simulating cellular behavior, and its most recent version—VCell 4.5—can simulate a number of cellular activities from ion diffusion to membrane transport to reaction kinetics. (Blinov et al. 2023, Loew et al. 2010, Moraru et al. 2008, Slepchenko et al. 2003).[79] A major challenge for these models, besides simulating more accurately and completely cellular functions and activities, is to make them more "accessible to a broader range of experimentalists, thereby progressively growing the area of computational systems biology beyond its theoretical level…and introducing more 'wet' experimentalists to power these 'dry' computational tools" (Kahlem and Birney 2006, p. 3).

Modeling and simulating biological, physiological, and pathological processes certainly have produced a profuse number of individual models, and the chief challenge for systems medicine and biology is to integrate these models to generate models that are accurately predictive (Kitano 2002a, Wolkenhauer et al. 2014). One of the main problems to meet this challenge is the "scaling-up" problem (Stalidzans et al. 2020). For example, to model and simulate metabolic pathways accurately involves larger scale models that include cellular entities, such as cellular organelles or even the cell itself (Mardinoglu and Nielsen 2012, Zang and Hua 2016). Resolving this problem then pertains to integrating biological, physiological, and pathological processes at multiple hierarchical levels. According to Anthony Finkelstein and colleagues, systems medicine and biology are "unlikely to produce a set of canonical models. Rather, a complex ecology of models embedded within a framework that enables debate and collaboration among contributors will arise" (Finkelstein et al. 2004, p. 30). Besides the spatial dimension, another significant challenge is the temporal dimension. Cellular processes can occur at different rates, from a fraction of a second to minutes, days, or even years. Overall, there is a crucial need to develop models that can simulate cell-to-cell interactions in terms of tissue and organ physiology and pathology.

Today, supercomputing can overcome traditional limits on computational speeds, but the requisite software to apply this technology to biological, physiological, and pathological systems needs to be developed or at least improved (Finkelstein et al. 2004, November 2012, Leonelli 2019, You 2004). For example, the computer language, Systems Biology Markup Language (SBML), has been very instrumental in developing disparate software tools

[79] The National Resource for Cell Analysis and Modeling sponsors VCell through funding to University of Connecticut (https://vcell.org/).

and models, although SBML often serves more as a *lingua franca* than as a universal language (Hucka et al. 2004). Accordingly,

> The SBML project is not an attempt to define a universal language for representing quantitative models; the fluid and rapidly evolving views of biological function, and the vigorous rate at which new computational techniques and individual tools are being developed today, are incompatible with a one-size-fits-all idea of a universal language. A more realistic alternative is to acknowledge the diversity of approaches and methods being explored by different software tool developers, and seek a common intermediate format—a lingua franca—enabling communication of the most essential aspects of the models (Hucka et al. 2004, pp. 41-42).

Moreover, computer language development represents a challenge to communicate data and results more effectively to both colleagues and the public.

Obviously, computational challenges certainly confront the integration of the physico-biomolecular P (P1), the psycho-cognitive P (P2), and the population-public P (P3) to operationalize and implement the personal P (P4) for the clinic. One means of addressing this challenge is through the metaverse associated with digital medicine (Garavand and Aslani 2022, Haleem et al. 2022, Sun et al. 2022, Volkov et al. 2021). As Mamon Alazab and colleagues note:

> The Metaverse is a confluence of multiple enabling technologies such as artificial intelligence, virtual reality, augmented reality, internet of medical devices, robotics, quantum computing, etc. through which new directions for providing quality healthcare treatment and services can be explored. The amalgamation of these technologies ensures immersive, intimate and personalized patient care (Chengoden et al. 2023, p. 12765).

Finally, artificial intelligence represents a computational means for integrating the various Ps to provide truly personalized healthcare that is precise and personal (Cesario et al. 2021, Kulikowski 2019). Specifically, cognitive artificial intelligence could provide the means for integrating the P2 component with the P1 and P3 components to forge the personal P (Laird et al. 2017, Sumari and Ahmad 2018).

3. Conceptual and Theoretical Challenges

Besides methodological challenges, systems medicine and biology also face significant conceptual and theoretical challenges (Clermont et al. 2009, Kirschner 2016, Tretter 2019, Vandamme et al. 2013, Van Speybroeck et al. 2005, Wolkenhauer et al. 2007). These latter challenges represent barriers or limitations that threaten to cripple the development and advancement of systems medicine and biology. And the present book represents a sustained effort to examine these challenges and to map the terrain by which to engage them and to pursue practical solutions. These conceptual and theoretical challenges in particular need to be addressed to ensure the future success of both systems medicine and biology. Moreover, these challenges are critical because their resolution provides the intellectual scaffolding necessary for structuring the concepts and theories required to understand and explain more adequately or completely biological, physiological, and pathological mechanisms and processes. In addition, according to Linda Van Speybroeck and collaborators, "the construction of a strong conceptual [and theoretical] framework [permits] interdisciplinary communication, infrastructures and publication channels into which scientific disciplines other than (molecular) biology can feed" (Van Speybroeck et al. 2005, p. 1305). In other words, with a robust conceptual and theoretical scaffolding both systems medicine and biology must be implemented through interdisciplinarity not only within the medical community but also within the social and political communities, which the COVID-19 pandemic made so painfully obvious.

One of the major theoretical challenges is whether systems medicine and biology are sufficiently definable conceptually to provide the necessary framework to guide future research in their respective fields (Bousquet et al. 2014, Kirschner 2016, Tretter 2019, Zanin et al. 2021). Evelyn Keller (2005), for example, thinks systems biology is not precisely definable and cites the lack of integration among the various biological and scientific disciplines that constitute systems biology. Although this lack of integration is certainly problematic, it appears not to be an insuperable barrier to defining systems biology (Friboulet and Thomas 2005, Ideker et al. 2007). For example, there are several functional definitions that provide a sufficient or practical framework for guiding systems biology research (Capobianco 2012, Kirschner 2005, Lisacek and Appel, 2007). Moreover, Edison Liu (2005) insists that systems biologists can supply a sufficient framework not only to direct biological research but that such direction makes systems biology a predictive science. Another important challenge with defining systems biology is the precise articulation of particular concepts like emergence and robustness, in order to construct models to simulate system behavior (Deguet et al. 2006, Kitano 2007a).

In terms of systems medicine, defining P7 systems medicine theoretically in terms of the four P-components and three P-actions is advantageous for medicine's advancement into the twenty-first century. Specifically, as detailed earlier the various P-components can be investigated with respect to omics technology (Table 2). For example, the physico-biomolecular P (P1) can be examined and quantitated through the technology associated with genomics/epigenomics, transcriptomics/proteomics, and metabolomics/nutrigenomics, through their corresponding systems sciences. Conceptually, from the entanglement of the P1-3 components emerges the personal P (P4), which is not reducible in terms of its properties to the properties of the P1-3 components. The three P-actions also enhance medical investigation through predicting possible health and disease issues (P5), soliciting the patient's participation (P6) in then preventing (P7) the issues. Overall, P7 systems medicine integrates the sum of medical research to provide the most comprehensive picture of the patient.

Another conceptual issue facing systems medicine and biology is whether they represent a Kuhnian paradigm shift, i.e., whether systems medicine and biology are incompatible or incommensurable with traditional biomedicine and biology conceptually (Bland et al. 2017, Maier 2017, Marcum 2009, Zhu et al. 2009). The resolution depends on whether the transition from biomedicine to systems medicine is revolutionary or evolutionary. If revolutionary in the traditional Kuhnian sense, then it represents a paradigm shift. If evolutionary then it does not. As evident in the literature and throughout this book, the transition has been revolutionary with respect to a conceptual shift from incommensurable concepts like biomedicine's reductionism to systems medicine's wholism (Ahn et al. 2006, Gatherer 2010, Ma'ayan 2017, Mazzocchi 2012). But this is from a global perspective. From a local perspective, however, the conceptual shift is evolutionary. For example, biomedicine and systems medicine do share the importance and necessity of biomolecular compounds in understanding and explaining disease mechanisms. And so systems medicine from a local conceptual context is the evolutionary product of traditional biomedicine.

The evolution of both systems medicine and biology from traditional biomedicine and biology can yield hybrid forms of medicine and biology, which are available for systems biologists. For example, Maureen O'Malley and John Dupré (2005) propose a pragmatic systems biology, which roughly equates to an evolutionary systems biology, and a theoretical systems biology, which roughly equates to a revolutionary systems biology (Marcum 2008c). Moreover, Martin Latterich (2005) goes on to assert that integrating these two hybrid forms of systems biology provides a more comprehensive picture of biological phenomena in that the data from them complement each other. The problem with such integration, however, is that often the concepts are incommensurable with one another, which might lead to possible constraints. For example, as noted earlier systems biomedicine is a very active field within systems medicine, but the issue that surfaces is whether the incommensurability associated with its conceptual basis might constrain its future development. In other words, is the hybrid systems biomedicine a sterile offspring of biomedicine and systems science?

Besides the two chief paradigms of biomedicine and systems medicine or even intermediate paradigms of systems medicine and biology, some commentators argue for a *tertium quid*. For example, Mihajlo Mesarović and colleagues proposed a "new" complex systems biology (or system of systems), based upon organizational or coordination principles that transcend not just traditional biology but also both network and systems biology (Mesarović et al. 2004, Mesarović and Sreenath 2005).[80] Moreover, Avi Ma'ayan (2017) has also proposed a "complex" systems biology based on various design principles. Probably one of the most important conceptual challenges for both systems medicine and biology, then, is to discover and formulate design and organizational principles (Berlin et al. 2017, Bruggeman and Westerhoff, 2007, Kohl and Noble 2009). These principles are critical for defining and clarifying complex systems investigated in either systems medicine or biology. Knowledge of these principles should provide robust ways for elucidating life and for creating therapeutic modalities to treat diseases, especially through combinatorial methods.

Finally, P7 systems medicine provides a means to address the conceptual and theoretical challenges facing systems medicine. Conceptually, the personal P (P4) represents an entanglement of the physio-biomolecular P (P1), psycho-cognitive P (P2), and population-public P (P3). This entanglement reflects a shift from biomedical's reductionism to system medicine's wholism, along with other concepts including new materialism, emergent synthesis, and nonlinear dynamics—among many others. Theoretically, P7 medicine depends on development not only in systems theory and science but also in

80 "For a conceptual breakthrough," argue Mesarović and Sreenath, "a new paradigm is needed for a complex biological phenomenon beyond the current parameters of networks and of systems" (2005, p. 33).

network theory and science, and it can provide guidance for them through the various P-components and P-actions. For example, the physio-biomolecular P can anchor network-based methods to connect genotype to phenotype associated with various pathologies (Ranea et al. 2022). P7 systems medicine also address other theoretical challenges such as complexity and chaos theories (Dandekar and Kunz 2023). For example, the three P-actions can be instrumental in terms of accounting for the variation in breast cancer patient's response to pharmaceutical treatments (Yu et al. 2021).

4. Social and Political Challenges

Although the methodological, technological, computational, and conceptual and theoretical challenges facing systems medicine are important, the social and political challenges are equally, if not more, important at times. One of the major challenges facing systems medicine is cooperation among scientists and clinicians within the biomedical community, especially through crowdsourcing (Khare et al. 2016, Wazny 2018). Unfortunately, such cooperation often runs counter to the traditional emphasis on individual scientists or clinicians as autonomous or independent agents. The model of independent agents within the biomedical community worked reasonably well under a reductionist view of science, when isolating components of physiological and pathological phenomena and describing them. However, this model began to fail, when scientists and clinicians tried to investigate complex phenomena in order to explain and manipulate them at higher-level order or scale. The investigation and explanation of complex phenomena requires not only cooperation and teamwork among community members but also integration of the different disciplines. In this section, the various social and political challenges facing systems medicine are examined in terms of disciplinary integration, attribution of credit for research or discovery, data ownership, extramural funding, information distribution, institutional structures, public policies, and the integration of biological and social determinants to explain pathological processes and phenomena. Resolving these challenges is critical for the future success of systems medicine.

Systems medicine generally requires disciplinary integration with respect to an interdisciplinary or a multidisciplinary approach to studying complex physiological and pathological phenomena (Marcum 2020, Morrison-Smith et al. 2022, Tretter and Löffler-Stastka 2019). It necessitates scientists and clinicians from traditional disciplines of biology, physics, chemistry, mathematics, engineering, and computer sciences to cooperate on projects of common interest. The single greatest challenge is how to integrate these various disciplines at the social level and to promote cooperation among its disciplinary members. "Medicine today is an extremely heterogeneous field of knowledge," write Felix Tretter and Henriette Löffler-Stastka, "based on clinical observations and action knowledge and on data from the biological, behavioral and social sciences" (2019, p. 1). The challenges associated with interdisciplinary or multidisciplinary are especially keen in terms of teamwork (Aderem 2005, Gohar et al. 2019, Smye and Frangi 2021). Interdisciplinary teamwork runs counter to the standard ethos and culture within the biomedical community, which portrays biomedical scientists as autonomous agents who pull back the cover that hides—or dis-covers—nature's secrets.[81]

Two related social and political challenges emerging from the challenge of interdisciplinary teamwork often involved in systems medicine include attribution of credit for research or discovery and data ownership. Attribution of credit for the research within a particular project or a novel discovery is a critical challenge for systems medicine, which relies on work across several independent disciplines (Hara et al. 2003, Perryman 2018). For the traditional model of biomedical research and its principal investigator, the question of credit is easy to answer politically—the person who is responsible for the research project and its funding or who makes the discovery. For interdisciplinary team members, however, who each contribute to the research project or discovery, the question of credit attribution is trickery to answer politically. One possibility is to attribute credit to the director of the project or to the principal investigator on the project's funding. This is often the common approach to this challenge. But as projects become more complex and involve directors of other disciplinary projects, identification of an individual or even a few individuals can be problematic. The second closely related challenge pertains to data ownership, especially for large sets of data (Dicuonzo et al. 2022, Kruse et al. 2016, Lipworth et al. 2017, Mifsud and Gavrilovici 2019). Again, this challenge is not so easily resolved under the current framework for practicing biomedical science, but the recent push towards public access of data certainly addresses this challenge (Belle et al. 2015, Rockhold et al. 2016).

[81] This image of the biomedical scientist is heavily laden with gender biases (Merchant 1980).

Extramural funding of systems medicine is an important social challenge for its success within the twenty-first century, particularly since it tackles the frontiers of clinical research and practice (Lemmen et al. 2021). Such funding is often obtained from both public and private granting agencies. For example, the US National Institutes of Health (https://www.nih.gov/grants-funding) and the National Institute of General Medical Sciences (https://www.nigms.nih.gov/grants/Pages/Home.aspx) actively fund various systems medicine initiatives throughout various medical schools, especially as it relates to precision and personalized medicine. In addition, private granting agencies provide funds to support systems medicine initiatives. For example, Hood and the Institute for Systems Biology received a $13 million grant from the Bill and Melinda Gates Foundation and Amgen for conducting systems medicine research (https://philanthropynewsdigest.org/news/gates-foundation-amgen-award-13-million-for-medical-research). However, more funding of both basic and clinical research remains a pressing challenge for the future of systems medicine.

Another social challenge for systems medicine is the distribution of its information, especially in terms of convincing both the medical community and the public that systems medicine is properly addressing if not resolving the problems or anomalies that traditional biomedicine has failed to resolve, especially chronic diseases like cancer and cardiovascular diseases. Traditional disciplines have outlets for such information in the form of professional and public books, as well as professional journals, along with institutions and their conferences. Since systems medicine spans several disciplines, a professional manuscript may not be possible to review if it incorporates technologies or concepts that are outside the expertise of a journal's reviewers. But this challenge is being addressed with the appearance of journals devoted to systems medicine. Such journals include, for example, *Systems Medicine* (Baumbach and Schmidt 2018), *Journal of Medical Systems* (https://www.springer.com/journal/10916), Systems Medicine series in *BMC Systems Biology* (https://www.biomedcentral.com/collections/sysmed), *Family Systems Medicine* (Bloch 1983), and *Families, System, & Health* (https://www.apa.org/pubs/journals/fsh). Besides journals, systems medicine also includes various textbooks and professional monographs on specialized topics. For example, Schmitz and Wolkenhauer's *Systems Medicine* (2016) is an excellent introduction to the discipline, while Wolkenhauer's 3-volume *Systems Medicine: Integrative, Qualitative and Computational Approaches* (2020) is a comprehensive introduction to systems medicine. Finally, professional societies and their conferences, such as the European Association of Systems Medicine (http://www.eisbm.org/projects/easym/), are instrumental in meeting the challenge of information dispersal.

Because systems medicine requires a change in the culture of medical research and practices, the chief challenge is generally how to organize systems medicine institutionally. Specifically, the challenge is whether to create formally a new institutional structure dedicated strictly to systems medicine or to maintain informally a loose association among various medical and research departments interested in the systems medicine. Obviously, advantages and disadvantages exist for both approaches to this challenge. For example, formal institutional approaches require more capital to initiate, but they do provide a single location for implementing systems medicine. Although informal approaches are less expensive, they do raise practical issues of how to integrate separate medical departments and specialties. An excellent example of an approach to institutionalizing systems medicine is Georgetown University's Systems medicine program (https://grad.georgetown.edu/systems-medicine-ms/#about-the-program). The program offers an M.S. degree in systems medicine that can be coupled to the M.D. degree. Other systems medicine programs include the Laboratory for Systems Medicine at the University of Florida (https://systemsmedicine.pulmonary.medicine.ufl.edu/), the Bioinformatics and Systems Medicine program at UTHealth Houston (https://sbmi.uth.edu/prospective-students/bism.htm), and Institute of Cellular and Systems Medicine at Taiwan's National Health Research Institutes (https://cs.nhri.org.tw/sample-page/). Finally, the recent advances in the metaverse in terms of augmented and virtual reality can help to address the social challenges facing systems medicine, particularly in terms of blockchain technology (Bhugaonkar et al. 2022, Supriya and Chattu 2021).

Another important social challenge for systems medicine, which is quite different from those previously discussed, involves the integration of social and biological components and determinants to explain pathological processes and phenomena (Best and Khushf 2006, Diez-Roux, 2007, Kelly et al. 2014, Schofield 2015). Instead of viewing biological factors as proximal causes and social factors as distal causal factors in explaining health and illness, according to Ana Diez-Roux (2007), a systems approach integrates both factors. Diez-Roux proposes a social-biologic interactionist model in contrast to a social factor-antecedent model or a gene-environment interaction model. According to her model, "social experience has the capacity to directly alter both the structure and functioning of biological systems" (Diez-Roux, 2007, p. 571). Thus, social determinants are not simply antecedents or just environmental to the expression of health or illness; rather, they are equally as important in explaining health and illness causally as genetic or other biological determinants. Diez-Roux proceeds to illustrate the proposed model with the obesity epidemic. A social factor-antecedent or gene-environment interaction model isolates the various biological and social factors independently of one another and conducts a regression analysis on them. Diez-Roux's systems model, however, includes in the analysis not only individual factors such as obesity predisposing genes or a person's or even a society's images of body but also the system's characteristics such as the production and distribution of food.

Finally, P7 systems medicine can address not only the various social challenges facing the future of systems medicine but more importantly the political challenges. As noted earlier, Ferrara (2017) introduced a P5 medicine that appends a political P to Hood's P4 medicine. What is particularly important is that the political challenge to systems medicine is addressed through the population-public P (P3), especially in terms of the public domain. Specifically, the P3 component protects the patient qua personal P (P4) by guarding the patient's data obtained from either physio-biomolecular P (P1) and psycho-cognitive P (P2) from being exploited for monetary gain. As for the social challenges, P7 medicine, for example, can contribute to exploring the biological or P1 component and the social or P3 component interactions, especially through the P-actions—particularly the participatory P (P6) action in terms of the patient being an active contributor to maintaining personal health or preventing illness. And each of the first three P-components can help to integrate the various medical, scientific, and social disciplines associated with them, especially in terms of composing the patient qua personal P (P4).

5. Ethical Challenges

Unfortunately, scant attention has been paid in the literature to the ethical issues and challenges specifically confronting systems medicine, although some attention has been paid to these issues facing systems biology. For example, in a "Target Article" published in *The American Journal of Bioethics*, O'Malley and collaborators proposed a socioethics approach and compared it to a bioethics approach, to address ethical issues associated with systems biology (O'Malley et al. 2007). Their socioethics approach integrates a wide variety of disciplines, from the biological sciences to the humanities, to achieve a comprehensive approach to ethical problems and challenges. Their approach can also serve to address ethical issues associated with systems medicine. Specifically, they identify four sets of ethical issues and challenges facing systems biology, and by implication systems medicine, and contrast their dynamic socioethical approach to the traditional static bioethical approach.

The first set of challenges concerns disease identification, especially in terms of privacy and discrimination (O'Malley et al. 2007). Although this set is comparable to that for bioethicists, socioethicists face the additional burden of sorting out the issues that emerge from the complex interactions between genes and their environment. For bioethicists, disease identification is reducible simply to genetic sequences and the tests used to identify relevant genetic information, especially in terms of genetic predisposition towards a disease. An important ethical challenge is how much of this genetic information should be publicly available (Lowrance and Collins 2007, McGuire and Gibbs 2006). Moreover, for socioethicists the genetic sequence is necessary but not sufficient for disease expression. A systems socioethics approach to disease, according to O'Malley and colleagues, diminishes the importance of genetic sequence information and thereby downplays privacy issues.

The next set of challenges is associated with personal identity and ancestry (O'Malley et al. 2007). For bioethicists, ethical issues concerning the nature of a person's identity are simply reducible to DNA. However, for socioethicists personal identity represents an emergent property of multilevel interactions, which complicates the ethical issues surrounding personal identity. Fundamentally, argue O'Malley and collaborators, a systems socioethics approach provides a new framework for a "cultural understanding" of personal identity, especially as it pertains to detecting predisposition towards expressing a disease later in life. The ethical issue is how best to proceed in treating patients predisposed to a genetic disease if genetic makers for that disease are available for testing. A well-publicized example is the BRCA gene for breast cancer, especially with direct-to-consumer testing (Gronowski and Budelier 2020). A dynamic socioethical approach, in contrast to a static bioethical approach, certainly helps to address that challenge by articulating holistically notions of personal identity and ancestry.

The third set of ethical challenges pertain to genetic modification or engineering and to the integrity of life itself (O'Malley et al. 2007). In recent decades since the Human Genome Project's completion and the introduction of CRISPR technology, genomic biology has issued in a spectre of genetically modified or engineered organisms along with the ethical challenge of the natural versus the unnatural (Baumann 2016, Mulvihill 2017). The practical issues of genetically modified tissues and patients pose greater challenges for socioethicists, especially in terms of the natural-unnatural divide, than for bioethicists (Adli 2018, Hirakawa et al. 2020). For example, the development of human enhancements using CRISPR technology raises ethical challenges to the distinction between therapy and enhancement itself (Gouw 2018). Moreover, such technology challenges the crux of human nature and the dignity of human personhood (de Araujo 2017, Raposo 2019). This situation leads to a variety of important ethical questions, especially for systems medicine. How should society view such genetic modifications, particularly in terms of treating patients? Are they unnatural or artificial? And if so, what limits, if any, should society place on them? These and other challenging questions demand answers, especially from advocates of systems medicine.

The final set of ethical challenges concerns the commercialization and ownership of genetic information (O'Malley et al. 2007). This set, according to bioethicists, revolves around the uniqueness of genetic sequences in terms of patenting them, which raises issues of ownership. However, according to socioethicists, genetic sequences are only a part of the overall information required for defining an individual's uniqueness. Therefore, patenting such information may not be as straightforward as simply patenting genetic sequences. O'Malley and collaborators identified several issues with such patenting efforts, such as compromising the integrity of life or depriving patients of their biological personhood. And these are serious issues for advocates of systems medicine (Yan 2011). On the one hand, greater information concerning patient genomics and other omics provides opportunity for advancing systems medicine technologically; but on the other hand, it deprives patients of their ownership of such information. For example, the National Institutes of Health's *All of Us* initiative fails to address the ethical issues over the data it is collecting (Sankar and Parker 2017).

Importantly, O'Malley and colleagues' "Target Article" prompted responses from several bioethicists that are relevant for the ethical challenges facing systems medicine (Drell 2007, Foster 2007, Robert 2007). One of the chief responses was that the list of challenges was not exhaustive. For example, Griffin Trotter identified several more challenges including:

> 1) enhanced precision in the characterization of traditional concepts and distinctions (including their practical implications); 2) enhanced ability to integrate useful elements of diverse and incompatible moral theories; 3) enhanced appreciation for the extent of plausible moral diversity; and

> 4) enhanced ability to distill out the nonsense that afflicts many prevalent value theories (2007, p. 84).

These additional ethical challenges are certainly relevant for systems medicine as it progresses into the twenty-first century. Finally, Lenny Moss (2007) cautions that a socioethics approach must take into consideration what constitutes the essential nature of human nature or risk the possibility of distorting it.

Robert Best and George Khushf make a similar plea as O'Malley and colleagues for the ethical challenges facing systems biology and medicine, but for nanomedicine:

> Consideration of ethical and other societal issues should in fact be made explicit early in the process to allow the highest possible degree of freedom in establishing systems. This is in contrast to the traditions where consideration of ethics only comes in at a late stage, after important developments in science and technology have taken place (2006, p. 738).

Their warning is crucial for twenty-first century systems medicine, if it is to avoid finding it has led society into a dire ethical conundrum from which it cannot recover. Moreover, Steffen Fleßa and colleagues develop an "innovation theory" to explore not simply the technical challenges but also the ethical challenges to the development of systems medicine (Fleßa et al. 2016).

Finally, P7 systems medicine, with its emphasis upon the personal P (P4), provides the means for addressing many of the above ethical challenges. For example, the issue of personal identity is not simply the result of a single factor, such as a person's genomics, but the compilation of other omics that define the physio-biomolecular P (P1), along with the factors composing the psycho-cognitive P (P2) and the population-public P (P3). The entanglement of the first three P-components to generate a unique personal P (P4) stresses that the integrity of the patients, as well as healthcare professionals, is critical for delivering not only ethical care but also quality care that yields the best clinical outcome. Moreover, the three P-actions also contribute to addressing the ethical challenges facing systems medicine. For example, the participatory P (P6) empowers patients to seek ownership over their personal healthcare data, ensuring their active contribution to clinical outcomes.

6. COVID-19 Pandemic

As often noted, and discussed throughout the book, the COVID-19 pandemic has certainly exposed the problems plaguing biomedicine and EBM (Shamasunder et al. 2020, Marcum and Tretter 2023, Tretter and Marcum 2023, Tretter et al. 2020, 2021, 2023). These problems range from the theoretical to the technological and empirical of severe acute respiratory syndrome coronavirus 2 (SARS-CoV-2) infection and from public policies to political and governmental management of the pandemic. One of the major problems has been providing sound quality medical science to treat patients safely, effectively, and efficiently and to reduce or eliminate the spread of SARS-CoV-2. Unfortunately, both the biomedical sciences and EBM have failed to resolve these problems in that they could not conduct the necessary randomized controlled trials and translate them readily into actionable clinical practices or public policies (Carley et al. 2020, Greenhalgh 2020).

What has been central to problems faced by biomedicine and EBM is that the mantra "follow the science" is just too simplistic for tackling the COVID-19 pandemic, especially with respect to public health policies and governmental management of the pandemic (Mercuri 2020, Stevens 2020). In other words, many of those policies were based on expert opinions and not on randomized clinical trials (Pfaff and Schmitt 2021). And even EBM^{+} has been criticized as ineffectual since mechanistic pathological explanations can be wrong or misleading (Solomon 2021). Systems medicine, particularly P7 systems medicine, provides an approach for resolving these problems by addressing the pandemic at the personal, populational, and planetary levels.

As discussed earlier, systems medicine is predicated on assumptions about health and disease that counter biomedicine and EBM. Specifically, it assumes wholist organicism in contrast to biomedicine and EBM's reductionist mechanism (Beresford 2010, Nunn 2012). In terms of the COVID-19 pandemic, biomedicine and EBM assume that knowing the pathological mechanisms is sufficient for treating patients with SARS-CoV-2 infection, as well as for curtailing or stopping the spread of the virus (Fairman 2022). Although this assumption permits the identification of several key components responsible for the pandemic and its impact on individuals and societies, it fails to deliver a robust personal and public health system to respond to the pandemic and to mitigate or even prevent future pandemics and other possible public health crises.

P7 systems medicine, with its wholist organicism approach, provides a framework for addressing and resolving the problems raised by the COVID-19 pandemic that has challenged both biomedicine and EBM (Rao 2021, Rehman et al. 2021). Specifically, it integrates the various levels associated with SARS-CoV-2 infection of individual patients and its spread throughout a population and global community. First, the physico-biomolecular P (P1) incorporates the basic systems and medical sciences, including systems virology, vaccinology, and epidemiology, along with systems physiology and pathology, to deal particularly with personal infection. Next, the psycho-cognitive P (P2) embraces systems psychology and psychiatry to address the mental and behavioral issues, such as compliance with masking, social distancing, and vaccination. The population-public P (P3) is also included and incorporates not just a specific population but also the planetary context as a whole in terms of the pandemic.

The above P1-3 components are entangled to generate the personal P (P4), which then can be guided by the three P-actions. First, the predictive P (P5) provides the information needed for a clinician to advise a patient qua personal P about the risks associated with SARS-CoV-2 infection or for an epidemiologist about the virus' spread. Next, the participatory P (P6) involves empowering the personal P to engage with the requisite agency to recover from viral infection. Lastly, the preventive P (P7) includes enlisting the personal P in activities to reduce viral infection and its spread. Importantly, P7 systems medicine provides a strategy for enhancing not only personal and public health but also planetary health.

In short, P7 systems medicine represents a conceptual framework to develop a robust personal, public, and planetary health system that can prevent or at least mitigate future pandemics by extending the focus from a reductionist mechanistic perspective to a wholist organicist one. Although P7 medicine shares with postgenomic P4 systems medicine's reliance on various omics defining the physico-biomolecular P (P1), including genomics, epigenomics, transcriptomics, and proteomics, it also includes other omics associated with the psycho-cognitive P (P2), such as connectomics and psychomics, as well as omics associated with the population-public P (P3), including environomics/enviromics, exposomics, and viromics. Finally, although P7 medicine shares with P4 systems medicine an emphasis on prediction of possible health problems based on biological factors, it also incorporates into the prediction calculus psychological, public, and planetary factors.

Conclusion

As noted in this chapter, systems medicine certainly faces a number of challenges as the twenty-first century progresses. The two biggest challenges for its future success are the big picture and the finer grain picture. The big picture challenge is making sense of the vast amounts of information generated by high throughput omics assays, or putting together Humpty-Dumpty or the patient, as Noble articles it.

> The last decades of the 20th century saw the immense success of the reductive approach. We have broken Humpty-Dumpty down into his smallest fragments: his genes and proteins. We now have the monumental task of putting him back together again. I see this as being one of the great challenges for biology in the 21st century (2003, p. 157).

This is certainly a colossal challenge but one that some advocates of system medicine are facing with confidence (An et al. 2007, Hood et al. 2004, Lemberger 2007Powell 2004, Van Der Greef 2011). To be truly transformative, systems medicine must expand its horizon to include the entire system.

Besides the overall picture of the patient, systems medicine also has important implications for treating specific diseases and medical disciplines—the finer grain picture. For example, it offers a novel means by which to transform oncology (Hornberg et al. 2006, Khalil and Hill 2005, Powathil et al. 2015, Wang et al. 2007). The challenge in the twenty-first century for oncologists is to expound new metaphysical categories (especially in terms of causation) and to identify organizational or coordination rules that complement or even possibly subsume the reductionist or genetic rules. Advocates of systems medicine must also develop methodological techniques (4-D and artificial tissue culture conditions and mathematical or computational and *in silico* models) to guide and drive the cognitive and material elements of scientific practices, which should capture more accurately and completely the complexity of carcinogenesis.

Thus, systems medicine is faced with what Michael Sporn (2006) calls a dichotomy. In other words, it is important not only to view the big picture but also the details or brush strokes for explaining the nature of complex diseases, like cancer, and especially for treating them. Importantly, according to Sporn, not only must the details of cancer biology be attended to, but those details must also be incorporated at a larger level or scale, such as the patient's lifestyle and society's strategies to support the patient, especially in terms of preventing disease. "We need a new, holistic approach to prevention," acknowledges Sporn, "that will include both chemoprevention *and* a better life-style, with cooperative efforts from people in both areas, directed toward a better quality of life for the patient" (2006, p. 371). Thus, systems medicine chief challenge is not simply disease prevention but enhancing the quality of life.

To address that challenge, P7 systems medicine provides the healthcare community with the means not only to meet Nobel's concern of putting Humpty-Dumpty or the patient back together again but also Sporn's concern of overcoming the dichotomy of the big picture and its brush strokes. Specifically, both the four P-components and three P-actions provide the big picture in terms of the personal P (P4), which is composed of the first three P-components. And the P-actions complete that picture in terms of how to operationalize the P-components. In other words, for the big picture, the personal P (P4) provides the information required for predicting the patient's health state (P5) and for determining what is required to prevent possible compromise to it (P7). Such information can be utilized to enlist the patient's participation (P6) to achieve the best possible outcome. In conclusion, P7 systems medicine provides healthcare with the conceptual structure for integrating organicism, emergence, and robustness.

Glossary

As for any discipline, systems medicine has a unique set of terms and keywords; but being interdisciplinary it shares a number of terms and keywords with other disciplines. The goal of this glossary is two-fold: to include as many salient terms and keywords as possible and to provide sufficient working definitions of them. For the best resource for systems medicine terminology see Zanin et al. (2021), while for contemporary philosophy of medicine see Marcum (2017b).

Analysis: conclusion or judgment entailed from premises with respect to formal or logical reasoning, which is often contrasted with synthesis.

Autonomy: bioethical principle concerned with patient's power or right for self-determination.

Biological system: system or network composed on biological agents and phenomena, such as gene-regulatory network, protein-interaction network, metabolic network, and signaling network.

Biomarker: measurable or detectable substance indicating possible incidence of disease or a possible clinical state of outcome.

Biopsychosocial model: George Engel's model of healthcare that incorporates the biological, psychological, and social factors into patient care.

Cancerome: module or network of specific interacting genes and proteins involved in the mechanism of tumor formation or carcinogenesis.

Causation: agency required to produce an effect, including the principle of causality that states every effect has a cause.

Chaos theory: although complex systems might appear random, closer analysis reveals patterns, such as fractals, and interactions, such as feedback loops, that are responsible for a systems behavior, especially self-organization.

Circular causality: sequence of cause and effect relationships in which original cause is modified causally by its successive effects through a feedback loop.

Clinical expertise: clinician's opinion based on education, skill, and experience.

Cognition: mental faculty involved in acquiring knowledge through perceiving and conceiving.

Cognomics: exploration of the connections among genes, brain anatomy and structure, and cognitive functions such as memory and language processing, including psychiatric disorders.

Complex adaptive system: complex system or network that adjusts to environmental perturbations and thereby retains its function.

Complex system: system or network composed of diverse components that often function in a nonlinear fashion.

Complexity theory: rational analysis of interacting components under nonlinear environmental conditions.

Connectomics: investigation of the structural and functional connections among the brain's neuronal cells.

Consciousness: facility to perceive or to be aware of either physical or mental phenomena.

Constitutive reductionism: belief that systems are constituted causally by lower-level systems.

Constraints: parameters or parametric conditions at one level that impose limits or inhibits function at another level, such as homeostatic constraints.

Cure: to restore physiological and/or mental function.

Determinism: belief that events are causally straightforward or decisive, given antecedent conditions, in contrast to stochasticity.

Diagnosis: determining a pathological condition based on clinical symptoms and evidence.

Digital health: physiological state based on digital technology, ranging from genomic sequencing to smartphone apps, which can generate a digital twin or virtual model of a patient's physiological or pathological state.

Dignity: having either intrinsic or extrinsic value or worth.

Disease: pathological dysfunction of the body or bodily part.

Diseasome: module or network of specific interacting genes and proteins involved in the mechanism of disease etiology.

Downward causation: causal relationship in which higher-level events and phenomena have a deterministic impact on shaping lower-level events and phenomena.

Drugome: specific drugs composing a therapeutic network.

Dualism: belief in two opposing realities, such as mind-body, which is often contrasted with monism.

Efficient cause: that which brings about an effect.

Emergence: process by which novel entities or properties appear that are not reducible to components entities or properties.

Emergent mechanism: belief that structure alone is not responsible for the appearance of novel or unpredictable entities or properties, in contrast to resultant mechanism.

Empiricism: belief that experience is sufficient to justify knowledge or belief, which is often contrasted with rationalism.

Entanglement: interactions that involve the emergence of causal agency.

Enviromics: branch of ecology that investigates the environmental factors involved in the functioning of biological organisms, also called environomics.

Environment: geological or geographical factors or conditions that can have an impact on biological organisms.

Epidemiology: study of population health and its determinants.

Epigeneticism: analysis of environmental or external factors on genome expression, particularly in terms of variability or plasticity of an organism's structure and function.

Epigenetics: modification of gene expression through environmental factors.

Epistemological reductionism: belief that explanation of higher-level phenomena in theoretical terms and laws used to explain lower-level phenomena.

Epistemological wholism: belief that explanation of higher-level phenomena in terms of an integrated system in which the system's integrity is not violated but maintained.

Epistemology: study of the scope and validity of knowledge, especially in terms of justified true belief.

Evidence: data or observations obtained from investigations.

Evidence-based medicine: clinical practice based on best available scientific and clinical evidence.

Evolvability: biological organism's ability to adapt to changing environmental conditions.

Explanation: statement or set of statements expounding or clarifying a phenomenon.

Exposomics: analysis of environment's impact on organism's behavior and function, especially in terms of organism's genetic and epigenetic components.

Fact: statement's veracity based on judgment of evidence.

Formal cause: that upon which an effect is structured.

Fragility: entity's sensitivity to changing environmental conditions in terms of its functional capacity, conceptually opposite to robustness.

Fragmentation: shattering an entity into its constitutive parts, which is often contrasted with wholeness.

Functionality: operable design responsible for a system's capacity for normal or standard behavior or state.

Geneticism: belief that an organism's genetic make-up dictates or determines its phenotype.

Genetics: study of genes as basic units or factors of heredity and their expression.

Genome: an organism's complete set of genes.

Genomic medicine: clinical care based on genomic information.

Genomics: study of genome and its expression.

Healing: to make whole by relieving suffering associated with illness or by finding meaning in illness.

Health: state of well-being and not simply absence of disease.

Heuristics: rules to facilitate problem solving or other cognitive activities.

Historicism: belief that historical laws govern human affairs.

Human Genome Project: international project that mapped and sequenced human and other species genomes.

Idealism: belief in mind-dependent reality, which is often contrasted with realism.

Illness: impact of disease's pathology on daily life.

Integration: analysis of how a system's parts are combined structurally and functionally.

Interactome: interactive network or system of a cell's molecular components, such as nucleic acids, proteins, or lipids.

Internet of Medical Things: connection of medical devices and services through the internet, which is based on Internet of Things.

Intuition: cognitive faculty of immediate apprehension or understanding.

Linear dynamics: rectilinear structure or temporal interaction of a mechanism's components such that a system and its properties are directly proportional to the summation of its parts and their properties.

Machine: entity composed of structured parts that define or explain it.

Material cause: that from which an effect is composed.

Materialism: belief that natural objects are composed of or reducible to matter, which is sufficient to account for natural objects.

Mechanism: linear series of causally related or adapted events, often contrasted with organicism.

Mechanistic evidence: evidence provided by the mechanism itself.

Mechanistic explanation: statement or set of statements expounding or clarifying the family resemblance with respect to a phenomenon's component parts and its operation.

Mechanistic reasoning: rational faculty that links a series of causally related or adapted parts or events into a mechanism.

Medical (therapeutic) nihilism: belief that medical or therapeutic interventions are often ineffective and generally do more harm than good clinically.

Medical pluralism: diversity of approaches to the nature and practice of medicine, whether Western medical specialties and/or complementary and alternative medicine.

Metabolomics: analysis of an organism's set of metabolites.

Metaphysics: philosophical domain investigating the essence of existence.

Methodological reductionism: belief that protocols or techniques are sufficient to investigate higher-level phenomena in terms of lower-level phenomena.

Methodological wholism: belief that protocols or techniques to investigate higher-level phenomena should maintain these phenomena's integrity within an environmental context.

Methodology: set of rules, procedures, or practices for investigating or analyzing natural phenomena.

Microbiomics: analysis of the community of microbes inhabiting an organism.

Molecular biology: study of biological processes and mechanisms at molecular or macromolecular level.

Molecular medicine: diagnosis and treatment at the molecular or macromolecular level.

Monism: belief in reality's singularity, which is often contrasted with dualism.

Nanotechnology: investigating or manipulating matter at nano (<100 nanometers) scale.

Narrative: spoken or written story of events.

Naturalism: belief that reality is result of natural causes, which is often contrasted with normativism.

Network medicine: graphical analysis of the relationships and interactions among various components of a medical system, particularly in terms of diagnosing and treating disease.

New materialism: belief that causal agency is located within matter itself.

Nonlinear dynamics: circuitous structure or temporal interaction of a mechanism's components such that a system and its properties are not directly proportional to the summation of its parts and their properties.

Normativism: belief that reality reflects social norms, which is often contrasted with naturalism.

Nutrigenomics: analysis of the interaction between an organism's nutritional requirements and its genome.

Objectivity: judgments made independent of subjective perspective, which is often contrasted to subjectivity.

Observational study: clinical observations are made under uncontrolled conditions, which is often contrasted to randomized clinical trial.

Ontological reductionism: belief that material or physical components are sufficient to make up natural phenomena.

Ontological wholism: belief that natural phenomena are not reducible material or physical parts but that the whole constitutes a metaphysical category.

Ontologies: formal analysis of knowledge or information within a particular specialty or domain.

Ontology: metaphysical study on the essence of being or existing.

Organicism: belief that an organism represents an integration of its component parts, and this integration is crucial for understanding life and its relationship to the environment, often contrasted with mechanism.

Organism: living entity composed of integrated parts.

P4 medicine: systems biology approach to clinical medicine that is predictive, preventive, personalized, and participatory.

Pathome: simulating or modelling human pathological states based on omics data.

Person-centered medicine: clinical healthcare focusing on nature of personhood.

Personalism: early twentieth century philosophical movement emphasizing importance of personhood for understanding self and reality.

Personalized medicine: diagnosis, treatment, and prognosis based on patient's genetic profile.

Personhood: state or condition of being a person.

Personome: simulating or modeling human personhood based on omics data.

Phenomenology: first-person viewpoint of intentional human consciousness.

Physicalism: belief that material and efficient causes sufficiently account for natural entities and phenomena.

Physiome: simulating or modeling human physiological states or conditions based on omics data.

Plasticity: system's or organism's capacity to respond to perturbations.

Pluralism: diversity of methods to investigate phenomena and of causes to explain them.

Precision medicine: approach to diagnosis and treatment based on the individual patient's specific molecular and clinical data.

Presupposition: assumption upon which a proposition or question is based.

Prognosis: to presage disease's course or outcome.

Proteomics: analysis of the protein interactions within a cell.

Psychiatome: simulating or modeling human psychiatric or psychological states or conditions.

Randomized clinical trial: clinical observations are made under randomized and controlled conditions, which is often contrasted with observational study.

Rationalism: reason is sufficient to justify knowledge or belief, which is often contrasted with empiricism.

Realism: reality is mind-independent, which is often contrasted with idealism.

Reductionism: investigation and explanation of complex events and processes in terms of their parts, which is often contrasted with wholism.

Resultant mechanism: belief that structure alone is responsible for the appearance of predictable entities or properties, in contrast to emergent mechanism.

Robustness: entity's insensitivity to changing environmental conditions in terms of its functional capacity, conceptually opposite of fragility.

Sickness: impact of pathology on patient's social role or life.

Standard: system's or protocol's accepted norm or average.

Stasis: system's or organism's stability with respect to its internal and external conditions or environment.

Stochasticity: belief that events are not causally straightforward or decisive, given antecedent conditions, in contrast to determinism.

Subjectivity: subjective perspective is essential for knowing, which is often contrasted with objectivity.

Suffering: patient's existential state of physical pain or mental discomfort.

Synthesis: conclusion or judgment inferred from informal or empirical reasoning, which is often contrasted with analysis.

Systems biology: biological research and practice based on systems science, bioinformatics, and big data.

Systems dynamics: modeling a system's complex structure and behavior in terms of interacting components.

Systems medicine: medical research and practice based on systems science, medical informatics, and big data.

Transcriptomics: analysis of an organism's transcription factors.

Translational medicine: clinical practice based on relevant biomedical research, i.e., "from laboratory bench to patient bedside."

Value: worth or importance of something or someone.

Vice: character trait that displays moral or epistemic blame or shame, which is often contrasted with virtue.

Virtue: character trait that displays moral or epistemic excellence, which is often contrasted with vice.

Wellbeing: physical and psychological wholeness.

Wholeness: state of being constitutionally complete or undivided, which is often contrasted with fragmentation.

Wholism: belief that property of the whole is greater than sum of the parts' individual properties.

Annotated Bibliography

The annotated bibliography lists the salient and relevant literature in both systems medicine and contemporary philosophy of medicine within the twenty-first century. Moreover, representative entries from bioethical and medico-sociological literature are also listed. Obviously, this bibliography is not exhaustive; but it does provide a starting point for investigating the various issues in systems medicine and contemporary philosophy of medicine. See Marcum (2014, 2017b) for comparable annotated bibliographies.

Accad, M. (2017). *Moving Mountains: A Socratic Challenge to the Theory and Practice of Population Medicine*. College Station, TX: Green Publishing House.
The author engages through a dialogue between the Greek philosopher, Socrates, and a founder of population medicine, Geoffrey Rose, in rather amusing criticisms of the hype surrounding the promises made by advocates of population medicine.

Aho, J., and Aho, K. (2008). *Body Matters: A Phenomenology of Sickness, Disease, and Illness*. Lanham, MD: Lexington Books.
The authors discuss phenomenological dimensions of disease and critique common assumptions about individual and social manifestations of disease to humanize medical therapies.

Al-Akiti, A., and Padela, A. I. (Eds.). (2022). *Islam and Biomedicine*. Cham, CH: Springer. https://doi.org/10.1007/978-3-030-53801-9.
These insightful essays explore the ontological, epistemological, and theological impact of modern biomedicine upon Islam, and they attempt to bridge the gap between the technological advances in biomedicine and the Islamic faith.

Ananth, M. (2012). *In Defense of an Evolutionary Concept of Health: Nature Norms and Human Biology*. Burlington, VT: Ashgate Publishing.
The author defends Boorse's naturalistic conception of health from an evolutionary perspective.

André, A. (Ed.). (2018). *Digital Medicine*. Cham, CH: Springer. https://doi.org/10.1007/978-3-319-98216-8.

The collection of essays explores the digital revolution in medicine, covering topics such as telemedicine, precision medicine, preventive medicine, regenerative medicine, artificial intelligence, biomarkers, eHealth, and omics technology.

Anjum, R. L., Copeland, S., and Rocca, E. (Eds.). (2020). *Rethinking Causality, Complexity and Evidence for the Unique Patient: A CauseHealth Resource for Healthcare Professionals and the Clinical Encounter.* Cham, CH: Springer. https://doi.org/10.1007/978-3-030-41239-5.
The volume is the product of an interdisciplinary project, CauseHealth (2015-2019), and it targets healthcare professionals exploring the philosophical issues associated with medical causality that influence clinical practice.

Atala, A., Lanza, R., Mikos, T., and Nerem, R. (Eds.). (2019). *Principles of Regenerative Medicine*, 3rd edition. London: Academic Press.
The edited volume covers the recent developments in regenerative medicine from biomolecular and cellular to the technical and ethical challenges facing its future.

Baer, H. A. (2004). *Toward an Integrative Medicine: Merging Alternative Therapies with Biomedicine*. Walnut Creek, CA: AltaMira Press.
The author chronicles the holistic health movement and its legitimization and impact on the delivery of healthcare vis-à-vis traditional biomedicine.

Bai, J. P. F., and Hur, J. (Eds.). (2022). *Systems Medicine*. New York: Humana Press. https://doi.org/10.1007/978-1-0716-2265-0.
The essays examine the recent scientific, medical, and pharmacological advances in systems medicine, as well as the development of technical tools and methodologies to further those advances.

Barro, S., and Marín, R. (Eds.). (2002). *Fuzzy Logic in Medicine*. New York: Springer, 2002. https://doi.org/10.1007/978-3-7908-1804-8.
These essays explore the application of fuzzy logic in medicine with respect to contemporary developments from its use in diagnosis of common diseases to monitoring anesthesia and analyzing medical data.

Bauer, B. A. (2017). *Mayo Clinic Guide to Integrative Medicine*. Rochester, MN: Mayo Clinic Press.
The Mayo Clinic's guidebook introduces the notion of integrative medicine for achieving and maintaining wellness through various techniques, including relaxation, meditation, guided imagery, acupuncture, herbs, massage therapy, and spirituality.

Beneduce, C., and Bertolaso, M. (Eds.). (2022). *Personalized Medicine in the Making: Philosophical Perspectives from Biology to Healthcare*. Cham, CH: Springer. https://doi.org/10.1007/978-3-030-74804-3.
The essays examine the nature of personalized medicine from a multidisciplinary perspective and explore its ethical and political challenges.

Berman, J. J. (2018). *Precision Medicine and the Reinvention of Human Disease*. London: Academic Press.
The author argues that precision medicine's goal is to identify precise diagnostic categories and to tailor highly effective treatments for them.

Bolton, D., and Gillett, G. (2019). *The Biopsychosocial Model of Health and Disease: New Philosophical and Scientific Developments*. Cham, CH: Palgrave Pivot. https://doi.org/10.1007/978-3-030-11899-0.
The authors recount the forty-year history of the biopsychosocial model, especially its various critics, and propose a revised model in terms of contemporary biomedicine, psychology, and sociology.

Boniolo, G., and Nathan, M. J. (Eds.). (2017). *Philosophy of Molecular Medicine: Foundational Issues in Research and Practice*. London: Routledge. https://doi.org/10.4324/9781315674162.
The collection of essays explores the origins, nature, and scope of molecular medicine, as well as how molecular medicine provides explanations for diseases and how to treat them.

Braude, H. D. (2012). *Intuition in Medicine: A Philosophical Defense of Clinical Reasoning*. Chicago: University of Chicago Press.
The author argues for a central role of intuition in clinical reasoning and decision-making, particularly in connecting medicine's technical and moral mandates not to harm or injure the patient.

Broadbent, A. (2019). *Philosophy of Medicine*. New York: Oxford University Press. https://doi.org/10.1093/oso/9780190612139.001.0001.
In two major parts of the book, the author sets out to answer what medicine is and the attitude both professionals and the public should have towards it.

Brody, H. (2003). *Stories of Sickness*, 2nd edition. New York: Oxford University Press.
First published in 1987, the author examines the nature of narrative medicine, as well as the types of stories patients tell, and the impact of illness and disability on a patient's daily life.

Brown, M. M., Brown, G. C., and Sharma, S. (2005). *Evidence-Based to Value-Based Medicine*. Chicago: American Medical Association Press.
The authors recount the development of value-based medicine, which takes into account the patient's values and how best to use those values to provide quality healthcare.

Brownson, R. C., Baker, E. A., Deshpande, A. D., and Gillespie, K. N. (2018). *Evidence-Based Public Health*, 3rd edition. New York: Oxford University Press.
The authors explore the use of evidence by public health practitioners, governmental policy makers, nongovernmental stakeholders, and population health researchers.

Brüne, M., and Schiefenhövel, W. (Eds.). (2019). *The Oxford Handbook of Evolutionary Medicine*. New York: Oxford University Press. https://doi.org/10.1093/oxfordhb/9780198789666.001.0001.

The collection of essays is concerned with the general principles of evolutionary medicine and with applying them to specific pathological systems along with exploring evolutionary medicine's future.

Bunge, M. (2013). *Medical Philosophy: Conceptual Issues in Medicine*. Singapore: World Scientific Publishing Co.

The author explores various concepts and topics relevant to contemporary philosophy of medicine, including disease and diagnosis, drugs and therapy, iatroethics, and the art or science of modern medicine.

Burri, R. V., and Dumit, J. (Eds.). (2007). *Biomedicine as Culture: Instrumental Practices, Technoscientific Knowledge, and New Modes of Life*. New York: Routledge.

The collection of essays explores biomedicine from a multitude of perspectives and disciplines, including cultural anthropology, history, and sociology.

Campaner, R. (2012). *Philosophy of Medicine: Causality, Evidence and Explanation*. Bologna: ArchetipoLibri.

The author discusses a variety of issues facing contemporary philosophy of medicine, including the nature of disease and the notions of causation, explanation, mechanism, and reductionism, as well as the complexities and uncertainties involved in clinical medicine.

Caplan, A. L., McCartney, J. J., and Sisti, D. A. (Eds.). (2004). *Health, Disease and Illness: Concepts in Medicine*. Washington, DC: Georgetown University Press.

The collection of essays analyzes the concepts of health, disease, and illness, from a historical perspective, as well as their clinical application.

Carel, H. (2013). *Illness: The Cry of the Flesh*, revised edition. Durham, UK: Acumen.

The author engages the philosophical issues concerning the nature of illness with respect to its individual and social dimensions, based on her own illness experience.

Carel, H., and Cooper, R. V. (Eds.). (2013). *Health, Illness and Disease: Philosophical Essays*. Durham, UK: Acumen.

The collection of essays examines the notions of health and disease with respect to organic pathology, as well as in terms of the patient's lived experience.

Cassell, E. J. (2004). *The Nature of Suffering and the Goals of Medicine*, 2nd edition. New York: Oxford University Press. https://doi.org/10.1093/acprof:oso/9780195156164.001.0001.

The author provides a convincing argument for the goal of medicine as the relief of suffering through a therapeutic patient-physician relationship.

Cassell, E. J. (2013). *The Nature of Healing: The Modern Practice of Medicine*. New York: Oxford University Press. https://doi.org/10.1093/acprof:oso/9780195369052.001.0001.

The author examines the nature of healing, particularly in terms of the sick and their illness narrative and the role of the clinician in forming a healing relationship with the patient.

Cassell, E. J. (2015). *The Nature of Clinical Medicine: The Return of the Clinician*. New York: Oxford University Press. https://doi.org/10.1093/acprof:oso/9780199974863.001.0001.

The author identifies the contemporary goals of medicine, from medical thinking to therapy, and how they relate to clinical practice.

Cerrato, P., and Halamka, J. (2018). *Realizing the Promise of Precision Medicine: The Role of Patient Data, Mobile Technology, and Consumer Engagement*. London: Academic Press.

The authors contrast population-based medicine's average or one-size-fits-all approach to precision medicine's tailored approach towards treating the individual patient.

Charon, R. (2006). *Narrative Medicine: Honoring the Stories of Illness*. New York: Oxford University Press.

The author examines the notion of narrative medicine, as well as the principles involved in its practice, and explores the dividends of narrative competence for clinical practice.

Charon, R., DasGupta, S., Hermann, N., Irvine, C., Marcus, E. R., Colsn, E. R., Spencer, D., and Spielgel, M. (2017). *The Principles and Practice of Narrative Medicine*. New York: Oxford University Press. https://doi.org/10.1093/med/9780199360192.001.0001.

The book discusses a range of principles that govern the practice of narrative medicine, such as intersubjectivity, personhood, creativity, and qualitative knowledge, and their importance in the practice of clinical medicine.

Chopra, D. (2000). *Perfect Health: The Complete Mind Body Guide*, revised edition. New York: Three Rivers Press.

The book, published originally in 1991, is a popular approach to integrating contemporary Western medicine with Indian Ayurveda medicine.

Collins, F. S. (2010). *The Language of Life: DNA and the Revolution in Personalized Medicine*. New York: Harper.

The author recounts the development of personalized medicine beginning with the completion of the Human Genome Project and illustrates its development from his own personal experience.

Cooper, R. (2005). *Classifying Madness: A Philosophical Examination of the Diagnostic and Statistical Manual of Mental Disorders*. New York: Springer. https://doi.org/10.1007/1-4020-3345-1.
The author first examines the philosophical and theoretical problems and disputes associated with the nature of mental disorders and then addresses the metaphysical question of whether they represent natural kinds.

Cooper, R. (2014). *Psychiatry and Philosophy of Science*. London: Routledge. https://doi.org/10.4324/9781315711843.
Using analytic philosophy of science, the author explores the various conceptual issues in psychiatry, especially the nature of mental illness.

Cooper, E. L., and Yamaguchi, N. (Eds.). (2004). *Complementary and Alternative Approaches to Biomedicine*. New York: Springer.
https://doi.org/10.1007/978-1-4757-4820-8.
After introducing evidence-based complementary and alternative medicine and its need globally, the essays first explore various national practices of complementary and alternative medicine and then examines complementary and alternative medicine approaches to a variety of diseases.

Corey, E. J., Czakó, B., and Kürti, L. (2007). *Molecules and Medicine*. Hoboken, NJ: John Wiley & Sons.
The authors provide an analysis of the "miracle molecules" that set off a revolution in contemporary medicine, representing over one hundred therapeutic molecules and drugs to treat a wide range of diseases.

Cullis, P. (2015). *The Personalized Medicine Revolution: How Diagnosing and Treating Disease are About to Change Forever*. Vancouver: Greystone Books.
The author examines from a semi-popular perspective the revolution in healthcare precipitated by genomics technology and then delves into personalized medicine's future—warts and all.

Cutter, M. A. G. (2003). *Reframing Disease Contextually*. New York: Springer. https://doi.org/10.1007/978-94-017-0155-6.
The author engages in a comprehensive survey of the debate surrounding the nature of disease in contemporary medicine and defends a context-dependent and value-laden notion of disease.

Dahl, E., Falke, C., and Thor Eirik Eriksen, T. E. (Eds.). (2019). *Phenomenology of the Broken Body*. New York: Routledge.
The edited volume of essays explores the body's vulnerability in terms of its weakness and subjectivity to violence and trauma, the body's suffering with respect to its brokenness, uncanniness, affectedness, pain, and fatigue, and the possible recovery of broken bodies.

Daly, J. (2005). *Evidence-Based Medicine and the Search for a Science of Clinical Care*. Berkeley: University of California Press.
The author discusses the achievements and limitations of evidence-based medicine (EBM) in clinical practice.

Danesi, M., and Zukowski, N. (2019). *Medical Semiotics. Medicine and Cultural Meaning*. Munich: Lincom Europa.
The book explores the nature of semiotics, particularly the meaning of basic medical terms, and how semiotics relates to medical practice, especially in terms of diagnosis and the patient-physician relationship.

Dawson, A. (Ed.). (2016). *The Philosophy of Public Health*. New York: Routledge.
Originally published in 2009 by Ashgate, the book has been republished and covers a wide range of philosophical, legal, and social topics in public health, from risk to HIV prevention.

Derkatch, C. (2016). *Bounding Biomedicine: Evidence and Rhetoric in the New Science of Alternative Medicine*. Chicago: University of Chicago Press.
The author explores the rhetorical devices involved in the debate over evidence for supporting complementary and alternative medicine in contrast to the dominant field of biomedicine.

Dolezal, L. (2015). *The Body and Shame: Phenomenology, Feminism, and the Socially Shaped Body*. Lanham, MD: Lexington Books.
The author engages the phenomenological issues from a feminist perspective surrounding bodily shame and the medical and social efforts to reshape the body.

Drew, K. (2021). *Complementary and Alternative Medicine: Containing and Expanding Therapeutic Possibilities*. New York: Routledge. https://doi.org/10.4324/9780429287176.
The author undertakes a sociological analysis of complementary and alternative medicine across institutions globally and their therapeutic spaces, especially as confronted by traditional Western medicine.

Engelhardt, Jr, H. T. (Ed.). (2000). *The Philosophy of Medicine: Framing the Field*. New York: Springer. https://doi.org/10.1007/0-306-47475-1.
The collected essays engage various philosophical and bioethical issues, ranging from the embodied person to the nature of death and euthanasia.

Evans, M., Louhiala, P., and Puustinen, R. (Eds.). (2004). *Philosophy for Medicine: Applications in a Clinical Context*. Oxford: Radcliffe Publishing.
The essays tackle not only the theoretical issues challenging medical science but also the practical issues facing its practice, especially the clinical encounter.

Fagot-Largeault, A. (2010). *Médecine et Philosophie*. Paris: Presses Universitaires de France.
The author, drawing on Georges Canguilhem's *Le Normal et le Pathologique* (1943), discusses various metaphysical, epistemological, and ethical issues involving modern medicine and its practice.

Foss, L. (2002). *The End of Modern Medicine: Biomedical Science under a Microscope*. New York: SUNY Press.
The author conducts a postmodern critique of the biomedical model and proposes a "psychobiological" model for disease ontology and etiology.

Fountoulakis, K. N. (2022). *Psychiatry: From Its Historical and Philosophical Roots to the Modern Face*. Cham, CH: Springer.
https://doi.org/10.1007/978-3-030-86541-2.
The author launches into the historical roots of psychiatry, beginning with the Greeks and ending with the early twenty-first century, and then unpacks the philosophical and scientific roots of the discipline, and concludes with the state of contemporary psychiatry and its future.

Frampton, S. B., and Charmel, P. A. (Eds.). (2009). *Putting Patients First: Best Practices in Patient-Centered Care*, 2nd edition. San Francisco: Wiley.
The book promotes the Planetree philosophy of patient-centered healthcare (https://planetree.org/), which stresses proactive healthcare.

Frankel, R. M., Quill, T. E., and McDaniel, S. H. (Eds.). (2003). *The Biopsychosocial Approach: Past, Present, and Future*. Rochester, NY: University Rochester Press.
The essays cover issues surrounding the implementation and practice of the biopsychosocial model, including its role in clinical research, medical administration, and medical education, as well as its historical and philosophical contexts.

Fulford, K. W. M., Peile, E., and Carroll, H. (2012). *Essential Values-Based Practice: Clinical Stories Linking Science with People*. New York: Cambridge University Press.
The book examines the role of values in clinical practice, with the goal of equipping the clinician with the necessary skill set to implement values in the clinical encounter.

Fulford, K. W. M., Davies, M., Gipps, R., Graham, G., Sadler, J., Stanghellini, G., and Thornton, T. (Eds.). (2013). *The Oxford Handbook of Philosophy and Psychiatry*. Oxford, UK: Oxford University Press. https://doi.org/10.1093/oxfordhb/9780199579563.001.0001.
The handbook is composed of over 70 chapters that explore not just the past but also the future of psychiatry over the next century, ranging in topics from the "contexts of care" for psychiatric disorders to explaining such disorders to their possible cure.

Ghaemi, S. N. (2010). *The Rise and Fall of the Biopsychosocial Model: Reconciling Art and Science in Psychiatry*. Baltimore, MD: The Johns Hopkins University Press.
The author insists that the biopsychosocial model failed to deliver the promised humanistic care and then proposes an alternative model to it.

Gideon, J. (Ed.). (2016). *Handbook on Gender and Health*. Northampton, MA: Edward Elgar Publishing. https://doi.org/10.4337/9781784710866.
The Handbook explores a variety of issues facing gender and health, including public policies, working conditions, migratory patterns, health systems, households, and social activism.

Gibbon, S., Prainsack, B., Hilgartner, S., and Lamoreaux, J. (Eds.) (2018). *Routledge Handbook of Genomics, Health and Society*, 2nd edition. New York: Routledge.
The *Handbook* focuses on four basic themes of genomics and health, specifically the globalization of genomics, the (in)stability of (post)genomics, the role of big data in genomic medicine, and the importance and value of genomic technology in optimizing health.

Gifford, F. (Ed.). (2011). *Philosophy of Medicine*. Oxford: Elsevier.
The essays cover a wide range of topics in the philosophy of medicine, from the theoretical, such as Boorse's essay on the nature of health and disease, and the practical, such as Lizza's essay on brain death, to traditional topics, such as medical experimentation and uncertainty.

Ginsburg, G. S., and Willard, H. F. (Eds.). (2010). *Essentials of Genomic and Personalized Medicine*. London: Academic Press.
The collection of essays discusses the various issues involved in implementing genomics into personalized medicine.

Glezerman, M. (2016). *Gender Medicine: The Groundbreaking New Science of Gender- and Sex-related Diagnosis and Treatment*. New York: Overlook.
The author examines the recent scientific developments associated with gender medicine, covering a range of topics from traditional reproductive physiology to gender pain, and concludes with the future of gender medicine and how best to promote and practice it.

Gluckman, P., Beedle, A., Buklijas, T., Low, F., and Hanson, M. (2016). *Principles of Evolutionary Medicine*. New York: Oxford University Press. https://doi.org/10.1093/acprof:oso/9780199663927.001.0001.
The authors identify the general principles of evolutionary biology, along with cultural evolution, and they then propose a framework for applying these principles to medicine and public health.

Goli, F. (Ed.). (2016). *Biosemiotic Medicine: Healing in the World of Meaning*. New York: Springer. https://doi.org/10.1007/978-3-319-35092-9.
This collection of essays roots the practice of medicine within contemporary biosemiotics—the successor of medical semiotics—as a meaning-generating system.

Goodman, K. W. (2003). *Ethics and Evidence-Based Medicine: Fallibility and Responsibility in Clinical Science*. New York: Cambridge University Press.
The author recounts the origins and history of EBM and provides an insightful examination of the ethical challenges facing it.

Gray, J. A. M. (2013). *How to Practice Population Medicine*. Oxford: Offox Press.
The author provides a practical exposition not only for practicing population medicine but also addresses the question of why twenty-first century clinicians should practice it.

Groopman, J. (2007). *How Doctors Think*. Boston, MA: Houghton Mifflin.
The author discusses the cognitive processes clinicians engage in to make clinical judgments, which he illustrates from his own clinical experience.

Gupta, M. (2014). *Is Evidence-Based Psychiatry Ethical?* New York: Oxford University Press. https://doi.org/10.1093/med/9780199641116.001.0001.
The author examines the relationship between EBM and the practice of psychiatry; and she concludes that evidence-based practice can benefit psychiatry ethically by cultivating moral and intellectual virtues in the discipline's practice.

Guyatt, G. H., Rennie, D., Meade, M. O., Cook, D. J. (Eds.). (2015). *Users' Guides to the Medical Literature: Essentials of Evidence-Based Clinical Practice*, 3rd edition. New York: McGraw-Hill. https://doi.org/10.1036/0071590382.
The Guide is a practical manual for EBM, with an introductory section providing the foundations of EBM and then six sections on implementing EBM clinically.

Halpern, J. (2001). *From Detached Concern to Empathy: Humanizing Medical Practice*. New York: Oxford University Press. https://doi.org/10.1093/acprof:osobl/9780195111194.001.0001.
The author contends for transition from the traditional emotionally detached concern for clinical practice to the inclusion of empathy, through emotional reasoning, in the patient-physician encounter.

Hannaway, C. (Ed.). (2008). *Biomedicine in the Twentieth Century: Practices, Policies, and Politics*. Amsterdam: IOS Press.
The collection of essays explores the history of the U.S. National Institutes of Health and its impact on the history of biomedicine in terms of its practices, politics, and policies.

Hays, P. (2022). *Advancing Healthcare Through Personalized Medicine*, 2nd edition. Cham, CH: Springer. https://doi.org/10.1007/978-3-030-80100-7.
The author examines how modern technologies issued in the era of personalized medicine and then explores the regulatory, economical, and ethical issues involved in implementing personalized medicine.

Heller, T., Lee-Treweek, F., Katz, J., Stone, J., Spurr, S., (Eds.). (2005). *Perspectives on Complementary and Alternative Medicine*. Abingdon, UK: Routledge.
The essays explore the public's changing perspective towards complementary and alternative medicine and the cultural and social issues associated with that change.

Higgs, J., Jones, M. A., Loftus, S., and Christensen, N. (Eds.). (2008). *Clinical Reasoning in the Health Professions*, 3rd edition. Boston: Elsevier.
Originally published in 1995, the third edition covers current trends in clinical reasoning and decision-making, as well as the role of communication in clinical practice.

Ho, D. (Ed.). (2017). *Philosophical Issues in Pharmaceutics: Developing, Dispensing, and Use*. New York: Springer. https://doi.org/10.1007/978-94-024-0979-6.
The essays cover important philosophical and ethical issues facing the pharmaceutical industry, including the development and dispensing of pharmaceutics and pharmaceutical usage.

Ho, D. (2019). *A Philosopher Goes to the Doctor: A Critical Look at Philosophical Assumptions in Medicine*. New York: Routledge. https://doi.org/10.4324/9781315626871.
In a rather ingenious approach, the author wrestles with the philosophical assumptions, from health to happiness, upon which modern medicine rests, especially for the lay patient.

Howick, J. H. (2011). *The Philosophy of Evidence-Based Medicine*. Hoboken, NJ: Wiley-Blackwell.
The author conducts a philosophical analysis of EBM's conceptual foundations, especially in terms of what constitutes good evidence, and then engages its critics.

Huneman, P., Lambert, G., and Silberstein, M. (Eds.). (2015). *Classification, Disease and Evidence: New Essays in the Philosophy of Medicine*. New York: Springer. https://doi.org/10.1007/978-94-017-8887-8.
The essays explore recent discussions on the nature and classification of disease, from genetic to psychiatric disorders, to provide guidance for best treatment and to maintain personal and public health.

Illari, P., and Russo, F. (2014). *Causality: Philosophical Theory Meets Scientific Practice*. Oxford: Oxford University Press.
The authors propose a "mosaic" model to unify the pluralistic theories of causation in the natural sciences, including the biomedical sciences.

Ip, K. T. (Ed.). (2009). *The Bioethics of Regenerative Medicine*. Dordrecht, NL: Springer. https://doi.org/10.1007/978-1-4020-8967-1.
The essays explore the ethical and moral issues and challenges associated with regenerative medicine from both Western and Eastern perspectives.

Jain, K. K. (2021). *Textbook of Personalized Medicine*, 3rd edition. New York: Springer. https://doi.org/10.1007/978-3-030-62080-6.

The textbook is an up-to-date resource for implementing personalized medicine into the clinic, especially in terms of various complex diseases, and concludes by discussing the challenges to its future.

James, J. E. (2016). *The Health of Populations: Beyond Medicine*. London: Academic Press.

The author argues for advancing healthcare beyond the biomedical model for achieving optimal health both physically and mentally.

Johansson, I., and Lynøe, N. (2008). *Medicine & Philosophy: A Twenty-First Century Introduction*. Frankfurt: Ontos.

The authors frame the book in terms of the philosophy of science and discuss traditional philosophical issues in contemporary philosophy of medicine from a biomedical perspective.

Karhausen, L. (2023). Analytic Philosophy of Clinical and Community Medicine, 2nd edition. Xlibris.

The author considers philosophy of medicine as a subset of philosophy of science and to that end, he engages in an "epistemological bottom-up" approach to it.

Kattan, M. W. (Ed.). (2009). *Encyclopedia of Medical Decision Making*. London: SAGE Publications. https://doi.org/10.4135/9781412971980.

The Encyclopedia explores diverse topics concerning medical decision-making from healthcare organizations to patients, especially in terms of how decisions are made under biased conditions, patient preferences, or social factors.

Keikhosrokiani, P. (Ed.). (2022). *Big Data Analytics for Healthcare: Datasets, Techniques, Life Cycles, Management, and Applications*. London: Elsevier.

These essays examine the role of big data analytics from theoretical and conceptual perspectives with respect to decision-making and healthcare intelligence for disease classification, diagnosis, treatment, prediction, and prognosis.

Kelner, M., and Wellman, B. (Eds.). (2003). *Complementary and Alternative Medicine: Challenge and Change*. London: Routledge. https://doi.org/10.4324/9781315080109.

The essays examine complementary and alternative medicine's impact on modern healthcare and its future, particularly in terms of medical pluralism and integrative health reform.

Kendler, K. S., and Parnas, J. (Eds.). (2008). *Philosophical Issues in Psychiatry: Explanation, Phenomenology, and Nosology*. Baltimore: Johns Hopkins University Press.

The chapters explore three themes: understanding and explaining the etiological factors involved in psychiatric disorders, the nosology of such disorders, and the phenomenological approaches to the practice of psychiatry.

Keyes, K. M., and Galea, S. (2016). *Population Health Science*. New York: Oxford University Press. https://doi.org/10.1093/med/9780190459376.001.0001.

The authors identify several principles for practicing population health science, including (1) population health represents a continuum and is causally multivariant and multilevel, (2) what benefits the many might not benefit the few, and (3) predicting population health more accurately than individual health.

Kincaid, H., and McKitrick, J. (Eds.). (2007). *Establishing Medical Reality: Essays in the Metaphysics and Epistemology of Biomedical Science*. New York: Springer. https://doi.org/10.1007/1-4020-5216-2.

These essays break with the myopia of bioethical issues associated with medicine and discuss the metaphysical and epistemological issues associated with the biomedical sciences.

Kleinman, A. (2020). *The Illness Narratives: Suffering, Healing and the Human Condition*. New York: Basic Books.

The book was originally published in 1988 and is now a classic on the subject. In it, the author argues for the inclusion of the patient's story into the treatment and management of chronic diseases.

Kligler, B., and Lee, R. (Eds.). (2013). *Integrative Medicine: Principles for Practice*. New York: McGraw-Hill.

The essays represent an introduction to the principles of integrative medicine—traditional biomedicine conjoined with complementary and alternative medicine—relevant for medical practice.

Kotsirilos, V., Vitetta, L., and Sali, A. (2011). *A Guide to Evidence-Based Integrative and Complementary Medicine*. Chatswood, NSW: Elsevier Australia.

The authors propose an evidence-based integrative and complementary medicine, and they then discuss precautions for practicing integrative and complementary medicine.

Kumar, D., and Antonarakis, S. (Eds.). (2016). *Medical and Health Genomics*. London: Academic Press.

The goal for the collection of essays is to explore the relevance of genomics for medicine, as well as public and population health.

Kumar, P., Kumar, Y., and Tawhid, M. A. (Eds.). (2021). *Machine Learning, Big Data, and IoT for Medical Informatics*. London: Academic Press.

The chapters explore the role of machine learning and Internet of Things for the field of medical informatics, covering topics ranging from blockchain technology to cloud computing.

Lee, K. (2012). *The Philosophical Foundations of Modern Medicine*. New York: Palgrave Macmillan. https://doi.org/10.1057/9780230353251.

The author examines a variety of themes in the philosophy of medicine, including health, disease, mechanism, and causation, especially as these themes are informed by contemporary philosophy of science.

Lieberman, D. E. (2013). *The Story of the Human Body: Evolution, Health, and Disease*. New York: Pantheon Books.

The author addresses the paradox facing modern humans—we live during one of the healthiest periods in human history, but chronic diseases are epidemic—and proposes an evolutionary approach to resolve the paradox.

Lock, M. M., and Nguyen, V. K. (2018). *An Anthropology of Biomedicine*, 2nd edition. Hoboken, NJ: Wiley-Blackwell.

First published in 2010, the book explores biomedicine as a "sociotechnical system" from an anthropological perspective, especially its drive to standardize the human body.

Loscalzo, J., Barabási, A. L., and Silverman, E. K. (Eds.). (2017). *Network Medicine: Complex Systems in Human Disease and Therapeutics*. Cambridge, MA: Harvard University Press.

In a series of essays, the "new paradigm" of network medicine is explored in terms of its basic principles and its application to particular diseases, especially cancer.

Loughlin, M. (Ed.). (2014). *Debates in Values-Based Practice: Arguments For and Against*. Cambridge, UK: Cambridge University Press.

The essays explore the advantages and disadvantages of values-based medicine from both philosophical and practical perspectives.

Lueddeke, G. R. (2016). *Global Population Health and Well-Being in the 21st Century: Toward New Paradigms, Policy, and Practice*. New York: Springer.

The author works through population health's history to the contemporary crises facing it, and he then proposes a new worldview for advancing population health.

Maier, B., and Shibles, W. A. (2011). *The Philosophy and Practice of Medicine and Bioethics: A Naturalistic-Humanistic Approach*. New York: Springer. https://doi.org/10.1007/978-90-481-8867-3.

The authors critically examine, from a naturalistic-humanistic perspective, the metaphors driving EBM.

Marcum, J. A. (2008). *An Introductory Philosophy of Medicine: Humanizing Modern Medicine*. New York: Springer. https://doi.org/10.1007/978-1-4020-6797-6.

The author constructs a metaphysical, ontological, epistemological, and ethical framework for humanizing scientific medicine.

Marcum, J. A. (2012). *The Virtuous Physician: The Role of Virtue in Medicine*. New York: Springer. https://doi.org/10.1007/978-94-007-2706-9.

The author explores the role of virtues and vices in the practice of modern medicine to resolve its quality of care and professionalism crises.

Marcum, J. A. (Ed.). (2017). *The Bloomsbury Companion to Contemporary Philosophy of Medicine*. London: Bloomsbury.
The Companion explores current research in contemporary philosophy of medicine, ranging from molecular and genomic medicine to patient-centered medicine, including the topics of health and disease, medical causation, and clinical reasoning, as well as new directions for scholarship in philosophy of medicine.

Marcum, J. A. (2020). *From Systems Biology to Systems Medicine*. New York: Nova Science Publishers.
The author reconstructs systems medicine's emergence from systems biology, during the latter half of the twenty century and the beginning of the twenty-first century, and its establishment as an independent discipline.

Marini, M. G. (2016). *Narrative Medicine: Bridging the Gap between Evidence-Based Care and Medical Humanities*. Cham, CH: Springer. https://doi.org/10.1007/978-3-319-22090-1.
The author uses a narrative approach to bridge the gap between EBM and humane practice to provide quality healthcare.

Meacham, D. (Ed.). (2015). *Medicine and Society, New Perspectives in Continental Philosophy*. New York: Springer. https://doi.org/10.1007/978-94-017-9870-9.
The essays explore a wide range of topics within medicine, including illness and eugenics, from a continental philosophical framework.

Mehl-Madrona, L. (2007). *Narrative Medicine: The Use of History and Story in the Healing Process*. Rochester, VT: Bear & Company.
The author acknowledges that patients are composed of physical material but at the same time they are comprised by their stories, which often reflect their culture.

Meza, J. P., and Passerman, D. S. (2011). *Integrating Narrative Medicine and Evidence-Based Medicine: The Everyday Social Practice of Healing*. London: Radcliffe.
The authors explore the social and philosophical issues associated with integrating evidence-based and narrative medicine, beginning with practical problems and culminating in theoretical challenges.

Micozzi, M. S. (2019). *Fundamentals of Complementary and Alternative Medicine*, 6th edition. St. Louis, MO: Elsevier Health Sciences.
The book is a comprehensive introduction to complementary and alternative medicine and covers topics ranging from quantum biology to mind-body physiology.

Minor, L., and Rees, M. (2020). *Discovering Precision Health: Predict, Prevent, and Cure to Advance Health and Well-Being*. Hoboken, NJ: John Wiley & Sons.
The authors identify a half-dozen key principles of precision medicine, including predictive and preventive, personalized and precise, person-centered, participatory, preeminent, and "high tech" and "high touch."

Miettinen, O. S. (2014). *Toward Scientific Medicine*. New York: Springer. https://doi.org/10.1007/978-3-319-01671-9.
The author insists that contemporary medicine is really pre-scientific and proposes a framework for transforming it into a scientific discipline.

Mol, A. (2002). *The Body Multiple: Ontology in Medical Practice*. Durham, NC: Duke University Press.
Drawing on the medical example of atherosclerosis, the author explores philosophical issues associated with the disease-objectivity and illness-subjectivity distinction.

Mol, A. (2008). *The Logic of Care: Health and the Problem of Patient Choice*. London: Routledge.
The author argues that healthcare should be based on a "logic of care" from those engaged in clinical encounters and not on patient as customer.

Montgomery, K. (2006). *How Doctors Think: Clinical Judgment and the Practice of Medicine*. New York: Oxford University Press.
The author contends that clinical judgment should involve Aristotelian phronesis and not the hypothetical-deductive method of positive science.

Morgan, A. (2022). *Continental Philosophy of Psychiatry: The Lure of Madness*. Cham, CH: Palgrave Macmillan. https://doi.org/10.1007/978-3-031-09334-0.
The author examines twentieth-century phenomenology's impact on psychiatry, especially in terms of understanding madness.

Moseley, D. D., and Gala, G. (Eds.). (2016). *Philosophy and Psychiatry: Problems, Intersections and New Perspectives*. New York: Routledge.
The essays focus on philosophical issues involved in psychiatric diagnosis and treatment, as well as the ethical issues that surface during psychiatric practice.

Mozes, B. (2010). *The Truth of Scientific Medicine*. Jerusalem: Hebrew University Magnes Press.
The author claims that contemporary scientific medicine is facing a credibility crisis and identifies six core concepts involved in medical truth to that end, including methods, borders, criteria, inferences, interpretations, and paradigms.

Nash, D. B., Fabius, R. J., Skoufalos, A., Clarke, J. L., and Horowitz, M. R. (2016). *Population Health: Creating a Culture of Wellness*, 2nd edition. Burlington, MA: Jones & Bartlett.
The book is a collection of essays that explore the nature of population health and the business and policy changes required to actualize optimum population health.

National Research Council. (2011). *Toward Precision Medicine: Building a Knowledge Network for Biomedical Research and a New Taxonomy of Disease*. Washington, DC: National Academies Press. https://doi.org/10.17226/13284.
The report canvases the biomedical research community's efforts to define disease at the molecular level and the implications for providing "a new taxonomy of human

disease" tailored to target the disease's molecular pathology and thereby improve healthcare outcomes.

Nelson, J. (2015). *More Than Medicine: A History of the Feminist Women's Health Movement*. New York: New York University Press.
The author recounts the historical changes, during the second half of the twentieth century, associated with the women's health movement and activists, specifically in the United States.

Pellegrino, E. D. (2008). *The Philosophy of Medicine Reborn: A Pellegrino Reader*. H. T. Engelhardt, Jr., and F. Jotterand (Eds.). Notre Dame, IN: University of Notre Dame Press.
The reader is a collection of Pellegrino's seminal essays, edited by two of his disciples, on contemporary philosophy of medicine, ranging from medical humanism to the role of virtues in medical practice.

Pereau, K. (2018). *The Digital Health Revolution*. Walnut Creek, CA: TranscendIT Health.
The author provides a layperson's account of the revolution in digital health, especially from his personal perspective and experience, and the shift in focus from healthcare providers at the center of the clinical encounter to healthcare consumers through digital technology in order to promote personal and public health.

Peteet, J. R. (Ed.). (2022). *The Virtues in Psychiatric Practice*. New York: Oxford University Press. https://doi.org/10.1093/med/9780197524480.001.0001.
The edited collection of essays explores the role of and the need for virtues in psychiatric practice to achieve human flourishing.

Pisanelli, D. M. (Ed.). (2004). *Ontologies in Medicine*. Amsterdam: IOS Press.
The essays cover the technology associated with managing medical knowledge, ranging from clinical guidelines to disease conditions.

Pollard, T. M. (2008). *Western Diseases: An Evolutionary Perspective*. New York: Cambridge University Press.
The author examines Western chronic diseases, like obesity, diabetes, and hypertension, in terms of evolutionary medicine.

Prainsack, B. (2017). *Personalized Medicine: Empowered Patients in the 21st Century?* New York: New York University Press. https://doi.org/10.18574/nyu/9781479814879.001.0001.
The author tackles the question of whether or how personalized medicine empowers the individual patient, especially in terms of the deluge of personal data and technological options.

Pržulj, N. (Ed.). (2019). *Analyzing Network Data in Biology and Medicine: An Interdisciplinary Textbook for Biological, Medical and Computational Scientists*. New York: Cambridge University Press.
The textbook introduces network theory, along with machine learning and cluster analysis, to analyze large sets of genetic, epigenetic, and protein-protein interaction data for clinical application.

Rabins, P. V. (2013). *The Why of Things: Causality in Science, Medicine, and Life*. New York: Columbia University Press.
The author confronts the questions concerning causality in the natural, biomedical, and social sciences, and then proposes a "three-facet" model of causality to answer them.

Radden, J., and Sadler, J. (2010). *The Virtuous Psychiatrist: Character Ethics in Psychiatric Practice*. New York: Oxford University Press. https://doi.org/10.1093/acprof:oso/9780195389371.001.0001.
The authors examine the notion of the virtuous psychiatrist in terms of the virtues required for virtuous practice, and they provide vivid case studies to illustrate such practice.

Rakel, D., and Minichiello, V. J. (2023). *Integrative Medicine*, 5th edition. Philadelphia: Elsevier.
Originally published in 2003, the book is a popular overview of integrative medicine, including chapters written by invited experts within their respective disciplines.

Ralston, D. C., and Ho, J. H. (Eds.). (2010). *Philosophical Reflections on Disability*. New York: Springer. https://doi.org/10.1007/978-90-481-2477-0.
The essays canvas specific issues surrounding disability, including quality of life, social justice, and public policy, with a final essay narrating the life of a "polio person."

Robertson, C., and Clegg, G. (Eds.). (2016). *Storytelling in Medicine: How Narrative can Improve Practice*. Boca Raton, FL: CRC Press. https://doi.org/10/1201.9781315381152.
The essays explore the power of narrated stories not only of patients but also of doctors, medical students, and even hospitals.

Robertson, D., and Williams, G. H. (Eds.). (2009). *Clinical and Translational Science: Principles of Human Research*. London: Academic Press.
The collection of essays covers the general principles guiding translational research and clinical trials, the methodology of translational research and its infrastructure, pedagogy and funding, human genetics and pharmacology, societal context of human research, and population-based research.

Robinson, D (2017). *Translationality: Essays in the Translational-Medical Humanities*. New York: Taylor & Francis.
The author proposes a notion of translationality to develop translational medical humanities through intersecting translational medicine with medical literature, hermeneutics, neuroscience, and phenomenology.

Rosen, D. H., and Hoang, U. B. (2017). *Patient-Centered Medicine: A Human Experience*. New York: Oxford University Press. https://doi.org/10.1093/med/9780190628871.001.0001.
The authors draw upon the biopsychosocial model of medicine and the patient's illness experience to forge a patient-centered medicine.

Runge, M. S., and Patterson, C. (Eds.). (2006). *Principles of Molecular Medicine*, 2nd edition. Totowa, NJ: Humana Press. https://doi.org/10.1007/978-1-59259-963-9.
Originally published in 1998, the new edition incorporates recent advances in understanding the molecular mechanisms of disease for designing molecular therapeutics.

Sadegh-Zadeh, K. (2015). *Handbook of Analytic Philosophy of Medicine*, 2nd edition. New York: Springer. https://doi.org/10.1007/978-94-017-9579-1.
To improve the clinical encounter, the author examines in the second edition—first published in 2012—the philosophical issues in the metaphysical, methodological, epistemological, logical, and ethical foundations of modern medicine.

Schmidt, H. H. H. W. (2022). *The End of Medicine as We Know It—And Why Your Health Has a Future*. Cham, CN: Springer. https://doi.org/10.1007/978-3-030-95293-8.
The author begins with the crisis facing modern medicine in terms of (not) understanding the causes of diseases and then offers hope to resolve the crisis through big data, digital medicine.

Schramme, T., and Edwards, S. (Eds.). (2017). *Handbook of the Philosophy of Medicine*. New York: Springer. https://doi.org/10.1007/978-94-017-8706-2.
The Handbook explores medicine not only philosophically in terms of its scientific dimension but also with respect to its ethical, political, and social dimensions.

Seifert, J. (2004). *The Philosophical Diseases of Medicine and Their Cure. Philosophy and Ethics of Medicine, Vol. 1: Foundations*. New York: Springer. https://doi.org/10.1007/978-1-4020-2871-7.
The author engages the philosophical "diseases" plaguing modern medicine, especially with its emphasis on the technological, and he then explores a "cure" of restoring the proper ends of medicine vis-à-vis the good of the patient.

Seising, R., and Tabacchi, M. E. (Eds.). (2013). *Fuzziness and Medicine: Philosophical Reflections and Application Systems in Health Care*. New York: Springer. https://doi.org/10.1007/978-3-642-36527-0.

The essays are a companion to the first edition of Sadegh-Zadeh's *Handbook of Analytic Philosophy of Medicine* and explore the intersection between logical fuzziness and medicine.

Shortliffe, E. H., and Cimino, J. J. (Eds.). (2014). *Biomedical Informatics: Computer Applications in Health Care and Biomedicine*, 4th edition. London: Springer. https://doi.org/10.1007/978-1-4471-4474-8.
The collection of essays deals with the theoretical and technological background of bioinformatics and covers topics including probabilistic reasoning, cognitive science, computer architecture, and software engineering, along with applying bioinformatics to the healthcare system and the clinic.

Slatman, J. (2014). *Our Strange Body: Philosophical Reflections on Identity and Medical Interventions*. Amsterdam: Amsterdam University Press.
The body entails a "strangeness," according to the author, which allows it to be reshaped through the interventions of medical technology without losing personal identity.

Smart, B. (2016). *Concepts and Causes in the Philosophy of Disease*. New York: Palgrave Macmillan. https://doi.org/10.1057/9781137552921.
The author explores the philosophical debate over the nature of disease as a pathological condition and its implications for practicing clinical medicine.

Smith, M. (2022). *Progress in Genomic Medicine: From Research to Clinical Application*. London: Academic Press.
The author provides a comprehensive analysis of genomic medicine, especially in terms of its clinical application.

Snyder, M. (2016). *Genomics and Personalized Medicine: What Everyone Needs to Know*. New York: Oxford University Press.
The book is a popular but authoritative look into genomic medicine in terms of treating patients at a personalized level.

Solomon, M. (2015). *Making Medical Knowledge*. New York: Oxford University Press. https://doi.org/10.1093/acprof:oso/9780198732617.001.0001.
The author explores the relationship between the art and science of medicine and the various approaches to medical knowledge production. Moreover, she proposes a pluralistic account to address the epistemological issues associated with the production of medical knowledge.

Solomon, M., Simon, J. R., and Kincaid, H. (Eds.). (2017). *The Routledge Companion to Philosophy of Medicine*. New York: Routledge.
The Companion engages various philosophical concepts in contemporary medicine, such as health, disease, and dying, as well as different philosophical perspectives towards medicine, such as biomedical, evolutionary, and phenomenological.

Stearns, S. C., and Koella, J. C. (Eds.). (2008). *Evolution in Health and Disease*, 2nd edition. Oxford, UK: Oxford University Press. https://doi.org/10.1093/acprof:oso/9780199207466.001.0001.

The second edition of the book—first published in 1999—examines a variety of medical topics, ranging from infectious to noninfectious diseases, from an evolutionary perspective.

Stegenga, J. (2018). *Care and Cure: An Introduction to Philosophy of Medicine*. Chicago: University of Chicago Press.

The author initially examines the concepts of health, disease, and death, before turning to notions of causation, holism and reductionism, and evidence and inference, and then concluding with issues in psychiatry and public health.

Stegenga, J. (2018). *Medical Nihilism*. New York: Oxford University Press. https://doi.org/10.1093/oso/9780198747048.001.0001.

In response to medical nihilism, the author proposes *la médicine douce*, or gentle medicine, in contrast to an aggressive medicine that is often common within the healthcare industry.

Steinhoff, G. (Ed.). (2016). *Regenerative Medicine—From Protocol to Patient*. 5 volumes, 3rd edition. Cham, CH: Springer.

The five edited volumes explore the most recent advances in regenerative medicine, ranging from basic biology to therapies.

Stewart, M., Brown, J. B., Weston, W. W., McWhinney, I. R., McWilliam, C. L., and Freeman, T. (Eds.). (2014). *Patient-Centered Medicine: Transforming the Clinical Method*, 3rd edition. Boca Raton, FL: CRC Press.

First published in 1995, the edited volume is the standard textbook for introducing the fundamental principles of patient-centered medicine and clinical research.

Stocum, D. L. (2018). *Foundations of Regenerative Biology and Medicine*. Bristol, UK: IOP Publishing.

The book recounts the history of regenerative biology and medicine and discusses its general concepts, and then covers topics such as fibrosis and wound repair, adult stem cell and non-stem cell regeneration, and vertebrate appendage regeneration, along with clinical research and application.

Stempsey, W. E. (2000). *Disease and Diagnosis: Value-Dependent Realism*. Dordrecht, NL: Kluwer. https://doi.org/10.1007/0-306-46874-3.

After exploring the fact-value distinction, the author proposes a "value-dependent" realism to account for the role of values in clinical diagnoses.

Sullivan, M. D. (2017). *The Patient as Agent of Health and Health Care: Autonomy in Patient-Centered Care for Chronic Conditions*. New York: Oxford University Press. https://doi.org/10.1093/med/9780195386585.001.0001.

According to the author, traditional medicine has failed to provide the necessary care for patients suffering from chronic diseases, and he argues for patient-centered medicine as the means for providing quality care.

Svenaeus, F. (2022). *The Hermeneutics of Medicine and the Phenomenology of Health: Steps towards a Philosophy of Medical Practice*, 2nd edition. Cham, CH: Springer. https://doi.org/10.1007/978-3-031-07281-9.
The author applies phenomenological hermeneutics of Heidegger, Gadamer, and Ricoeur, to explore the nature of health and illness and the practice of clinical medicine.

Taboada, P., Cuddeback, K. F., and Donohue-White, P. (Eds.). (2002). *Person, Society and Value: Towards a Personalist Concept of Health*. Dordrecht, NL: Kluwer. https://doi.org/10.1007/978-94-017-2570-5.
The thesis of the edited essays is that health can be framed from a phenomenological personalist perspective and then operationalized clinically.

Taylor, P. (2006). *From Patient Data to Medical Knowledge: The Principles and Practice of Health Informatics*. Oxford: Blackwell.
The author explores the notion of health informatics and the challenges facing its implementation clinically, especially in terms of producing medical knowledge.

Tekin, Ş., and Bluhm, R. (Eds.). (2019). *The Bloomsbury Companion to Philosophy of Psychiatry*. London: Bloomsbury.
The Companion is a collection of original essays that examine key issues in psychiatry from a philosophical perspective, including the intersection of psychiatry with the philosophy of mind and science, phenomenology, ethics, social and political philosophy, metaphysics and epistemology, and finally philosophy of medicine.

Thompson, R. P., and Ross E. G., and Upshur, R. E. G. (2018). *Philosophy of Medicine: An Introduction*. New York: Routledge.
The authors discuss various topics in contemporary medicine, such as health and disease, theories and models, materialism and reductionism, causality and induction, randomized controlled trials and meta-studies, phenomenology, and clinical reasoning, along with EBM, evolutionary medicine, precision and personalized medicine, and alternative medicine.

Thornton, T. (2007). *Essential Philosophy of Psychiatry*. New York: Oxford University Press. https://doi.org/10.1093/med/9780199228713.001.1.
The author examines three dimensions of psychiatric clinical judgment, including the impact of values on clinical judgment in psychiatry, how meanings are constructed from a first-person perspective, and what constitutes good evidence for psychiatric practice.

Tomasi, D. L. (2016). *Medical Philosophy: A Philosophical Analysis of Self-Perception in Diagnostics and Therapy*. Stuttgart, Germany: Ibidem-Verlag.
The author initially explores the history of medical philosophy before examining the role of philosophy in medical practice, especially in terms of reasoning in clinical diagnosis and judgment.

Toombs, S. K. (Ed.). (2001). *Handbook of Phenomenology and Medicine*. New York: Springer. https://doi.org/10.1007/978-94-010-0536-4.
The aim of the collection of essays is to explore topics in modern medicine, such as the body in illness and the patient's lived experience, from a phenomenological perspective.

Topol, E. (2013). *The Creative Destruction of Medicine: How the Digital Revolution Will Create Better Human Health Care*. New York: Basic Books.
The author examines the radical transformation from traditional biomedicine to digital medicine, especially in terms of *Homo digitus*, and the benefits digital medicine with respect to quality healthcare.

Trent, R. (2012). *Molecular Medicine: Genomics to Personalized Healthcare*, 4th edition. London: Academic Press.
The new edition emphasizes the impact molecular medicine on realizing the goals of personalized medicine and includes updates and new additions to the field of molecular medicine.

Trevathan, W., Smith, E. O., and McKenna, J. J (Eds.). (2008). *Evolutionary Medicine and Health: New Perspectives*. New York: Oxford University Press.
The essays explore various research topics in evolutionary medicine from an anthropological perspective, such as nutrition and diet, sex and reproduction, and the evolutionary role of environment and ecology in health and disease.

Tsou, J. Y. (2021). *Philosophy of Psychiatry*. New York: Cambridge University Press. https://doi.org/10.1017/9781108588485.
The author explores various philosophical issues confronting psychiatry from a naturalistic and realist perspective, and he defends the position that mental illnesses represent naturalistic biological kinds with associative injurious consequences.

Tutton, R. (2014). *Genomics and the Reimagining of Personalized Medicine*. Farnham, UK: Ashgate. https://doi.org/10.4324/9781315584317.
The author explores the role of genomics in birthing personalized medicine and discusses its limits and future.

Valles, S. A. (2018). *Philosophy of Population Health: Philosophy for a New Public Health Era*. London: Routledge. https://doi.org/10.4324/9781315163307.
The author formulates a "blueprint" for a philosophy of/for population health, concerning the meaning of health for population health science, the pertinent causes and effects of population health, and population health inequities.

Venkatapuram, S., and Broadbent, A. (Eds.). (2023). *The Routledge Handbook of Philosophy of Public Health.* London: Routledge. https://doi.org/10.4324/9781315675411.

These essays canvas a broad set of philosophical topics, ranging from fundamental concepts of public health to its ethical and social implications.

Verma, M., and Barh, D. (Eds.). (2016). *Progress and Challenges in Precision Medicine.* Amsterdam: Elsevier.

These essays explore precision medicine's potential with respect to the application of genomic technologies to population health and primary medicine, as well as its future development.

Watts, J. H. (2016). *Gender, Health and Healthcare: Women's and Men's Experience of Health and Working in Healthcare Roles*. London: Routledge.

The author explores the role of gender in receiving healthcare and uses a social constructionist perspective to analyze the impact of social norms about gender on the nature of health and on the provision of healthcare.

Wehling, M. (Ed.). (2021). *Principles of Translational Science in Medicine: From Bench to Bedside*, 3rd edition. London: Academic Press.

The edited volume introduces the field of translational medicine and then examines topics such as omics technology, tissue banks and animal models, biomarkers, clinical trial designs, toxicology, biostatistics and modelling, and legal issues.

Weil, A. (2004). *Health and Healing: The Philosophy of Integrative Medicine and Optimum Health*, revised edition. New York: Houghton Mifflin.

First published in 1983, the author lays out a popular approach to integrating complementary and alternative medicine into traditional Western medicine.

West, B. J. (2006). *Where Medicine Went Wrong: Rediscovering the Path to Complexity.* Hackensack, NJ: World Scientific Publishing Co. https://doi.org/10.1142/6175

According to the author, contemporary scientific medicine made a wrong turn in pursuing the average of various physiological functions to define health and argues for its reorientation in terms of complexity science and fractal physiology.

West, D. M., and Miller, E. A. (2009). *Digital Medicine: Health Care in the Internet Era.* Washington, DC: Brookings Institution Press.

The authors investigate information technology's impact on healthcare in terms of its individual, professional, social, and political dimensions.

Wisneski, L. (2017). *The Scientific Basis of Integrative Health*, 3rd edition. Boca Raton, FL: CRC Press.

This edition represents an updated version of the classic textbook on the scientific basis of the integrative approach to health, including chapters by several guest authors discussing topics germane to an integrative approach to health.

Wolkenhauer, O. (Ed). (2020). *Systems Medicine: Integrative, Qualitative and Computational Approaches*, 3 volumes. Cambridge, MA: Academic Press.
The 3-volume set covers recent advances within contemporary systems medicine, including tools and techniques for generating and analyzing big omics datasets; the application of systems medicine to oncology and immunology, and neurodegenerative, metabolic, and cardiovascular diseases; and the recent advances in computational systems medicine such as network modelling, medical informatics, telemedicine and e-health.

World Health Organization. (2006). *Constitution of the World Health Organization*. Geneva, CH: World Health Organization. https://apps.who.int/gb/bd/PDF/bd47/EN/constitution-en.pdf.
The Constitution defines health as "a state of complete physical, mental and social well-being and not merely the absence of disease or infirmity."

Zaner, R. M. (2004). *Conversations on the Edge: Narratives of Ethics and Illness*. Washington DC: Georgetown University Press.
The author examines a variety of narratives, particularly from his own experience as a healthcare professional, concerning death and dying and the philosophical lessons learned from them.

Zeiler, K., and Käll, L. (Eds.). (2014). *Feminist Phenomenology and Medicine*. New York: SUNY Press.
The essays explore the various conceptual and methodological perspectives involved in the intersection between medical practices and feminist phenomenology.

References

Abarbanel, H. D. I. (1996). *Analysis of Observed Chaotic Data*. New York: Springer.

Ackermann, R. J. (1976). *The Philosophy of Karl Popper*. Amherst, MA: University of Massachusetts Press.

Adams, S. A., and Petersen, C. (2016). Precision medicine: Opportunities, possibilities, and challenges for patients and providers. *Journal of the American Medical Informatics Association* 23(4): 787-790. https://doi.org/10.1093/jamia/ocv215.

Aderem, A. (2005). Systems biology: Its practices and challenges. *Cell* 121: 511-513. https//doi.org/10.1016/j.cell.2005.04.020.

Adli, M. (2018). The CRISPR tool kit for genome editing and beyond. *Nature Communications* 9(1): 1911. https://doi.org/10.1038/s41467-018-04252-2.

Agarwal, S., Zhou, X., Ye, F., He, Q., Chen, G. C., Soo, J., Boey, F., Zhang, H., and Chen, P. (2010). Interfacing live cells with nanocarbon substrates. *Langmuir*, *26*(4), 2244-2247. https://doi.org/10.1021/la9048743.

Agazzi, E., and Montecucco, L. (Eds.). (2002). *Complexity and Emergence*. Singapore: World Scientific Publishing.

Aggarwal, K., and Lee K. H. (2003). Functional genomics and proteomics as a foundation for systems biology. *Briefings in Functional Genomics and Proteomics* 2: 175-184. https://doi.org/10.1093/bfgp/2.3.175.

Aguirre, L. A., and Letellier, C. (2009). Modeling nonlinear dynamics and chaos: A review. *Mathematical Problems in Engineering* 2009: 238960. https://doi.org/10.1155/2009/238960.

Agutter, P. S., and Wheatley, D. N. (2007). *About Life: Concepts in Modern Biology*. New York: Springer.

Ahn, A. C., Tewari, M., Poon, C. S., and Phillips, R. S. (2006). The limits of reductionism in medicine: Could systems biology offer an alternative? *PLoS Medicine* 3(7): e209. https://doi.org/10.1371/journal.pmed.0030209.

Ahrens, C. H., Wagner, U., Rehrauer, H. K., Türker, C., and Schlapbach, R. (2007). Current challenges and approaches for the synergistic use of systems biology data in the scientific community. In Plant Systems Biology, (pp. 277-307), S. Baginsky and A. R. Fernie (Eds.). Basel: Birkhäuser. https://doi.org/10.1007/978-3-7643-7439-6_12.

Akram, P., and Liao, L. (2019). Prediction of comorbid diseases using weighted geometric embedding of human interactome. *BMC Medical Genomics* 12(7): 161. https://doi.org/10.1186/s12920-019-0605-5.

Alexander, S. (1920). *Space, Time, and Deity*. London: Macmillan.

Alexander, C. Y. (2006). Methods in biomedical ontology. *Journal of Biomedical Informatics* 39(3): 252-266. https://doi.org/10.1016/j.jbi.2005.11.006.

All of Us Research Program Investigators. (2019). The "All of Us" research program. *New England Journal of Medicine* 381(7): 668-676. https://doi.org/10.1056/NEJMsr1809937.

Allen, G. E. (1984). The roots of biological determinism. *Journal of the History of Biology* 17(1): 141-145. https://doi.org/10.1007/BF00397505.

Allen, G. E. (2018). Mechanism, organicism, and vitalism. In *The Routledge Handbook of Mechanisms and Mechanical Philosophy* (pp. 59-73), S. Glennan and P. Illari (Eds.). New York: Routledge. https://doi.org/10.4324/9781315731544.

Allis, C. D., and Jenuwein, T. (2016). The molecular hallmarks of epigenetic control. *Nature Reviews Genetics* 17(8): 487-500. https://doi.org/10.1038/nrg.2016.59.

Almeida, J., Dress, A., Kühne, T., and Parida, L. (2013). ICT strategies for bridging biology and precision medicine. *Dagstuhl Reports* 3(8): 87-135.

Alon, U. (2019). *An Introduction to Systems Biology: Design Principles of Biological Circuits*, 2nd edition. New York: Chapman and Hall. https://doi.org/10.1201/9780429283321.

Alon, U. (2023). *Systems Medicine: Physiological Circuits and the Dynamics of Disease*. New York: Chapman and Hall.

Alper, J. S. (1977). Biological determinism. *Telos* 1977(31): 164-172. https://doi.org/10.3817/0377031164.

Alper, J. S., and Beckwith, J. (1993). Genetic fatalism and social policy: The implications of behavior genetics research. *Yale Journal of Biology and Medicine* 66(6): 511-524.

Álvarez, Z., Kolberg-Edelbrock, A. N., Sasselli, I. R., Ortega, J. A., Qiu, R., Syrgiannis, Z., Mirau, P. A., Chen, F., Chin, S. M., Weigand, S., and Kiskinis, E. (2021). Bioactive scaffolds with enhanced supramolecular motion promote recovery from spinal cord injury. *Science* 374(6569): 848-856. https://doi.org/10.1126/science.abh3602.

Alyass, A., Turcotte, M., and Meyre, D. (2015). From big data analysis to personalized medicine for all: Challenges and opportunities. *BMC Medical Genomics* 8(1): 33. https://doi.org/10.1186/s12920-015-0108-y.

An, G., Hunt, C. A., Clermont, G., Neugebauer, E., and Vodovotz, Y. (2007). Challenges and rewards on the road to translational systems biology in acute illness: Four case reports from interdisciplinary teams. *Journal of Critical Care* 22: 169-175. https://doi.org/10.1016/j.jcrc.2006.12.011.

Andersen, H. (2001). The history of reductionism versus holism approaches to scientific research. *Endeavor* 25: 153-156. https://doi.org/10.1016/S0160-9327(00)01387-9.

Andersen, H. K. (2017). Reductionism in the biomedical sciences. In *The Routledge Companion to Philosophy of Medicine* (pp. 81-88), M. Solomon, J. R. Simon, and H. Kincaid (Eds.). New York: Routledge. https://doi.org/10.4324/9781315720739.

Anderson, P. W. (1972). More is different. *Science* 177(4047): 393-396. https://doi.org/10.1126/science.177.4047.393.

Andrews, S. S., Dinh, T., and Arkin, A. P. (2009). Stochastic models of biological processes. In *Encyclopedia of Complexity and Systems Science* (pp. 8730-8749), R.A. Meyers (Ed.). New York: Springer.

Anjum, R. L., Copeland, S., and Rocca, E. (2020). Medical scientists and philosophers worldwide appeal to EBM to expand the notion of 'evidence.' *BMJ Evidence-Based Medicine* 25(1): 6-8. https://dx.doi.org/10.1136/bmjebm-2018-111092.

Annas, G. J. (2014). Personalized medicine or public health? Bioethics, human rights, and choice. *Revista Portuguesa de Saúde Pública* 32: 158-163. https://doi.org/10.1016/j.rpsp.2014.04.003.

Anscombe, E. (2001). Causality and determination. In *Agency and Responsibility* (pp. 57-73), L.W. Ekstrom (Ed.). New York: Routledge.

Anstey, P. R., (2000). *The Philosophy of Robert Boyle*. New York: Routledge.

Anthony, J. C. (2001). The promise of psychiatric enviromics. *British Journal of Psychiatry* 178(S40), s8-s11. https://doi.org/10.1192/bjp.178.40.s8.

Antony, P. M. A., Balling, R., and Vlassis, N. (2012). From systems biology to systems biomedicine. *Current Opinion in Biotechnology* 23(4): 604-608. https://doi.org/10.1016/j.copbio.2011.11.009.

Apweiler, R., Beissbarth, T., Berthold, M. R., Blüthgen, N., Burmeister, Y., Dammann, O., Deutsch, A., Feuerhake, F., Franke, A., Hasenauer, J., and Hoffmann, S. (2018). Whither systems medicine? *Experimental & Molecular Medicine* 50(3): e453-e453. https://doi.org/10.1038/emm.2017.290.

Arikha, N. (2007). *Passions and Tempers: A History of the Humours*. New York: HarperCollins Publishers.

Aristotle. (1979). *Aristotle's Metaphysics*, H.G. Apostle, trans. Des Moines, IA: Peripatetic Press.

Aristotle. (1993). *De Anima: Books II and III*, D.W. Hamlyn, trans. New York: Oxford University Press.

Aronson, J. K., Auker-Howlett, D., Ghiara, V., Kelly, M. P., and Williamson, J. (2021). The use of mechanistic reasoning in assessing coronavirus interventions. *Journal of Evaluation in Clinical Practice* 27(3): 684-693. https://doi.org/10.1111/jep.13438.

Arribas-Ayllon, M. (2016). After geneticization. *Social Science & Medicine* 159: 132-139. https://doi.org/10.1016/j.socscimed.2016.05.011.

Aschebrook-Kilfoy, B., Zakin, P., Craver, A., Shah, S., Kibriya, M. G., Stepniak, E., Ramirez, A., Clark, C., Cohn, E., Ohno-Machado, L., and Cicek, M. (2022). An overview of cancer in the first 315,000 *All of Us* participants. *PloS One* 17(9): e0272522. https://doi.org/10.1371/journal.pone.0272522.

Ashley, E. A. (2015). The precision medicine initiative: A new national effort. *Journal of the American Medical Association* 313(21): 2119-2120. https://doi.org/10.1001/jama.2015.3595.

Ashley, E. A. (2016). Towards precision medicine. *Nature Reviews Genetics* 17(9): 507-522. https://doi.org/10.1038/nrg.2016.86.

Assmus, H. H., Herwig, R., Cho, K. H., and Wolkenhauer, O., (2006). Dynamics of biological systems: Role of systems biology in medical research. *Expert Review of Molecular Diagnostics* 6: 891-902. https://doi.org/10.1586/14737159.6.6.891.

Åström, K. J., and Murray, R. M. (2021). *Feedback Systems: An Introduction for Scientists and Engineers*, 2nd edition. Princeton. NJ: Princeton University Press.

Au, L. (2021). Recent scientific/intellectual movements in biomedicine. *Social Science & Medicine* 278: 113950. https://doi.org/10.1016/j.socscimed.2021.113950.

Auffray, C., Chen, Z., and Hood, L. (2009). Systems medicine: the future of medical genomics and healthcare. *Genome Medicine* 1(1): 2. https://doi.org/10.1186/gm2.

Auletta, G., Ellis, G. F., and Jaeger, L. (2008). Top-down causation by information control: From a philosophical problem to a scientific research programme. *Journal of the Royal Society Interface* 5(27): 1159-1172. https://doi.org/10.1098/rsif.2008.0018.

Aurich, M. K., and Thiele, I. (2016). Computational modeling of human metabolism and its application to systems biomedicine. In *Systems Medicine* (pp. 253-281), U. Schmitz and O. Wolkenhauer (Eds.). New York: Humana Press. https://doi.org/10.1007/978-1-4939-3283-2_12.

Auyang, S. Y. (1999). *Foundations of Complex-System Theories: Economics, Evolutionary Biology, and Statistical Physics*. New York: Cambridge University Press.

Avery, O. T., MacLeod, C. M., and McCarty, M. (1944). Studies on the chemical nature of the substance inducing transformation of pneumococcal types. *Journal of Experimental Medicine* 79: 137-158.

Ayala, F. Y. (1974). Introduction. In *Studies in the Philosophy of Biology: Reductionism and Related Problems* (pp. vii-xvi), F. J. Ayala and T. Dobzhansky (Eds.). Berkeley, CA: University of California Press.

Ayers, D., and Day, P. J. (2015). Systems medicine: The application of systems biology approaches for modern medical research and drug development. *Molecular Biology International* 2015: 698169. https://doi.org/10.1155/2015/698169.

Azimzadeh Jamalkandi, S., Mozhgani, S. H., Gholami Pourbadie, H., Mirzaie, M., Noorbakhsh, F., Vaziri, B., Gholami, A., Ansari-Pour, N., and Jafari, M. (2016). Systems biomedicine of rabies delineates the affected signaling pathways. *Frontiers in Microbiology* 7: 1688. https://doi.org/10.3389/fmicb.2016.01688.

Baas, N. A., and Emmeche, C. (1997). On emergence and explanation. *Intellectica* 25: 67-83. https://www.persee.fr/doc/intel_0769-4113_1997_num_25_2_1558.

Babu, M., and Snyder, M. (2023). Multi-omics profiling for health. *Molecular & Cellular Proteomics* 22(6): 100561. https://doi.org/10.1016/j.mcpro.2023.100561.

Bacon, F. (1994) *Novum Organum*, P. Urbach and J. Gibson, trans. Chicago, IL: Open Court.

Baedke, J. (2018). *Above the Gene, Beyond Biology: Toward a Philosophy of Epigenetics*. Pittsburgh, PA: University of Pittsburgh Press.

Bai, J. P. F., and Hur, J. (Eds.). (2022). *Systems Medicine*. New York: Humana Press. https://doi.org/10.1007/978-1-0716-2265-0.

Baigrie, B. S. (1996). Descartes's scientific illustrations and 'la grande mécanique de la nature.' In *Picturing Knowledge: Historical and Philosophical Problems Concerning the Use of Art in Science* (pp. 86-134), B.S. Baigrie (Ed.). Toronto, CA: University of Toronto Press.

Bakhoum, S. F., and Landau, D.A. (2017). Chromosomal instability as a driver of tumor heterogeneity and evolution. *Cold Spring Harbor Perspectives in Medicine* 7: a029611. https://doi.org/10.1101/cshperspect.a029611.

Ballereau S., Glaab, E., Kolodkin, A., and Chaiboonchoe, A. (2013). Functional genomics, proteomics, metabolomics and bioinformatics for systems biology. In *Systems Biology* (pp. 3-41), A. Prokop and B. Csukás (Eds.). Dordrecht, NL: Kluwer. https://doi.org/10.1007/978-94-007-6803-1_1.

Balling, R. (2007). From mouse genetics to systems biology. *Mammalian Genome* 18: 383-388. https://doi.org/10.1007/s00335-007-9044-2.

Barabási, A. L. (2016). *Network Science*. New York: Cambridge University Press.

Barabási, A. L., Gulbahce, N., and Loscalzo, J. (2011). Network medicine: A network-based approach to human disease. *Nature Reviews Genetics* 12(1): 56-68. https://doi.org/10.1038/nrg2918.

Barad, K. (2007). *Meeting the Universe Halfway: Quantum Physics and the Entanglement of Matter and Meaning*. Durham, NC: Duke University Press.

Barkai, N., and Leibler, S. (1997). Robustness in simple biochemical networks. *Nature* 387: 913-917. https://doi.org/10.1038/43199.

Barton, S. (2000). Which clinical studies provide the best evidence? The best RCT still trumps the best observational study. *British Medical Journal* 321(7256): 255-256. https://doi.org/10.1136/bmj.321.7256.255.

Bastarache, L., Denny, J. C., and Roden, D. M. (2022). Phenome-wide association studies. *Journal of the American Medical Association* 327(1): 75-76. https://doi.org/10.1001/jama.2021.20356.

Bates, S. (2010). Progress towards personalized medicine. *Drug Discovery Today* 15(3-4): 115-120. https://doi.org/10.1016/j.drudis.2009.11.001.

Bates, S. E. (2020). Epigenetic therapies for cancer. *New England Journal of Medicine* 383(7): 650-663. https://doi.org/10.1056/NEJMra1805035.

Bates, B. R., Templeton, A., Achter, P. J., Harris, T. M., and Condit, C. M. (2003). What does "a gene for heart disease" mean? A focus group study of public understandings of genetic risk factors. *American Journal of Medical Genetics Part A* 119(2): 156-161. https://doi.org/10.1002/ajmg.a.20113.

Bateson, W. (1909). *Mendel's Principles of Heredity*. Cambridge, UK: Cambridge University Press.

Batra, R., Baloni, P., Alcaraz, N., Hauschild, A. C., and Cervera, A. (2022). Computational systems biomedicine. *Frontiers in Genetics* 13: 1047760. https://doi.org/10.3389/fgene.2022.1047760.

Batterman, R. W. (2002). *The Devil in the Details: Asymptotic Reasoning in Explanation, Reduction, and Emergence*. New York: Oxford University Press. https://doi.org/10.1093/0195146476.001.0001.

Baumann, M. (2016). CRISPR/Cas9 genome editing—New and old ethical issues arising from a revolutionary technology. *NanoEthics* 10: 139-159. https://doi.org/10.1007/s11569-016-0259-0.

Baumbach, J., and Schmidt, H. H. (2018). The end of medicine as we know it: Introduction to the new journal, *Systems Medicine*. *Systems Medicine* 1(1): 1-2. https://doi.org/10.1089/sysm.2017.28999.jba.

Bawden, H. H. (1904). What is pragmatism? *Journal of Philosophy, Psychology and Scientific Methods* 1(16): 421-427. https://doi.org/10.2307/2011902.

Bayertz, K. (2015). Materialism. In *The Oxford Handbook of German Philosophy in the Nineteenth Century* (pp. 607-621), M. N. Forster and K. Gjesdal (Eds.). New York: Oxford University Press. https://doi.org/10.1093/oxfordhb/9780199696543.013.0031.

Baylin, S. B., and Jones, P. A. (2011). A decade of exploring the cancer epigenome-Biological and translational implications. *Nature Reviews Cancer* 11: 726-734. https://doi.org/10.1038/nrc3130.

Beaney, M. (2014). Analysis. In *Stanford Encyclopedia of Philosophy, E. N. Zalta (Ed.).* https://plato.stanford.edu/archives/sum2021/entries/analysis/.

Bechtel, W. (2006). *Discovering Cell Mechanisms: The Creation of Modern Cell Biology.* New York: Cambridge University Press.

Bechtel, W. (2007). Biological mechanisms: Organized to maintain autonomy. In *Systems Biology: Philosophical Foundations* (pp. 269-302), F. C. Boogerd, F. J.

Bruggeman, J. H. S. Hofmeyr, and H. V. Westerhoff (Eds.). Amsterdam, NL: Elsevier. https://doi.org/10.1016/B978-044452085-2/50014-0.

Bechtel, W., and Abrahamsen, A. (2005). Explanation: A mechanistic alternative. *Studies in History and Philosophy of the Biological and Biomedical Sciences 36: 421-441.* https://doi.org/10.1016/j.shpsc.2005.03.010.

Beckner, M. (1974). Reductionism, hierarchies and organicism. In *Studies in the Philosophy of Biology: Reductionism and Related Problems* (pp. 163-177), F. J. Ayala and T. Dobzhansky (Eds.). Berkeley, CA: University of California Press. https://doi.org/10.1007/978-1-349-01892-5_10.

Beckner, M. (2006). Organismic biology. In *Encyclopedia of Philosophy*, 2nd edition, volume 7 (pp. 36-39), D. M. Borchert (Ed.). Detroit, MI: Thomson Gale.

Bedau, M. A. (1997). Weak emergence. In *Philosophical Perspectives: Mind, Causation, and World*, volume 11 (pp. 375-399), J. Tomberlin (Ed.). Malden, MA: Blackwell. https://doi.org/10.1111/0029-4624.31.s11.17.

Bedau, M. A. (2002). Downward causation and the autonomy of weak emergence. *Principia* 6: 5-50. https://doi.org/10.5007/%25x.

Bedau, M. A. (2010). Weak emergence and context-sensitive reduction. In *Emergence in Science and Philosophy* (pp. 60-77), A. Corradini and T. O'Connor (Eds.). New York: Routledge.

Bedau, M. A. (2013). Weak emergence drives the science, epistemology, and metaphysics of synthetic biology. *Biological Theory* 8(4): 334-345. https://doi.org/10.1007/s13752-013-0139-6.

Beebee, H., Hitchcock, C., and Menzies, P. (Eds). (2009). *The Oxford Handbook Causation*. New York: Oxford University Press.

Belle, A., Thiagarajan, R., Soroushmehr, S. M., Navidi, F., Beard, D. A., and Najarian, K. (2015). Big data analytics in healthcare. *BioMed Research International* 2015: 370194. https://doi.org/10.1155/2015/370194.

Belling, K., Russo, F., Jensen, A. B., Dalgaard, M. D., Westergaard, D., Rajpert-De Meyts, E., Skakkebæk, N. E., Juul, A., and Brunak, S. (2017). Klinefelter syndrome comorbidities linked to increased X chromosome gene dosage and altered protein interactome activity. *Human Molecular Genetics* 26(7): 1219-1229. https://doi.org/10.1093/hmg/ddx014.

Benison, S., Barger, A. C., and Wolfe, E. L. (1987). *Walter B. Cannon: The Life and Times of a Young Scientist*. Cambridge, MA: Harvard University Press.

Benning, T. B. (2015). Limitations of the biopsychosocial model in psychiatry. *Advances in Medical Education and Practice* 6: 347-352. https://dx.doi.org/10.2147/AMEP.S82937.

Beresford, M. J. (2010). Medical reductionism: Lessons from the great philosophers. *QJM: An International Journal of Medicine* 103: 721-724. https://doi.org/10.1093/qjmed/hcq057.

Berger, S. L., Kouzarides, T., Shiekhattar, R., and Shilatifard, A. (2009). An operational definition of epigenetics. *Genes & Development* 23(7): 781-783. https://dx.doi.org/10.1101/gad.1787609.

Berlin, R., Gruen, R., and Best, J. (2017). Systems medicine—Complexity within, simplicity without. *Journal of Healthcare Informatics Research* 1(1): 119-137. https://doi.org/10.1007/s41666-017-0002-9.

Berlin, R., Gruen, R., and Best, J. (2018). Systems medicine disease: Disease classification and scalability beyond networks and boundary conditions. *Frontiers in Bioengineering and Biotechnology* 6: 112. https://doi.org/10.3389/fbioe.2018.00112.

Berman, J. J. (2018). *Precision Medicine and the Reinvention of Human Disease*. London: Academic Press.

Bernard, C. (1957). *An Introduction to the Study of Experimental Medicine*. New York: Dover Publications.

Berntson, G. G., and Cacioppo, J. T. (2007). Integrative physiology: Homeostasis, allostasis, and the orchestration of systemic physiology. In *Handbook of Psychophysiology* (pp. 433–452), J. T. Cacioppo, L. G. Tassinary, and G. G. Berntson (Eds.). Cambridge: Cambridge University Press. https://doi.org/10.1017/CBO9780511546396.019.

Berrondo, M., and Sandoval, M. (2016). Defining emergence: Learning from flock behavior. *Complexity* 21(S1), 69-78. https://doi.org/10.1002/cplx.21711.

Berryman, S. (2003). Ancient automata and mechanical explanation. *Phronesis* 48(4): 344-369. https://brill.com/view/journals/phro/48/4/article-p344_3.xml.

Bersini, H., Stano, P., Luisi, P. L., and Bedau, M. A. (2012). Philosophical and scientific perspectives on emergence. *Synthese* 185(2): 165-169. https://doi.org/10.1007/s11229-010-9718-2.

Bertalanffy, L. von. (1974). *General Systems Theory: Foundations, Development, Applications*, revised edition. New York: Braziller.

Bertolaso, M., Serrelli, E., and Caianiello, S. (2018). Introduction: Issues about robustness in the practice of biological sciences. In *Biological Robustness: Emerging Perspectives from within the Life Sciences* (pp. 1-22), M. Bertolaso, S. Caianiello, and E. Serrelli (Eds.). Cham, CH: Springer. https://doi.org/10.1007/978-3-030-01198-7_1.

Best, R., and Khushf, G. (2006). The social conditions for nanomedicine: disruption, systems, and lock-in. *Journal of Law, Medicine & Ethics* 34: 733-740. https://doi.org/10.1111/j.1748-720X.2006.00093.x.

Bhugaonkar, K., Bhugaonkar, R., and Masne, N. (2022). The trend of metaverse and augmented & virtual reality extending to the healthcare system. *Cureus*, 14(9): e29071. https://doi.org/10.7759/cureus.29071.

Bich, L., Mossio, M., Ruiz-Mirazo, K., and Moreno, A. (2016). Biological regulation: Controlling the system from within. *Biology & Philosophy* 31(2): 237-265. https://doi.org/10.1007/s10539-015-9497-8.

Billiard, S., and Alvergne, A. (2018). Stochasticity in cultural evolution: A revolution yet to happen. *History and Philosophy of the Life Sciences* 40(1): 9. https://doi.org/10.1007/s40656-017-0173-y.

Billman, G. E. (2013). Homeostasis: The dynamic self-regulatory process that maintains health and buffers against disease. In *Handbook of Systems and Complexity in Health* (pp. 159-170), J. P. Sturmberg and C. M Martin (Eds.). New York: Springer. https://doi.org/10.1007/978-1-4614-4998-0_10.

Billman, G. E. (2020). Homeostasis: The underappreciated and far too often ignored central organizing principle of physiology. *Frontiers in Physiology* 11: 200. https://doi.org/10.3389/fphys.2020.00200.

Bird, A. P. (1986). CpG-rich islands and the function of DNA methylation. *Nature* 321(6067): 209-213. https://doi.org/10.1038/321209a0.

Bird, A. (2007). Perceptions of epigenetics. *Nature* 447: 396-398. https://doi.org/10.1038/nature05913.

Birnstiel, M. L. (1996). The genetic revolution 1950–1996: An introduction. *European Review* 4(4): 333-334. https://doi.org/10.1002/(SICI)1234-981X(199610)4:4<333::AID-EURO147>3.0.CO;2-Y.

Bizzarri, M., Palombo, A., and Cucina, A. (2013). Theoretical aspects of systems biology. *Progress in Biophysics and Molecular Biology* 112(1-2): 33-43. https://doi.org/10.1016/j.pbiomolbio.2013.03.019.

Bizzarri, M., Naimark, O., Nieto-Villar, J., Fedeli, V., and Giuliani, A. (2020). Complexity in biological organization: Deconstruction (and subsequent restating) of key concepts. *Entropy* 22(8): 885. https://doi.org/10.3390/e22080885.

Blackburn, G. L. (2011). Medicalizing obesity: Individual, economic, and medical consequences. *AMA Journal of Ethics* 13(12), 890-895. https://doi.org/10.1001/visualmentor.2013.13.12.pfor1-1112.

Bland, J. S., Minich, D. M., and Eck, B. M. (2017). A systems medicine approach: Translating emerging science into individualized wellness. *Advances in Medicine* 2017: 1718957. https://doi.org/10.1155/2017/1718957.

Blinov, M. L., Moraru, I. I., Schaff, J. C., and Loew, L. M. (2023). Virtual cell modeling and simulation software. *Biophysical Journal* 122(3): 414a. https://doi.org/10.1016/j.bpj.2022.11.2249.

Bliss, M. (1982). *The Discovery of Insulin*. Chicago, IL: University of Chicago Press.

Blitz, D. (1992). *Emergent Evolution: Qualitative Novelty and the Levels of Reality*. Dordrecht, NL: Kluwer. https://doi.org/10.1007/978-94-015-8042-7.

Blobel, B., and Ruotsalainen, P. (2019). Healthcare transformation towards personalized medicine - Chances and challenges. In *pHealth* (pp. 3-21), B. Blobel and M. Giacomini (Eds.). Amsterdam: IOS Press. https://doi.org/10.3233/978-1-61499-975-1-3.

Bloch, D. A. (1983). Family systems medicine: The field and the journal. *Family Systems Medicine* 1(1): 3. https://doi.org/10.1037/h0090105.

Bock, G. R., and Goode, J. A. (Eds.). (1998). *The Limits of Reductionism in Biology*. London: John Wiley.

Bohm, D. (2005). *Wholeness and the Implicate Order*. London: Taylor & Francis.

Boissel, J. P., Auffray, C., Noble, D., Hood, L., and Boissel, F. H. (2015). Bridging systems medicine and patient needs. *CPT: Pharmacometrics & Systems Pharmacology* 4(3): 135-145. https://doi.org/10.1002/psp4.26.

Bokulich, P. (2011). Hempel's Dilemma and domains of physics. *Analysis* 71(4): 646-651. https://doi.org/10.1093/analys/anr087.

Bolton, D., and Gillett, G. (2019). *The Biopsychosocial Model of Health and Disease: New Philosophical and Scientific Developments*. Cham, CH: Palgrave Pivot. https://doi.org/10.1007/978-3-030-11899-0.

Boniolo, G., and Nathan, M. J. (Eds.), (2017). *Philosophy of Molecular Medicine: Foundational Issues in Research and Practice*. London: Routledge. https://doi.org/10.4324/9781315674162.

Boniolo, G., Campaner, R., and Carrara, M. (2021). Patient similarity in the era of precision medicine: A philosophical analysis. *Erkenntnis*. https://doi.org/10.1007/s10670-021-00483-w.

BonJour, L. (2010). Against materialism. In *The Waning of Materialism* (pp. 3-24), R. C. Koons and G. Bealer (Eds.). New York: Oxford University Press. https://doi.org/10.1093/acprof:oso/9780199556182.003.0001.

Boogerd, F. C., Bruggeman, F. J., Richardson, R. C., Stephan, A., and Westerhoff, H. V. (2005). Emergence and its place in nature: A case study of biochemical networks. *Synthese* 145: 131-164. https://doi.org/10.1007/s11229-004-4421-9.

Boogerd, F. C., Bruggeman, F. J., Hofmeyr, J. H. S., and Westerhoff, H. V. (2007a). Towards a philosophical foundation of systems biology: Introduction. In *Systems Biology: Philosophical Foundations* (pp. 3-19), F. C. Boogerd, F. J.

Bruggeman, J. H. S. Hofmeyr, and H. V. Westerhoff (Eds.). Amsterdam, NL: Elsevier. https://doi.org/10.1016/B978-044452085-2/50003-6.

Boogerd, F. C., Bruggeman, F. J., Hofmeyr, J. H. S., and Westerhoff, H. V. (2007b). Afterthoughts as foundations for systems biology. In *Systems Biology:*

Philosophical Foundations (pp. 321-336), F. C. Boogerd, F. J. Bruggeman, J. H. S. Hofmeyr, and H. V. Westerhoff (Eds.). Amsterdam, NL: Elsevier. https://doi.org/10.1016/B978-044452085-2/50016-4.

Boogerd, F. C., Bruggeman, F. J., and Richardson, R. C. (2013). Mechanistic explanations and models in molecular systems biology. *Foundations of Science* 18: 725-744. https://doi.org/10.1007/s10699-012-9302-y.

Boorse, C. (2014). A second rebuttal on health. *Journal of Medicine and Philosophy* 39(6): 683-724. https://doi.org/10.1093/jmp/jhu035.

Boran, A. D., and Iyengar, R. (2010). Systems pharmacology. *Mount Sinai Journal of Medicine: A Journal of Translational and Personalized Medicine* 77(4): 333-344. https://doi.org/10.1002/msj.20191.

Borck, C. (2020). Negotiating epistemic hierarchies in biomedicine: The rise of evidence-based medicine. In *Weak Knowledge: Forms, Functions, and Dynamics* (pp. 449–482), M. Epple, A. Imhausen, and F. Müller (Eds.). Frankfurt: Campus Verlag.

Bose, B. (2013). Systems biology: A biologist's viewpoint. *Progress in Biophysics and Molecular Biology* 113(3): 358-368. https://doi.org/10.1016/j.pbiomolbio.2013.07.001.

Botz-Bornstein, T. (2020). *Micro and Macro Philosophy: Organicism in Biology, Philosophy and Politics*. Leiden: Brill. https://doi.org/10.1163/9789004440425.

Bourget, D., and Chalmers, D. J. (2014). What do philosophers believe? *Philosophical Studies* 170(3): 465-500. https://doi.org/10.1007/s11098-013-0259-7.

Bousquet, J., Jorgensen, C., Dauzat, M., Cesario, A., Camuzat, T., Bourret, R., Best, N., M Anto, J., Abecassis, F., Aubas, P., and Avignon, A. (2014). Systems medicine approaches for the definition of complex phenotypes in chronic diseases and ageing. From concept to implementation and policies. *Current Pharmaceutical Design* 20(38): 5928-5944. https://dx.doi.org/10.2174/1381612820666140314115505.

Bowler, P. J., and Morus, I. R. (2020). *Making Modern Science: A Historical Survey*, 2nd edition. Chicago, IL: University of Chicago Press.

Bracken, J. A. (1984). Authentic subjectivity and genuine objectivity. *Horizons* 11(2): 290-303. https://doi.org/10.1017/S0360966900033703.

Bracken, P., Thomas, P., Timimi, S., Asen, E., Behr, G., Beuster, C., Bhunnoo, S., Browne, I., Chhina, N., Double, D., and Downer, S. (2012). Psychiatry beyond the current paradigm. *British Journal of Psychiatry* 201(6): 430-434. https://doi.org/10.1192/bjp.bp.112.109447.

Bragazzi, N. L. (2013a). Rethinking psychiatry with OMICS science in the age of personalized P5 medicine: Ready for psychiatome? *Philosophy, Ethics, and Humanities in Medicine* 8: 4. https://doi.org/10.1186/1747-5341-8-4.

Bragazzi, N. L. (2013b). From P0 to P6 medicine, a model of highly participatory, narrative, interactive, and "augmented" medicine: Some considerations on Salvatore Iaconesi's clinical story. *Patient Preference and Adherence* 7: 353-359. https://doi.org/10.2147/PPA.S38578.

Bragazzi, N. L., and Del Puente, G. (2013). Why P6 medicine needs clinical psychology and a trans-cultural approach. *Health Psychology Research* 1: 5. https://doi.org/10.4081/hpr.2013.e5.

Brandt, A. M. (2020). *No Magic Bullet: A Social History of Venereal Disease in the United States Since 1880*, 35th anniversary edition. New York: Oxford University Press.

Brémaud, P. (2020). *Probability Theory and Stochastic Processes*. Cham, CH: Springer. https://doi.org/10.1007/978-3-030-40183-2.

Brenner, P. (2004). The dangers of geneticism. *Journal of Midwifery & Women's Health* 49(3): 260-262. https://doi.org/10.1016/j.jmwh.2004.02.012.

Brigandt, I., and Love, A. (2017). Reductionism in biology. In *Stanford Encyclopedia of Philosophy, E. N. Zalta (Ed.).* https://plato.stanford.edu/archives/spr2017/entries/reduction-biology/.

Brigandt, I., Green, S., and O'Malley, M. A. (2017). Systems biology and mechanistic explanation. In *The Routledge Handbook of Mechanisms and Mechanical Philosophy* (pp. 362-374), S. Glennan and P. Illari (Eds.). New York: Routledge.

Brighton, B., Bhandari, M., Tornetta, P., and Felson, D. T. (2003). Hierarchy of evidence: From case reports to randomized controlled trials. *Clinical Orthopaedics and Related Research* 413: 19-24. https://doi.org/10.1097/01.blo.0000079323.41006.12.

Brin, M., and Stuck, G. (2002). *Introduction to Dynamical Systems*. New York: Cambridge University Press.

Broad, C. D. (1925). *The Mind and Its Place in Nature*. New York: Harcourt, Brace & Co.

Brodersen, J. (2017). Overdiagnosis: An unrecognised and growing worldwide problem in healthcare. *Slovenian Journal of Public Health* 56(3): 147-149. https://doi.org/10.1515/sjph-2017-0019.

Brody, H. (1973). The systems view of man: Implications for medicine, science, and ethics. *Perspectives in Biology and Medicine* 17(1): 71-92. https://doi.org/10.1353/pbm.1973.0007.

Brooks, D. S., DiFrisco, J., and Wimsatt, W. C. (Eds.). (2021). *Levels of Organization in the Biological Sciences*. Cambridge, MA: MIT Press.

Brown, G. G., and Ladyman, J. (2019). *Materialism: A Historical and Philosophical Inquiry*. New York: Routledge.

Brown, D. G., Wobst, H. J., Kapoor, A., Kenna, L. A., and Southall, N. (2022). Clinical development times for innovative drugs. *Nature Reviews Drug Discovery* 21: 793-794. *https://doi.org/10.1038/d41573-021-00190-9.*

Brücher, B. L., and Jamall, I. S. (2016). Somatic mutation theory—Why it's wrong for most cancers. *Cellular Physiology and Biochemistry* 38(5): 1663-1680. https://doi.org/10.1159/000443106.

Bruggeman, F. J., and Westerhoff, H. V. (2007). The nature of systems biology. *Trends in Microbiology* 15: 45-50. https://doi.org/10.1016/j.tim.2006.11.003.

Bruton, M., and O'Dwyer, N. (2018). Synergies in coordination: a comprehensive overview of neural, computational, and behavioral approaches. *Journal of Neurophysiology* 120(6): 2761-2774. https://doi.org/10.1152/jn.00052.2018.

Buchman, T. G. (2002). The community of the self. *Nature* 420: 246-251. https://doi.org/10.1038/nature01260.

Buchman, T. G. (2004). Nonlinear dynamics, complex systems, and the pathobiology of critical illness. *Current Opinion in Critical Care* 10(5): 378-382. https://doi.org/10.1097/01.ccx.0000139369.65817.b6.

Buiatti, M., and Longo, G. (2013). Randomness and multilevel interactions in biology. *Theory in Biosciences* 132(3): 139-158. https://doi.org/10.1007/s12064-013-0179-2.

Bunge, M. (1977). *Treatise on Basic Philosophy, Volume 3: Ontology I: The Furniture of the World*. Dordrecht, NL: Reidel. https://doi.org/10.1007/978-94-010-9924-0.

Bunge, M. (1979). *Treatise on Basic Philosophy, Volume 4: Ontology II: A World of Systems*. Dordrecht, NL: Reidel. https://doi.org/10.1007/978-94-009-9392-1.

Bunge, M. (1981). *Scientific Materialism*. Dordrecht, NL: Reidel. https://doi.org/10.1007/978-94-009-8517-9.

Bunge, M. (2017). *Causality and Modern Science*, 4th edition. New York: Routledge.

Burian, R. (2005). *The Epistemology of Development, Evolution, and Genetics*. New York: Cambridge University Press.

Burrage, K., Hood, L., and Ragan, M. A. (2006). Advanced computing for systems biology. *Briefings in Bioinformatics* 7: 390-398. https://doi.org/10.1093/bib/bbl033.

Bushev, M. (1994). *Synergetics: Chaos, Order, Self-Organization*. Singapore: World Scientific Publishing. https://doi.org/10.1142/1929.

Buskell, A., Enquist, M., and Jansson, F. (2019). A systems approach to cultural evolution. *Palgrave Communications* 5(1): 131. https://doi.org/10.1057/s41599-019-0343-5.

Buzzoni, M., Tesio, L., and Stuart, M. T. (2022). Holism and reductionism in the illness/disease debate. In *From Electrons to Elephants and Elections: Exploring the Role of Content and Context* (pp. 743-778), S. Wuppuluri and I. Stewart (Eds.). Cham, CH: Springer. https://doi.org/10.1007/978-3-030-92192-7_39.

Calude, C. S., and Longo, G. (2016). Classical, quantum and biological randomness as relative unpredictability. *Natural Computing* 15(2): 263-278. https://doi.org/10.1007/s11047-015-9533-2.

Cambrosio, A., and Keating, P. (2001). History and sociology of biomedical sciences and technology. In *International Encyclopedia of the Social and Behavioral Sciences*, volume 2 (pp. 1222-1226), N. J. Smelser and P. B. Baltes (Eds.). Amsterdam, NL: Pergamon Press.

Campbell, D. T. (1974). 'Downward causation' in hierarchically organized biological systems. In *Studies in the Philosophy of Biology: Reductionism and Related Problems* (pp. 179-186), F. J. Ayala and T. Dobzhansky (Eds.). London: Palgrave. https://doi.org/10.1007/978-1-349-01892-5_11.

Campbell, R. J., and Bickhard, M. H. (2011). Physicalism, emergence and downward causation. *Axiomathes* 21(1): 33-56. https://doi.org/10.1007/s10516-010-9128-6.

Cannon, B. (1994). Walter Bradford Cannon: reflections on the man and his contributions. *International Journal of Stress Management* 1: 145-158. https://doi.org/10.1007/BF01857608.

Cannon, W. B. (1926). Physiological regulation of normal states: some tentative postulates concerning biological homeostatics. In *À Charles Richet: Ses Amis, Ses Collègues, Ses Élèves* (pp. 91-93), A. Pettit (Ed.). Paris: Les Editions Médicales.

Cannon, W. B. (1929). Organization for physiological homeostasis. *Physiological Reviews* 9: 399-431. https://doi.org/10.1152/physrev.1929.9.3.399.

Cannon, W. B. (1939). *The Wisdom of the Body*, revised edition. New York: Norton.

Cantor, M., Chimento, M., Smeele, S. Q., He, P., Papageorgiou, D., Aplin, L. M., and Farine, D. R. (2021). Social network architecture and the tempo of cumulative cultural evolution. *Proceedings of the Royal Society B* 288(1946): 20203107. https://doi.org/10.1098/rspb.2020.3107.

Capobianco, E. (2012). Ten challenges for systems medicine. *Frontiers in Genetics* 3: 193. https://doi.org/10.3389/fgene.2012.00193.

Capobianco, E., and Lió, P. (2014). Advances in translational biomedicine from systems approaches. *Frontiers in Genetics* 5: 273. http://doi.org/10.3389/fgene.2014.00273.

Cardinal-Fernández, P., Nin, N., Ruíz-Cabello, J., and Lorente, J. A. (2014). Systems medicine: a new approach to clinical practice. *Archivos de Bronconeumología* 50(10): 444-451. https://doi.org/10.1016/j.arbr.2014.09.001.

Carley, S., Horner, D., Body, R., and Mackway-Jones, K. (2020). Evidence-Based Medicine and COVID-19: What to believe and when to change. *Emergency Medicine Journal* 37: 572-575. https://doi.org/10.1136/emermed-2020-210098.

Carlson, J.M., and Doyle, J. (2002). Complexity and robustness. *Proceedings of the National Academy of Science USA* 99: 2538-2545. https://doi.org/10.1073/pnas.012582499.

Cartwright, N. (1999). *The Dappled World: A Study of the Boundaries of Science*. New York: Cambridge University Press.

Cartwright, N. (2007). Are RCTs the gold standard? *BioSocieties* 2(1): 11-20. https://doi.org/10.1017/S1745855207005029.

Carusi, A. (2014). Validation and variability: Dual challenges on the path from systems biology to systems medicine. *Studies in History and Philosophy of Science Part C: Studies in History and Philosophy of Biological and Biomedical Sciences* 48: 28-37. https://doi.org/10.1016/j.shpsc.2014.08.008.

Cary, M. P., Bader, G. D., and Sander, C. (2005). Pathway information for systems biology. *FEBS Letters* 579: 1815-1820. https://doi.org/10.1016/j.febslet.2005.02.005.

Cassell, E. J. (2004). *The Nature of Suffering and the Goals of Medicine*, 2nd edition. New York: Oxford University Press. https://doi.org/10.1093/acprof:oso/9780195156164.001.0001.

Catanzaro, M., Fagiani, F., Racchi, M., Corsini, E., Govoni, S., and Lanni, C. (2020). Immune response in COVID-19: Addressing a pharmacological challenge by targeting pathways triggered by SARS-CoV-2. *Signal Transduction and Targeted Therapy* 5(1): 84. https://doi.org/10.1038/s41392-020-0191-1.

Catillon, M. (2017). Medical knowledge synthesis: A brief overview. Research Report. Harvard University and National Bureau of Economic Research. https://www2.nber.org/aging/valmed/WhitePaper-Catillon10.2017.pdf.

Cawadias, A. P. (1952). The Mid-Nineteenth Century Clinical School of Paris. *Proceedings of the Royal Society of Medicine* 45(5): 306-310.

Cazaly, E., Charlesworth, J., Dickinson, J. L., and Holloway, A. F. (2015). Genetic determinants of epigenetic patterns: Providing insight into disease. *Molecular Medicine* 21(1): 400-409. https://doi.org/10.2119/molmed.2015.00001.

Cerrone, M., Remme, C.A., Tadros, R., Bezzina, C. R., and Delmar, M. (2019). Beyond the one gene–one disease paradigm: Complex genetics and pleiotropy in inheritable cardiac disorders. *Circulation* 140(7): 595-610. https://doi.org/10.1161/CIRCULATIONAHA.118.035954.

Cesario, A., D'Oria, M., Bove, F., Privitera, G., Boškoski, I., Pedicino, D., Boldrini, L., Erra, C., Loreti, C., Liuzzo, G., and Crea, F. (2021). Personalized clinical phenotyping through systems medicine and artificial intelligence. *Journal of Personalized Medicine* 11(4): 265. https://doi.org/10.3390/jpm11040265.

Chalmers, D. J. (2006). Strong and weak emergence. In *The Re-Emergence of Emergence: The Emergentist Hypothesis from Science to Religion* (pp. 244-254), P. Clayton and P. Davies (Eds.). New York: Oxford University Press. https://doi.org/10.1093/acprof:oso/9780199544318.003.0011.

Chamberlain, L. L, and Bütz, M. R. (2013). *Clinical Chaos: A Therapist's Guide to Nonlinear Dynamics and Therapeutic Change*. New York: Routledge.

Champneys, A. R. (2006). A twenty-first century guidebook for applied dynamical systems. *Journal of Computational and Nonlinear Dynamics* 1: 279-282. https://doi.org/10.1115/1.2338663.

Chan, S. Y., and Loscalzo, J. (2012). The emerging paradigm of network medicine in the study of human disease. *Circulation Research* 111(3): 359-374. https://doi.org/10.1161/CIRCRESAHA.111.258541.

Chase, J. G., Preiser, J. C., Dickson, J. L., Pironet, A., Chiew, Y. S., Pretty, C. G., Shaw, G. M., Benyo, B., Moeller, K., Safaei, S., and Tawhai, M. (2018). Next-generation, personalised, model-based critical care medicine: A state-of-the art review of in silico virtual patient models, methods, and cohorts, and how to validation them. *BioMedical Engineering OnLine* 17(1): 24. https://doi.org/10.1186/s12938-018-0455-y.

Chattu, V. K. (2021). A review of artificial intelligence, big data, and blockchain technology applications in medicine and global health. *Big Data and Cognitive Computing* 5(3): 41. https://doi.org/10.3390/bdcc5030041.

Chen, L. (2019). Computational systems biology for omics data analysis. *Journal of Molecular Cell Biology* 11(8): 631-632. https://doi.org/10.1093/jmcb/mjz095.

Chen, R., and Snyder, M. (2013). Promise of personalized omics to precision medicine. *Systems Biology and Medicine* 5(1): 73-82. https://doi.org/10.1002/wsbm.1198.

Chen, F. C., Liao, Y. C., Huang, J. M., Lin, C. H., Chen, Y. Y., Dou, H. Y., and Hsiung, C. A. (2014). Pros and cons of the tuberculosis drugome approach–an empirical analysis. *PloS One* 9(6): e100829. https://doi.org/10.1371/journal.pone.0100829.

Chengoden, R., Victor, N., Huynh-The, T., Yenduri, G., Jhaveri, R. H., Alazab, M., Bhattacharya, S., Hegde, P., Maddikunta, P. K. R., and Gadekallu, T. R. (2023). Metaverse for healthcare: A survey on potential applications, challenges and future directions. *IEEE Access* 11: 12765-12795. https://doi.org/10.1109/ACCESS.2023.3241628.

Cherny, N. I., De Vries, E. G., Emanuel, L., Fallowfield, L., Francis, P. A., Gabizon, A., Piccart, M. J., Sidransky, D., Soussan-Gutman, L., and Tziraki, C. (2014). Words matter: Distinguishing "personalized medicine" and "biologically personalized therapeutics." *Journal of the National Cancer Institute* 106(12): dju321. https://doi.org/10.1093/jnci/dju321.

Chibbaro, S., Rondoni, L., and Vulpiani, A. (2014). *Reductionism, Emergence and Levels of Reality: The Importance of Being Borderline*. New York: Springer. https://doi.org/10.1007/978-3-319-06361-4.

Chiras, D. D. (2015). *Human Biology*, 8th edition. Burlington, MA: Jones & Bartlett.

Chisholm, R. M. (1973). Parts as essential to their wholes. *Review of Metaphysics* 26(4): 581-603.

Choat, S. (2018). Science, agency and ontology: A historical-materialist response to new materialism. *Political Studies* 66: 1027-1042. https://doi.org/10.1177/0032321717731926.

Chodasewicz, K. (2014). Evolution, reproduction and definition of life. *Theory in Biosciences* 133(1): 39-45. https://doi.org/10.1007/s12064-013-0184-5.

Chong, L., and Ray, L. B. (2002). Whole-istic biology. *Science* 295: 1661. https://doi.org/10.1126/science.295.5560.1661.

Choquet, D., and Triller, A. (2013). The dynamic synapse. *Neuron* 80(3): 691-703. https://dx.doi.org/10.1016/j.neuron.2013.10.013.

Choudhuri, S. (2011). From Waddington's epigenetic landscape to small noncoding RNA: Some important milestones in the history of epigenetics research. *Toxicology Mechanisms and Methods* 21(4): 252-274. https://dx.doi.org/10.3109/15376516.2011.559695.

Christensen, C. M., Grossman, J. H., and Hwang, J. (2009). *The Innovator's Prescription: A Disruptive Solution for Health Care*. New York: McGraw-Hill.

Claridge, J. A., and Fabian, T. C. (2005). History and development of evidence-based medicine. *World Journal of Surgery* 29(5): 547-553. https://doi.org/10.1007/s00268-005-7910-1.

Clarke, A. E. (2014). Biomedicalization. In *Wiley Blackwell Encyclopedia of Health, Illness, Behavior, and Society*, (pp. 137-142), W. C. Cockerham, R. Dingwall, and S. R. Quah (Eds.). London: Wiley-Blackwell. https://doi.org/10.1002/9781118410868.wbehibs083.

Clarke, B., and Russo, F. (2017). Mechanisms and biomedicine. In *The Routledge Handbook of Mechanisms and Mechanical Philosophy* (pp. 319-331), S. Glennan and P. Illari (Eds.). New York: Routledge. https://doi.org/10.4324/9781315731544-24.

Clarke, A. E., Shim, J. K., Mamo, L., Fosket, J. R., and Fishman, J. R. (2003). Biomedicalization: Technoscientific transformations of health, illness, and U.S. biomedicine. *American Sociological Review 68*(2): 161-194. https://doi.org/10.1515/9780822391258-005.

Clarke, A. E., Jeske, M., Mamo, L., and Shim, J. K. (2021). Biomedicalization revisited. In *The Wiley Blackwell Companion to Medical Sociology* (pp. 125-149), W. C. Cockerham (Ed.). London: Wiley-Blackwell. https://doi.org/10.1002/9781119633808.ch7.

Claussnitzer, M., Cho, J. H., Collins, R., Cox, N. J., Dermitzakis, E. T., Hurles, M. E., Kathiresan, S., Kenny, E. E., Lindgren, C. M., MacArthur, D. G., and North, K. N. (2020). A brief history of human disease genetics. *Nature* 577(7789): 179-189. https://doi.org/10.1038/s41586-019-1879-7.

Clayton, P. (2006). Conceptual foundations of emergence theory. In *The Re-Emergence of Emergence: The Emergentist Hypothesis from Science to Religion* (pp. 1-31), P. Clayton and P. Davies (Eds.). New York: Oxford University Press. https://doi.org/10.1093/acprof:oso/9780199544318.003.0001.

Clements, C. D. (1976). Stasis: The unnatural value. *Ethics* 86(2): 136-144.

Clermont, G., Auffray, C., Moreau, Y., Rocke, D. M., Dalevi, D., Dubhashi, D., Marshall, D. R., Raasch, P., Dehne, F., Provero, P., and Tegner, J. (2009). Bridging the gap between systems biology and medicine. *Genome Medicine* 1(9): 88. https://doi.org/10.1186/gm88.

Coffey, D. S. (1998). Self-organization, complexity and chaos: The new biology for medicine. *Nature Medicine* 4(8): 882-885. https://doi.org/10.1038/nm0898-882.

Coffman, J. A. (2006). Developmental ascendency: From bottom-up to top-down control. *Biological Theory* 1: 165-178. https://doi.org/10.1162/biot.2006.1.2.165.

Cohen, I. B. (1985). *Revolution in Science*. Cambridge, MA: Belknap Press.

Cohen, A. M., Stavri, P. Z., and Hersh, W. R. (2004). A categorization and analysis of the criticisms of evidence-based medicine. *International Journal of Medical Informatics* 73(1): 35-43. https://doi.org/10.1016/j.ijmedinf.2003.11.002.

Cohen, Z. D., Ashar, Y. K., and DeRubeis, R, J. (2019). Moving beyond "one size fits all." In *Evidence-Based Practice in Action: Bridging Clinical Science and Intervention* (pp. 111-132), S. Dimidjian (Ed.). New York: Guilford Press.

Collingwood, R. G. (1998). *An Essay on Metaphysics*, revised edition. Oxford, UK: Clarendon Press.

Collins, F. S., and Varmus, H. (2015). A new initiative on precision medicine. *New England Journal of Medicine* 372(9): 793-795. https://doi.org/10.1056/NEJMp1500523.

Conrad, P. (2007). *The Medicalization of Society: On the Transformation of Human Conditions into Treatable Disorders*. Baltimore, MD: Johns Hopkins University Press.

Conrad, P., Mackie, T., and Mehrotra, A. (2010). Estimating the costs of medicalization. *Social Science & Medicine* 70(12), 1943-1947. https://doi.org/10.1016/j.socscimed.2010.02.019.

Cooper, S. J. (2008). From Claude Bernard to Walter Cannon. Emergence of the concept of homeostasis. *Appetite* 51(3): 419-427. https://doi.org/10.1016/j.appet.2008.06.005.

Corning, P. A. (2012). The re-emergence of emergence, and the causal role of synergy in emergent evolution. *Synthese* 185(2): 295-317. https://doi.org/10.1007/s11229-010-9726-2.

Cornish-Bowden, A. (1995). Metabolic control analysis in theory and practice. *Advances in Molecular and Cell Biology* 11: 21-64. https://doi.org/10.1016/S1569-2558(08)60247-7.

Corradini, A., and O'Connor, T. (Eds.) (2010). *Emergence in Science and Philosophy*. New York: Routledge.

Cosentino, C., and Bates, D. (2019). *Feedback Control in Systems Biology*. Boca Raton, FL: CRC Press.

Coskun, A. F., and Ozcan, A. (2014). Computational imaging, sensing and diagnostics for global health applications. *Current Opinion in Biotechnology* 25: 8-16. https://doi.org/10.1016/j.copbio.2013.08.008.

Costa, J. (2012). Systems pathology: A critical review. *Molecular oncology* 6(1): 27-32. https://doi.org/10.1016/j.molonc.2011.11.007.

Coulter, H. L. (2000). *Divided Legacy, A History of the Schism in Medical Thought. Volume II, The Origins of Western Medicine: J. B. Van Helmont to Claude Bernard*. Berkeley, CA: North Atlantic Books.

Coveney, P. V., and Fowler, P. W. (2005). Modelling biological complexity: A physical scientist's perspective. *Journal of the Royal Society Interface* 2: 267-280. https://doi.org/10.1098/rsif.2005.0045.

Crafford, F. S. (1946). *Jan Smuts: A Biography*, 2nd edition. Oxford: Borodino Books.

Crane, T., and Farkas, K. (2004). Introduction. In *Metaphysics: A Guide and Anthology* (pp. 369-379), T. Crane and K. Farkas (Eds.). New York: Oxford University Press.

Crane, T., and Mellor, D. H. (1990). There is no question of physicalism. *Mind* 99: 185-206. https://doi.org/10.1093/mind/XCIX.394.185.

Craver, C. F., and Bechtel, W. (2007). Top-down causation without top-down causes. *Biology & Philosophy* 22(4): 547-563. https://doi.org/10.1007/s10539-006-9028-8.

Craver, C. F., and Darden, L. (2005). Introduction. *Studies in the History and Philosophy of Biological and Biomedical Sciences* 36: 233-244. https://doi.org/10.1016/j.shpsc.2005.03.001.

Creanza, N., Kolodny, O., and Feldman, M. W. (2017). Cultural evolutionary theory: How culture evolves and why it matters. *Proceedings of the National Academy of Sciences* 114(30): 7782-7789. https://doi.org/10.1073/pnas.1620732114.

Crespi, E., Burnap, R., Chen, J., Das, M., Gassman, N., Rosa Jr, E., Simmons, R., Wada, H., Wang, Z. Q., Xiao, J., and Yang, B. (2021). Resolving the rules of robustness and resilience in biology across scales. *Integrative and Comparative Biology* 61: 2163-2179. https://doi.org/10.1093/icb/icab183.

Crick, F. (1970). Central dogma of molecular biology. *Nature* 227: 561-563. https://doi.org/10.1038/227561a0.

Crowell, B. (2003). *Newtonian Physics*. Fullerton, CA: Light and Matter.

Csete, M. E., and Doyle, J. C. (2002). Reverse engineering of biological complexity. *Science* 295: 1664-1669. https://doi.org/10.1126/science.1069981.

Csete, M. E., and Doyle, J. C. (2004). Bow-tie, metabolism and disease. *Trends in Biotechnology* 22: 446-450. https://doi.org/10.1016/j.tibtech.2004.07.007.

Culliton, B. (1995). Molecular medicine in a changing world. *Nature Medicine* 1: 1. https://doi.org/10.1038/nm0195-1.

Cunningham, B. (2001). The reemergence of' 'emergence.' *Philosophy of Science* 68(S3): S62-S75. https://doi.org/10.1086/392898.

Dahabreh, I. J., Hayward, R., and Kent, D. M. (2016). Using group data to treat individuals: Understanding heterogeneous treatment effects in the age of precision medicine and patient-centred evidence. *International Journal of Epidemiology* 45(6): 2184-2193. https://doi.org/10.1093/ije/dyw125.

Dandekar, T., and Kunz, M. (2023). *Bioinformatics: An Introductory Textbook*. Berlin: Springer. https://doi.org/10.1007/978-3-662-65036-3.

Daniels, B. C., Chen, Y. J., Sethna, J. P., Gutenkunst, R. N., and Myers, C. R. (2008). Sloppiness, robustness, and evolvability in systems biology. *Current Opinions in Biotechnology* 19: 389-395. https://doi.org/10.1016/j.copbio.2008.06.008.

Darden, L. (2006). *Reasoning in Biological Discoveries: Essays on Mechanisms, Interfiled Relations, and Anomaly Resolution*. New York: Cambridge University Press.

Darden, L., Kundu, K., Pal, L. R., and Moult, J. (2018). Harnessing formal concepts of biological mechanism to analyze human disease. *PLoS Computational Biology* 14(12): e1006540. https://doi.org/ 10.1371/journal.pcbi.1006540.

Daschner,. A. (2019). The doctor in the face of scientific determinism. In *Medicina Evolucionista. Aportaciones Pluridisciplinares*, volume V (pp. 67-80), A. Daschner, J.-L. Gómez-Pérez, and M. J. Trujillo-Tiebas (Eds.). MedEvo.

Daskalaki, A. (Ed.). (2009). *Handbook of Research on Systems Biology Applications in Medicine*, 2 volumes. Hershey, PA: IGI Global. https://doi.org/10.4018/978-1-60566-076-9.

Davidov, E. J., Holland, J. M., Marple, E. W., and Naylor, S. (2003). Advancing drug discovery through systems biology. *Drug Discovery Today* 8: 175-183. https://doi.org/10.1016/S1359-6446(03)02600-X.

Davies, P. C. W. (2006). The physics of downward causation. In *The Re-Emergence of Emergence: The Emergentist Hypothesis from Science to Religion* (pp. 35-51), P. Clayton and P. Davies (Eds.). New York: Oxford University Press. https://doi.org/10.1093/acprof:oso/9780199544318.003.0002.

Davies, K. J. (2016). Adaptive homeostasis. *Molecular Aspects of Medicine* 49: 1-7. https://doi.org/10.1016/j.mam.2016.04.007.

Davis, G. W. (2006). Homeostatic control of neural activity: From phenomenology to molecular design. *Annual Review of Neuroscience* 29: 307-323. https://doi.org/10.1146/annurev.neuro.28.061604.135751.

Davis, A., Gao, R., and Navin, N. (2017). Tumor evolution: Linear, branching, neutral or punctuated? *Biochimica et Biophysica Acta* 1867(2): 151-161. https://doi.org/10.1016/j.bbcan.2017.01.003.

Dawkins, R. (1976). *The Selfish Gene*. New York: Oxford University Press.

Dawson, M. A. (2017). The cancer epigenome: Concepts, challenges, and therapeutic opportunities. *Science* 355: 1147-1152. https://doi.org/10.1126/science.aam7304.

Deacon, T. W. (2006). Emergence: The hole at the wheel's hub. In *The Re-Emergence of Emergence: The Emergentist Hypothesis from Science to Religion* (pp. 111-150), P. Clayton and P. Davies (Eds.). New York: Oxford University Press. https://doi.org/10.1093/acprof:oso/9780199544318.003.0005.

Deacon, B. J. (2013). The biomedical model of mental disorder: A critical analysis of its validity, utility, and effects on psychotherapy research. *Clinical Psychology Review* 33(7): 846-861. https://doi.org/10.1016/j.cpr.2012.09.007.

Deans, C., and Maggert, K. A. (2015) What do you mean, "Epigenetic"? *Genetics* 199: 887-896. https://doi.org/10.1534/genetics.114.173492.

de Araujo, M. (2017). Editing the genome of human being: CRISPR-Cas9 and the ethics of genetic enhancement. *Journal of Ethics and Emerging Technologies* 27(1): 24-42. https://doi.org/10.55613/jeet.v27i1.65.

Deese, J. (1985). *American Freedom and the Social Sciences*. New York: Columbia University Press.

Deguet, J., Demazeau, Y., and Magnin, L. (2006). Elements about the emergence issue: A survey of emergence definitions. *ComPlexUs* 3: 24-31. https://doi.org/10.1159/000094185.

Deichmann, U. (2016). Epigenetics: The origins and evolution of a fashionable topic. *Developmental Biology* 416(1): 249-254. https://doi.org/10.1016/j.ydbio.2016.06.005.

De Klerk, G. J. M. (1979). Mechanism and vitalism: A history of the controversy. *Acta Biotheoretica* 28: 1-10. https://doi.org/10.1007/BF00054676.

DeLanda, M. (2021). *Materialist Phenomenology: A Philosophy of Perception*. London: Bloomsbury.

Delcuve, G. P., Rastegar, M., and Davie, J. R. (2009). Epigenetic control. *Journal of Cellular Physiology* 219(2): 243-250. https://doi.org/10.1002/jcp.21678.

Delker, R. K., and Mann, R. S. (2017). From reductionism to holism: Toward a more complete view of development through genome engineering. In *Precision Medicine, CRISPR, and Genome Engineering: Moving from Association to Biology and Therapeutics* (pp. 45-74), S. H. Tsang (Ed.). Cham, CH: Springer. https://doi.org/10.1007/978-3-319-63904-8_3.

Denny, J. C., and Collins, F. S. (2021). Precision medicine in 2030—Seven ways to transform healthcare. *Cell* 184(6): 1415-1419. https://doi.org/10.1016/j.cell.2021.01.015.

Descartes, R. (1998). *The World and Other Writings*. New York: Cambridge University Press.

Des Chene, D. (2001). *Spirits and Clocks: Machine and Organism in Descartes*. Ithaca, NY: Cornell University Press.

De Solla Price, D. J. (1964). Automata and the origins of mechanism and mechanistic philosophy. *Technology and Culture* 5: 9-23.

Dethier, J., Drion, G., Franci, A., and Sepulchre, R. (2015). A positive feedback at the cellular level promotes robustness and modulation at the circuit level. *Journal of Neurophysiology* 114(4): 2472-2484. https://doi.org/10.1152/jn.00471.2015.

Deutscher, D., Meilijson, I., Schuster, S., and Ruppin, E. (2008). Can single knockouts accurately single out gene functions? *BMC Systems Biology* 2(1): 50. https://doi.org/10.1186/1752-0509-2-50.

Deville, Y., Gilbert, D., van Helden, J., and Wodak, S. J. (2003). An overview of data models for the analysis of biochemical pathways. *Briefings in Bioinformatics* 4: 246-259. https://doi.org/10.1093/bib/4.3.246.

DeWeerdt, S. (2016). Genetics: clues in the code. *Nature* 540(7634): S104-S105. https://doi.org/10.1038/540S104a.

Dhar, P. K., Zhu, H., and Mishra, S. K. (2004). Computational approach to systems biology: From fraction to integration and beyond. *IEEE Transactions on Nanobioscience* 3: 144-152. https://doi.org/10.1109/TNB.2004.833699.

Dicuonzo, G., Galeone, G., Shini, M., and Massari, A. (2022). Towards the use of big data in healthcare: A literature review. *Healthcare* 10: 1232. https://doi.org/10.3390/healthcare10071232.

Diez-Roux, A. V. (2007). Integrating social and biologic factors in health research: A systems view. *Annals of Epidemiology* 17: 569-574. https://doi.org/10.1016/j.annepidem.2007.03.001.

Dijksterhuis, E. J. (1986). *Mechanization of the World Picture: Pythagoras to Newton*. Princeton, NJ: Princeton University Press.

Dinicola, S., D'Anselmi, F., Pasqualato, A., Proietti, S., Lisi, E., Cucina, A., and Bizzarri, M. (2011). A systems biology approach to cancer: Fractals, attractors, and nonlinear dynamics. *Omics: A Journal of Integrative Biology* 15(3): 93-104. https://doi.org/10.1089/omi.2010.0091.

Dizadji-Bahmani, F., Frigg, R., and Hartmann, S. (2010). Who's afraid of Nagelian reduction? *Erkenntnis* 73(3): 393-412. https://doi.org/10.1007/s10670-010-9239-x.

Dolphijn, R., and Van Der Tuin, I. (2012). *New Materialism: Interviews & Cartographies*. Ann Arbor, MI: Open Humanities Press. https://doi.org/10.3998/ohp.11515701.0001.001.

Doob, J. L. (1942). What is a stochastic process? *American Mathematical Monthly* 49(10): 648-653. https://doi.org/10.1080/00029890.1942.11991300.

Dopson, S., Locock, L., Gabbay, J., Ferlie, E., and Fitzgerald, L. (2003). Evidence-based medicine and the implementation gap. *Health* 7(3): 311-330. https://doi.org/10.1177/1363459303007003004.

Dove, G. (2018). Redefining physicalism. *Topoi* 37(3): 513-522. https://doi.org/10.1007/s11245-016-9405-0.

Downie, R. S. (1975). Determinism. *Journal of Medical Ethics* 1(1): 49-50. https://doi.org/10.1136/jme.1.1.49.

Doyle, III, F. J. (2008). Robust control in biology: From genes to cells to systems. *Proceedings of the 17th IFAC World Congress* 17: 3470-3479. https://doi.org/10.3182/20080706-5-KR-1001.00588.

Doyle, J. C., Alderson, D. L., Li, L., Low, S., Roughan, M., Shalunov, S., Tanaka, R., and Willinger, W. (2005). The "robust yet fragile" nature of the Internet. *Proceedings of the National Academy of Sciences USA* 102: 14497-14502. https://doi.org/10.1073/pnas.0501426102.

Drell, D. (2007). The relation of ethics and science: a commentary on "The Study of Socioethical Issues in Systems Biology." *American Journal of Bioethics* 7: 79-80. https://doi.org/10.1080/15265160701221327.

Driesch, H. (1908). *The Science and Philosophy of the Organism*, volume 2. London: Adam and Charles Black.

Du, W., Wang, Y., Luo, Q., and Liu, B. F., (2006). Optimal molecular imaging for systems biology: From molecule to organism. *Analytic and Bioanalytic Chemistry* 386: 444-457. https://doi.org/10.1007/s00216-006-0541-z.

Dubitzky, W. (2016). Computational systems biomedicine. *Briefings in Bioinformatics* 17(3): 367. http://doi.org/10.1093/bib/bbw038.

Dubow, S. (2008). Smuts, the United Nations and the rhetoric of race and rights. *Journal of Contemporary History* 43(1): 45-74. https://doi.org/10.1177/0022009407084557.

Ducheyne, S. (2011). *The Main Business of Natural Philosophy: Isaac Newton's Natural-Philosophical Methodology*. New York: Springer. https://doi.org/10.1007/978-94-007-2126-5.

Duffin, J. M. (1986). The medical philosophy of R. T. H. Laennec (1781-1826). *History and Philosophy of the Life Sciences* 8: 195-219. http://www.jstor.org/stable/23328661.

Duffy, D. J. (2016). Problems, challenges and promises: Perspectives on precision medicine. *Briefings in Bioinformatics* 17(3): 494-504. https://doi.org/10.1093/bib/bbv060.

Duijndam, S., and Denollet, J. (2019). Social inhibition in population-based and cardiac patient samples: Robustness of inhibition, sensitivity and withdrawal as distinct facets. *General Hospital Psychiatry* 58: 13-23. https://doi.org/10.1016/j.genhosppsych.2019.02.004.

Dupré, J. (1993). *The Disorder of Things: Metaphysical Foundations of the Disunity of Science*. Cambridge, MA: Harvard University Press.

Dupré, J. (2020). Life as process. *Epistemology & Philosophy of Science* 57(2): 96-113. https://doi.org/10.5840/eps202057224.

Dyson, F. (1999). *Origins of Life*, 2nd edition. New York: Cambridge University Press.

Earman, J. (1986). *A Primer on Determinism*. Dordrecht, NL: Reidel.

Eberl, G. (2018). Robustness in living organisms is homeostasis. *Seminars in Immunology* 36: 56-57. https://doi.org/10.1016/j.smim.2017.12.007.

Edwards, D., Forster, J. W., Chagné, D., and Batley, J. (2007). What Are SNPs? In N. C. Oraguzie, E. H. A. Rikkerink, S. E. Gardiner, and H. N. De Silva (Eds.), *Association*

Mapping in Plants, (pp. 41-52). New York: Springer. https://doi.org/10.1007/978-0-387-36011-9_3.

Efroni, S. (2013). Introducing Systems Biomedicine. *Systems Biomedicine* 1(1): 1. http://doi.org/10.4161/sysb.26099.

Egger, G., Liang, G., Aparicio, A., and Jones, P. A. (2004). Epigenetics in human disease and prospects for epigenetic therapy. *Nature* 429(6990): 457-463. https://doi.org/10.1038/nature02625.

Eils, R., and Athale, C. (2003). Computational imaging in cell biology. *Journal of Cell Biology* 161: 477-481. https://doi.org/10.1083/jcb.200302097.

Elder-Vass, D. (2005). Emergence and the realist account of cause. *Journal of Critical Realism* 4(2): 315-338. https://doi.org/10.1558/jocr.v4i2.315.

El-Hani, C. N. (2007). Between the cross and the sword: The crisis of the gene concept. *Genetics and Molecular Biology* 30: 297-307. https://doi.org/10.1590/S1415-47572007000300001.

El-Hani, C. N., and Emmeche, C. (2000). On some theoretical grounds for an organism-centered biology: Property emergence, supervenience, and downward causation. *Theory in Biosciences* 119: 234-275. https://doi.org/10.1007/s12064-000-0018-0.

Ellis, G. F. R. (2005a). Physics and the real world. *Physics Today* 58: 49-54. https://doi.org/10.1063/1.2012463.

Ellis, G. F. R. (2005b). Physics, complexity and causality. *Nature* 435: 743. https://doi.org/10.1038/435743a.

Ellis, G. F. R. (2006). On the nature of emergent reality. In *The Re-Emergence of Emergence: The Emergentist Hypothesis from Science to Religion* (pp. 79-107), P. Clayton and P. Davies (Eds.). New York: Oxford University Press. https://doi.org/10.1093/acprof:oso/9780199544318.003.0004.

Ellis, G. F. R. (2020). The causal closure of physics in real world contexts. *Foundations of Physics* 50(10): 1057-1097. https://doi.org/10.1007/s10701-020-00366-0.

Ellis, G. F., and Kopel, J. (2019). The dynamical emergence of biology from physics: Branching causation via biomolecules. *Frontiers in Physiology* 9: 1966. https://doi.org/10.3389/fphys.2018.01966.

Elpidorou, A. (2018). Introduction: The character of physicalism. *Topoi* 37(3): 435-455. https://doi.org/10.1007/s11245-017-9488-2.

Elsassar, W. M. (1998). *Reflections on a Theory of Organisms: Holism in Biology.* Baltimore, MD: The Johns Hopkins University Press.

Emerich, D. F., and Thanos, C. G. (2003). Nanotechnology and medicine. *Expert Opinion on Biological Therapy* 3(4): 655-663. https://doi.org/10.1517/14712598.3.4.655.

Emerson, A. E. (1954). Dynamic homeostasis: a unifying principle in organic, social, and ethical evolution. *Scientific Monthly* 78: 67-85. http://www.jstor.org/stable/21188.

Emmeche, C., Køppe, S., and Stjernfelt, F., (2000). Levels, emergence, and three versions of downward causation. In *Downward Causation: Minds, Bodies, and Matter* (pp. 13-34), P. B. Andersen, C. Emmeche, N. O. Finnemann, and P. V. Christiansen (Eds.). Oakville, CN: Aarhus University Press.

Emmert-Streib, F., Tripathi, S., Simoes, R. D. M., Hawwa, A. F., and Dehmer, M. (2013). The human disease network: Opportunities for classification, diagnosis, and prediction of disorders and disease genes. *Systems Biomedicine* 1(1): 20-28. http://doi.org/10.4161/sysb.22816.

Endler, J. A. (1982). Alternative hypotheses in biogeography: Introduction and synopsis of the symposium. *American Zoologist* 22(2): 349-354. https://doi.org/10.1093/icb/22.2.349.

Engel, G. L. (1977). The need for a new medical model: A challenge for biomedicine. *Science* 196(4286): 129-136. https://doi.org/10.1126/science.847460.

Engen, S., Wright, J., Araya-Ajoy, Y. G., and Sæther, B. E. (2020). Phenotypic evolution in stochastic environments: The contribution of frequency-and density-dependent selection. *Evolution* 74(9): 1923-1941. https://doi.org/10.1111/evo.14058.

Epstein, R. J. (2003). *Human Molecular Biology: An Introduction to the Molecular Basis of Health and Disease*. New York: Cambridge University Press.

Esfeld, M. (1999). Physicalism and ontological holism. *Metaphilosophy* 30: 319-337. https://doi.org/10.1111/1467-9973.00141.

Esfeld, M. (2008). Cartwright on wholism. In *Nancy Cartwright's Philosophy of Science* (pp. 324-338), S. Hartmann, C. Hoefer, and L. Bovens (Eds.). New York: Routledge.

Esfeld, M. (2009). Philosophical holism. In *Unity of Knowledge in Transdisciplinary Research for Sustainability* (pp. 110-127), G. H. Hardon (Ed.). Oxford, UK: Eolss Publishers.

Eskov, V. M., Khadartsev, A. A., Eskov, V. V., Filatova, O. E., and Filatova, D. U. (2013). Chaotic approach in biomedicine: Individualized medical treatment. *Journal of Biomedical Science and Engineering* 6(8): 35655. https://doi.org/10.4236/jbise.2013.68103.

Eskov, V. M., Filatova, O. E., Eskov, V. V., and Gavrilenko, T. V. (2017). The evolution of the idea of homeostasis: Determinism, stochastics, and chaos—self-organization. *Biophysics* 62(5): 809-820. https://doi.org/10.1134/S0006350917050074.

Estrada, E., and Knight, P. (2015). *A First Course in Network Theory*. New York: Oxford University Press.

Ewis, A. A., Zhelev, Z., Bakalova, R., Fukuoka, S., Shinohara, Y., Ishikawa, M., and Baba, Y. (2005). A history of microarrays in biomedicine. *Expert Review of Molecular Diagnostics* 5(3): 315-328. http://dx.doi.org/10.1586/14737159.5.3.315.

Fairman, K. A. (2022). Pandemics, policy, and the power of paradigm: Will COVID-19 lead to a new scientific revolution? *Annals of Epidemiology* 69: 17-23. https://doi.org/10.1016/j.annepidem.2022.02.005.

Falzer, P. R. (2021). Evidence-based medicine's curious path: From clinical epidemiology to patient-centered care through decision analysis. *Journal of Evaluation in Clinical Practice* 27(3): 631-637. https://doi.org/10.1111/jep.13466.

Fang, F. C., and Casadevall, A. (2011). Reductionistic and holistic science. *Infection and Immunity* 79(4): 1401-1404. https://doi.org/10.1128/iai.01343-10.

Fangerau, H., and Badura-Lotter, G. (2019). Biomedicine and bioethics. In *Handbook of Popular Culture and Biomedicine* (pp. 41-55), A. Görgen, G. Nunez, and H. Fangerau (Eds.). Cham, CH: Springer. https://doi.org/10.1007/978-3-319-90677-5_4.

Fanos, V. (2016). *Metabolomics and Microbiomics: Personalized Medicine from the Fetus to the Adult*. New York: Academic Press.

Faratian, D., Clyde, R. G., Crawford, J. W., and Harrison, D. J. (2009). Systems pathology—taking molecular pathology into a new dimension. *Nature Reviews Clinical Oncology* 6(8): 455-464. https://doi.org/10.1038/nrclinonc.2009.102.

Farnsworth, K. D., Ellis, G. F. R., and Jaeger, L. (2017). Living through downward causation: From molecules to ecosystems. In *From Matter to Life: Information and Causality* (pp. 303-333), S. I. Walker, P. C. W. Davies, and G. F. R. Ellis (Eds.). New York: Cambridge University Press.

Farre, A., and Rapley, T. (2017). The new old (and old new) medical model: Four decades navigating the biomedical and psychosocial understandings of health and illness. *Healthcare* 5(4): 88. https://doi.org/10.3390/healthcare5040088.

Fearon, E. R., and Vogelstein, B. (1990). A genetic model for colorectal tumorigenesis. *Cell* 61(5): 759-767. https://doi.org/10.1016/0092-8674(90)90186-I.

Feero, W. G., and Guttmacher, A. E. (2014). Genomics, personalized medicine, and pediatrics. *Academic Pediatrics* 14(1): 14-22. https://doi.org/10.1016/j.acap.2013.06.008.

Federoff, H. J., and Gostin, L. O. (2009). Evolving from reductionism to holism: Is there a future for systems medicine? *Journal of the American Medical Association* 302(9): 994-996. https://doi.org/10.1001/jama.2009.1264.

Feil, R. (2008). Epigenetics, an emerging discipline with broad implications. *C.R. Biologies* 331: 837-843. https://doi.org/10.1016/j.crvi.2008.07.027.

Feinberg, A. P. (2014). Epigenetic stochasticity, nuclear structure and cancer: the implications for medicine. *Journal of Internal Medicine* 276(1): 5-11. https://doi.org/10.1111/joim.12224.

Feinberg, T. E., and Mallatt, J. (2016). The nature of primary consciousness. A new synthesis. *Consciousness and Cognition* 4:113-127. https://doi.org/10.1016/j.concog.2016.05.009.

Feinberg, A. P., Koldobskiy, M. A., and Göndör, A. (2016). Epigenetic modulators, modifiers and mediators in cancer aetiology and progression. *Nature Reviews Genetics* 17(5): 284-299. https://doi.org/10.1038/nrg.2016.13.

Felsenfeld, G. (2014). A brief history of epigenetics. *Cold Spring Harbor Perspectives in Biology* 6(1): a018200. https://doi.org/10.1101/cshperspect.a018200.

Félix, M. A., and Barkoulas, M. (2015). Pervasive robustness in biological systems. *Nature Reviews Genetics* 16(8): 483-496. https://doi.org/10.1038/nrg3949.

Fell, D. A. (2005). Metabolic control analysis. In *Systems Biology: Definitions and Perspectives* (pp. 69-80), L. Alberghina and H. Westerhoff (Eds.). Berlin: Springer. https://doi.org/10.1007/b137745 69-80.

Fernald, G. H., Capriotti, E., Daneshjou, R., Karczewski, K. J., and Altman, R. B. (2011). Bioinformatics challenges for personalized medicine. *Bioinformatics* 27(13): 1741-1748. https://doi.org/10.1093/bioinformatics/btr295.

Fernández, N., Maldonado, C., and Gershenson, C. (2014). Information measures of complexity, emergence, self-organization, homeostasis, and autopoiesis. In *Guided self-organization: Inception* (pp. 19-51), M. Prokopenko (Ed.). Berlin: Springer. https://doi.org/10.1007/978-3-642-53734-9_2.

Fernandez-Leon, J. A. (2014). Robustness as a non-localizable relational phenomenon. *Biological Reviews* 89(3), 552-567. https://doi.org/10.1111/brv.12067.

Ferrara, S. D. (2017). P5 medicine and justice: The future is now. *International Journal of Legal Medicine* 131(4): 897-899. https://doi.org/10.1007/s00414-017-1624-4.

Ferrell, Jr., J. E. (2009). Systems biology. *Journal of Biology* 8: 2. https://doi.org/10.1186/jbiol107.

Feyerabend, P. K. (1962). Explanation, reduction, and empiricism. In *Scientific Explanation, Space, and Time* (pp. 28-97), M. Feigl and G. Maxwell (Eds.). Minneapolis, MN: University of Minnesota Press.

Findlay, S. D., and Thagard, P. (2012). How parts make up wholes. *Frontiers in Physiology* 3: 455. https://doi.org/10.3389/fphys.2012.00455.

Finkelstein, A., Hetherington, J., Li, L., Margoninski, O., Saffrey, P., Seymour, R., and Warner, A. (2004). Computational challenges of systems biology. *Computer* 37: 26-33. https://doi.org/10.1109/MC.2004.1297236.

Flack, J. C. (2017). Coarse-graining as a downward causation mechanism. *Philosophical Transactions of the Royal Society A: Mathematical, Physical and Engineering Sciences* 375(2109): 20160338. https://doi.org/10.1098/rsta.2016.0338.

Flatt, T. (2005). The evolutionary genetics of canalization. *Quarterly Review of Biology* 80(3): 287-316. https://doi.org/10.1086/432265.

Fleming, D. (1984). Walter B. Cannon and homeostasis. *Social Research* 51: 609-640. https://www.jstor.org/stable/40970955.

Fleßa, S., Thum, C., Raths, S., Fischer, T., Erdmann, P., and Langanke, M. (2016). Systems medicine: Hype or revolution? *Personalized Medicine* 13(5): 441-453. https://doi.org/10.2217/pme-2016-0039.

Fletcher, J. M. (1921). Geneticism as a heuristic principle in psychology. *Journal of Philosophy* 18(16): 421-433. https://doi.org/10.2307/2939317.

Floridi, L. (2016). On human dignity as a foundation for the right to privacy. *Philosophy & Technology* 29(4): 307-312. https://doi.org/10.1007/s13347-016-0220-8.

Floyd, R. L., and Carson, E. R. (1993). *Dealing with Complexity: An Introduction to the Theory and Application of Systems Science*, 2nd edition. New York: Springer. https://doi.org/10.1007/978-1-4757-2235-2.

Foo, J., Leder, K., and Michor, F. (2011). Stochastic dynamics of cancer initiation. *Physical Biology* 8(1): 015002. http://dx.doi.org/10.1088/1478-3975/8/1/015002.

Forster, A. C., and Church, G. M. (2006). Towards synthesis of a minimal cell. *Molecular Systems Biology* 2: e45. https://doi.org/10.1038/msb4100090.

Foss, L. (2002). *The End of Modern Medicine: Biomedical Science under a Microscope*. New York: SUNY Press.

Foster, M. W. (2007). Everything old is new again, including systems biology. *American Journal of Bioethics* 7: 85-86. https://doi.org/10.1080/15265160701221350.

Fowler, S., Roush, R., and Wise, J. (2017). *Concepts of Biology*. Houston, TX: OpenStax.

Fox, K. (2020). The illusion of inclusion—The "All of Us" research program and indigenous peoples' DNA. *New England Journal of Medicine* 383(5): 411-413. https://doi.org/10.1056/NEJMp1915987.

Fox, N. J., and Alldred, P. (2018) New materialism. In: *The SAGE Encyclopedia of Research Methods*, P. Atkinson, S. Delamont, A. Cernat, J. W. Sakshaug, and R. A. Williams (Eds.). London: SAGE. http://dx.doi.org/10.4135/9781526421036768465.

Freeman, M. (2000). Feedback control of intercellular signaling in development. *Nature* 408: 313-319. https://doi.org/10.1038/35042500.

Freire, S. L. S., and Wheeler, A. R. (2006). Proteome-on-a-chip: Mirage, or on the horizon? *Lab on a Chip* 6: 1415-1423. http://dx.doi.org/10.1039/B609871A.

Friboulet, A., and Thomas, D. (2005). Systems biology—an interdisciplinary approach. *Biosensors and Bioelectronics* 20: 2404-2407. https://doi.org/10.1016/j.bios. 2004.11.014.

Friedlander, T., Mayo, A. E., Tlusty, T., and Alon, U. (2015). Evolution of bow-tie architectures in biology. *PLoS Computational Biology* 11(3): e1004055. https://doi.org/10.1371/ journal.pcbi.1004055.

Friedman, A. A., Letai, A., Fisher, D. E., and Flaherty, K. T. (2015). Precision medicine for cancer with next-generation functional diagnostics. *Nature Reviews Cancer* 15(12): 747-756. https://doi.org/10.1038/nrc4015.

Fujiwara, M., and Takada, T. (2017). Environmental stochasticity. In *eLS*, Chichester, UK: John Wiley & Sons. http://doi.org/10.1002/9780470015902.a0021220.pub2.

Fuller, J. (2017). The new medical model: A renewed challenge for biomedicine. *Canadian Medical Association Journal* 189(17): E640-E641. https://doi.org/10.1503/ cmaj.160627.

Funkhouser, E. (2002). Three varieties of causal overdetermination. *Pacific Philosophical Quarterly* 83(4): 335-351. https://doi.org/10.1111/1468-0114.00154.

Gagliasso, E. (2003). The metamorphosis of holism. In *Determinism, Holism, and Complexity* (pp. 339-348), V. Benci, P. Cerrai, P. Freguglia, G. Israel, and C. Pellegrini (Eds.). New York: Plenum.

Gaines, A. D., and Davis-Floyd, R. (2004). On biomedicine. In *Encyclopedia of Medical Anthropology* (pp. 95-109), C. Ember and M. Ember (Eds.). Boston, MA: Springer. https://doi.org/10.1007/0-387-29905-X_11.

Gallagher, R., and Appenzeller, T. (1999). Beyond reductionism. *Science* 284: 79. https://doi.org/10.1126/science.284.5411.79.

Galperin, M., and Ellison, M. J. (2006). Systems biology: Sprint or marathon? *Current Opinion in Biotechnology* 17: 437-439. https://doi.org/10.1016/j.copbio.2006.08.008.

Gamble, C. N., Hanan, J. S., and Nail, T. (2019). What is new materialism? *Angelaki* 24(6): 111-134. https://doi.org/10.1080/0969725X.2019.1684704.

Gannett, L. (2008). The Human Genome Project. In *Stanford Encyclopedia of Philosophy,* E. N. Zalta (Ed.). https://plato.stanford.edu/entries/human-genome/.

Gánti, T. (2003). *The Principles of Life*. New York: Oxford University Press. https://doi.org/10.1093/acprof:oso/9780198507260.001.0001.

Gao, X., Yang, L., Petros, J. A., Marshall, F. F., Simons, J. W., and Nie, S. (2005). In vivo molecular and cellular imaging with quantum dots. *Current Opinion in Biotechnology* 16: 63-72. https://doi.org/10.1016/j.copbio.2004.11.003.

Garavand, A., and Aslani, N. (2022). Metaverse phenomenon and its impact on health: A scoping review. *Informatics in Medicine Unlocked* 32: 101029. https://doi.org/ 10.1016/j.imu.2022.101029.

Garber, D. (2002). Descartes, mechanics, and the mechanical philosophy. *Midwest Studies in Philosophy* 26: 185-204. https://doi.org/10.1111/1475-4975.261061.

Garcia, R. (2014). Closing in on causal closure. *Journal of Consciousness Studies* 21(1-2): 96-109.

Garrett, L. (1994) *The Coming Plague: Newly Emerging Diseases in a World Out of Balance*. New York: Farrar, Straus and Giroux.

Gatenby, R., and Brown, J. (2018). The evolution and ecology of resistance in cancer therapy. *Cold Spring Harbor Perspectives in Medicine* 8(3): a033415. https://doi.org/10.1101/cshperspect.a033415.

Gatherer, D. (2010). So what do we really mean when we say that systems biology is holistic? *BMC Systems Biology* 4(1): 22. https://doi.org/10.1186/1752-0509-4-22.

Gaukroger, S. (2006). *The Emergence of a Scientific Culture: Science and the Shaping of Modernity, 1210-1685*. Oxford: Clarendon Press.

Gawande, A. (2002). *Complications: A Surgeon's Notes on an Imperfect Science*. New York: Picador.

Geronikolou, S. A., Pavlopoulou, A., Cokkinos, D., and Chrousos, G. (2017). Interactome of obesity: Obesidome: Genetic obesity, stress induced obesity, pathogenic obesity interaction. In *GeNeDis 2016: Genetics and Neurodegeneration* (pp. 233-241), P. Vlamos (Ed.). Cham, CH: Springer. https://doi.org/10.1007/978-3-319-57379-3_21.

Gershon, E. S., and Goldin, L. R. (1986). Clinical methods in psychiatric genetics: I. Robustness of genetic marker investigative strategies. *Acta Psychiatrica Scandinavica* 74(2): 113-118. https://doi.org/10.1111/j.1600-0447.1986.tb10594.x.

Ghaemi, S. N. (2017). Biomedical reductionist, humanist, and biopsychosocial models in medicine. In *Handbook of the Philosophy of Medicine* (pp. 773-791), T. Scharamme and S. Edwards (Eds.). Amsterdam, NL: Springer. https://doi.org/10.1007/978-94-017-8706-2_38-1.

Ghosh Roy, G., He, S., Geard, N., and Verspoor, K. (2021). Bow-tie architecture of gene regulatory networks in species of varying complexity. *Journal of the Royal Society Interface* 18(179): 20210069. https://doi.org/10.1098/rsif.2021.0069.

Gibb, S. (2015). The causal closure principle. *Philosophical Quarterly* 65(261): 626-647. https://doi.org/10.1093/pq/pqv030.

Gibson, G., and Lacek, K. A. (2020). Canalization and robustness in human genetics and disease. *Annual Review of Genetics* 54: 189-211. https://doi.org/10.1146/annurev-genet-022020- 022327.

Gilbert, S. F., and Sarkar, S. (2000). Embracing complexity: Organicism for the 21st century. *Developmental Dynamics* 219: 1-9. https://doi.org/10.1002/1097-0177(2000)9999:9999<::AID-DVDY1036>3.0.CO;2-A.

Gillett, C. (2006). Samuel Alexander's emergentism: Or, higher causation for physicalists. *Synthese* 153: 261-296. https://doi.org/10.1007/s11229-005-5470-4.

Gillett, C. (2016). *Reduction and Emergence in Science and Philosophy*. New York: Cambridge University Press.

Gillett, C., and Loewer, B. (Eds.). (2001). *Physicalism and its Discontents*. New York: Cambridge University Press.

Ginsburg, G. S., and McCarthy, J. J. (2001). Personalized medicine: Revolutionizing drug discovery and patient care. *TRENDS in Biotechnology* 19(12): 491-496. https://doi.org/10.1016/S0167-7799(01)01814-5.

Ginsburg, G. S., and Phillips, K. A. (2018). Precision medicine: From science to value. *Health Affairs* 37(5): 694-701. https://doi.org/10.1377/hlthaff.2017.1624.

Giroux, É. (2020). Is personalized medicine humanist? *Archives de Philosophie* 83(4): 59-82. https://doi.org/10.3917/aphi.834.0059.

Givens, P., and Reiss, M. J. (2002). *Human Biology and Health Studies*, 2nd edition. Cheltenham, UK: Nelson Thornes.

Gjuvsland, A. B., Vik, J. O., Beard, D. A., Hunter, P. J., and Omholt, S. W. (2013). Bridging the genotype–phenotype gap: what does it take? *Journal of Physiology* 591(8): 2055-2066. https://doi.org/10.1113/jphysiol.2012.248864.

Glauer, R. D. (2012). *Emergent Mechanisms: Reductive Explanation for Limited Beings.* Münster, DE: Mentis.

Glennan, S. (1996). Mechanism and the nature of causation. *Erkenntnis* 44: 49-71. https://doi.org/10.1007/BF00172853.

Glennan, S. (2002). Rethinking mechanistic explanation. *Philosophy of Science* 69: S342-S353. https://doi.org/10.1086/341857.

Glennan, S. (2017). *The New Mechanical Philosophy.* New York: Oxford University Press. https://doi.org/10.1093/oso/9780198779711.001.0001.

Goetz, L. H., and Schork, N. J. (2018). Personalized medicine: Motivation, challenges, and progress. *Fertility and Sterility* 109(6): 952-963. https://doi.org/10.1016/j.fertnstert.2018.05.006.

Goh, K. I., and Choi, I. G. (2012). Exploring the human diseasome: The human disease network. *Briefings in Functional Genomics* 11(6): 533-542. https://doi.org/10.1093/bfgp/els032.

Gohar, F., Maschmeyer, P., Mfarrej, B., Lemaire, M., Wedderburn, L. R., Roncarolo, M. G., and van Royen-Kerkhof, A. (2019). Driving medical innovation through interdisciplinarity: Unique opportunities and challenges. *Frontiers in Medicine* 6: 35. https://doi.org/10.3389/fmed.2019.00035.

Goldberg, B. (2017). Epigenesis and the rationality of nature in William Harvey and Margaret Cavendish. *History and Philosophy of the Life Sciences, 39*(2): 8. https://doi.org/10.1007/s40656-017-0134-5.

Goldberger, A. L. (1996). Non-linear dynamics for clinicians: Chaos theory, fractals, and complexity at the bedside. *Lancet* 347(9011): 1312-1314. https://doi.org/10.1016/S0140-6736(96)90948-4.

Goldberger, A. L. (2001). Heartbeats, hormones, and health: Is variability the spice of life? *American Journal of Respiratory and Critical Care Medicine* 163(6): 1289-1290. https://doi.org/10.1164/ajrccm.163.6.ed1801a.

Goldstein, J. (1999). Emergence as a construct: History and issues. *Emergence* 1: 49-72. https://doi.org/10.1207/s15327000em0101_4.

Golubewa, L., Rehman, H., Kulahava, T., Karpicz, R., Baah, M., Kaplas, T., Shah, A., Malykhin, S., Obraztsov, A., Rutkauskas, D., and Jankunec, M. (2020). Macro-, micro- and nano-roughness of carbon-based interface with the living cells: Towards a versatile bio-sensing platform. *Sensors* 20(18): 5028. https://doi.org/10.3390/s20185028.

Gouw, A. M. (2018). Challenging the therapy/enhancement distinction in CRISPR gene editing. In *The Palgrave Handbook of Philosophy and Public Policy* (pp. 493-508).

D. Boonin (Ed.), Cham, CH: Palgrave Macmillan. https://doi.org/10.1007/978-3-319-93907-0_38.

Goy, I. (2018). Was Aristotle the 'father' of the epigenesis doctrine? *History and Philosophy of the Life Sciences* 40(2): 28. https://doi.org/10.1007/s40656-018-0193-2.

GRADE Working Group. (2004). Grading quality of evidence and strength of recommendations. *British Medical Journal* 328(7454): 1490-1494. https://doi.org/10.1136/bmj.328.7454.1490.

Green, S. (2017). Philosophy of systems and synthetic biology. In *Stanford Encyclopedia of Philosophy,* E. N. Zalta (Ed.). *https://plato.stanford.edu/entries/systems-synthetic-biology/.*

Green, S. (2018). Scale dependency and downward causation in biology. *Philosophy of Science* 85(5): 998-1011. https://doi.org/10.1086/699758.

Greenhalgh, T. (2018). *How to Implement Evidence-Based Healthcare.* Hoboken, NJ: John Wiley & Sons.

Greenhalgh, T. (2020). Will COVID-19 be evidence-based medicine's nemesis? *PLoS Medicine* 17(6): e1003266. https://doi.org/10.1371/journal.pmed.1003266.

Greenhalgh, T., Howick, J., and Maskrey, N. (2014). Evidence based medicine: A movement in crisis? *British Medical Journal* 348: g3725. https://doi.org/10.1136/bmj.g3725.

Greenhalgh, T., Schmid, M. B., Czypionka, T., Bassler, D., and Gruer, L. (2020). Face masks for the public during the COVID-19 crisis. *British Medical Journal* 369: 1-4. https://doi.org/10.1136/bmj.m1435.

Greenhalgh, T., Fisman, D., Cane, D. J., Oliver, M., and Macintyre, C. R. (2022). Adapt or die: How the pandemic made the shift from EBM to EBM+ more urgent. *BMJ Evidence-Based Medicine* 27(5): 253-260. http://dx.doi.org/10.1136/bmjebm-2022-111952.

Gregersen, N. H. (2006). Emergence and complexity. In *The Oxford Handbook of Religion and Science* (pp. 767-783), P. Clayton (Ed.). New York: Oxford University Press. https://doi.org/10.1093/oxfordhb/9780199543656.003.0046.

Gregory, F. (1977). *Scientific Materialism in Nineteenth Century Germany.* Dordrecht, NL: Reidel. https://doi.org/10.1007/978-94-010-1173-0.

Griffiths, P. E., and Stotz, K. (2006). Genes in the postgenomic era. *Theoretical Medicine and Bioethics* 27: 499-521. https://doi.org/10.1007/s11017-006-9020-y.

Griffiths, A. J. F., Gelbart, W. M., Miller, J. H., and Lewontin, R. C. (1999). *Modern Genetic Analysis.* New York: W.H. Freeman.

Grigoriu, M. D. (2021). *Linear Dynamical Systems.* Cham, CH: Springer. https://doi.org/10.1007/978-3-030-64552-6.

Gronowski, A. M., and Budelier, M. M. (2020). The ethics of direct-to-consumer testing. *Clinics in Laboratory Medicine 40*(1): 93-103. https://doi.org/10.1016/j.cll.2019.11.001.

Grossman, J., and Mackenzie, F. J. (2005). The randomized controlled trial: Gold standard, or merely standard? *Perspectives in Biology and Medicine* 48(4): 516-534. https://doi.org/10.1353/pbm.2005.0092.

Grosz, E. (2017). *The Incorporeal: Ontology, Ethics, and the Limits of Materialism*. New York: Columbia University Press.

Grundeis, F., Ansems, K., Dahms, K., Thieme, V., Metzendorf, M. I., Skoetz, N., Benstoem, C., Mikolajewska, A., Griesel, M., Fichtner, F. and Stegemann, M. (2023). Remdesivir for the treatment of COVID-19. *Cochrane Database of Systematic Reviews* Issue 1: CD014962. https://doi.org/10.1002/14651858.CD014962.pub.

Guchet, X. (2022). Exposomics in the era of personalized medicine: A critical analysis. In *Personalized Medicine in the Making: Philosophical Perspectives from Biology to Healthcare* (pp. 207-225), C. Beneduce and M. Bertolaso (Eds.). Cham, CH: Springer. https://doi.org/10.1007/978-3-030-74804-3_11.

Guicciardini, N. (2009). *Isaac Newton on Mathematical Certainty and Method*. Cambridge, MA: MIT Press.

Guilger-Casagrande, M., De Barros, C. T., Antunes, V. A., De Araujo, D. R., Lima, R. (2021). Perspectives and challenges in the fight against COVID-19: The role of genetic variability. *Frontiers in Cellular and Infection Microbiology* 11: 598875. https://doi.org/10.3389/fcimb.2021.598875.

Gustafsson, M., Nestor, C. E., Zhang, H., Barabási, A. L., Baranzini, S., Brunak, S., Chung, K. F., Federoff, H. J., Gavin, A. C., Meehan, R. R., and Picotti, P. (2014). Modules, networks and systems medicine for understanding disease and aiding diagnosis. *Genome Medicine* 6: 82. https://doi.org/10.1186/s13073-014-0082-6.

Guthrie, W. K. C. (1965). *A History of Greek Philosophy: Volume II, The Presocratic Tradition from Parmenides to Democritus*. New York: Cambridge University Press.

Guyatt, G., Cairns, J., Churchill, D., Cook, D., Haynes, B., Hirsh, J., Irvine, J., Levine, M., Levine, M., Nishikawa, J., and Sackett, D. (1992). Evidence-based medicine: A new approach to teaching the practice of medicine. *Journal of American Medical Association* 268(17): 2420-2425. https://doi.org/10.1001/jama.1992.03490170092032.

Guyatt, G. H., Oxman, A. D., Kunz, R., Vist, G. E., Falck-Ytter, Y., and Schünemann, H. (2008). GRADE: What is "quality of evidence" and why is it important to clinicians? *British Medical Journal* 336(7651): 995-998. https://doi.org/10.1136/bmj.39490.551019.BE.

Guyatt, G. H., Rennie, D., Meade, M. O., Cook, D. J. (Eds.). (2015). *Users' Guides to the Medical Literature: Essentials of Evidence-Based Clinical Practice*, 3rd edition. New York: McGraw-Hill. https://doi.org/10.1036/0071590382.

Guyton, A. C., and Hall, J. E. (2005) *Textbook of Medical Physiology*, 11th edition. Philadelphia, PA: W.B. Saunders Company.

Hacking, I. (1983). Nineteenth century cracks in the concept of determinism. *Journal of the History of Ideas* 44(3): 455-475. https://doi.org/10.2307/2709176.

Hackshaw, A. (2009). *A Concise Guide to Clinical Trials*. Hoboken, NJ: John Wiley & Sons.

Häfner, S. J., and Lund, A. H. (2016). Great expectations–Epigenetics and the meandering path from bench to bedside. *Biomedical Journal* 39(3): 166-176. https://doi.org/10.1016/j.bj.2016.01.008.

Hagen, J. B. (2021). *Life Out of Balance: Homeostasis and Adaptation in a Darwinian World*. Tuscaloosa, AL: University of Alabama Press.

Haidt, J. (2007). The new synthesis in moral psychology. *Science* 316(5827): 998-1002. https://doi.org/10.1126/science.1137651.

Hájek, A. (2007). The reference class problem is your problem too. *Synthese 156*(3): 563-585. https://doi.org/10.1007/s11229-006-9138-5.

Haken, H. (2020). *Synergetics*, 2nd edition. New York: Springer. https://doi.org/10.1007/978-1-0716-0421-2.

Haleem, A., Javaid, M., Singh, R. P., and Suman, R. (2022). Medical 4.0 technologies for healthcare: Features, capabilities, and applications. *Internet of Things and Cyber-Physical Systems* 2: 12-30. https://doi.org/10.1016/j.iotcps.2022.04.001.

Hall, T. S. (1975a). *History of General Physiology: 600 B.C. to A.D. 1900. Volume 1: From Pre-Socratic Times to the Enlightenment*. Chicago, IL; University of Chicago Press.

Hall, T. S. (1975b). *History of General Physiology: 600 B.C. to A.D. 1900. Volume 2: From the Enlightenment to the End of the Nineteenth Century*. Chicago, IL; University of Chicago Press.

Hall, C. W. (1995). *The Age of Synthesis: A Treatise and Sourcebook*. New York: Peter Lang.

Hammerstein, P., Hagen, E. H., Herz, A. V. M., and Herzel, H. (2006). Robustness: A key to evolutionary design. *Biological Theory* 1: 90-93. https://doi.org/10.1162/biot.2006.1.1.90.

Hanahan, D., and Weinberg, R. A. (2000). The hallmarks of cancer. *Cell* 100: 57-70. https://doi.org/10.1016/S0092-8674(00)81683-9.

Hannaway, C., and La Berge, A. (Eds.). (1998). *Constructing Paris Medicine*. Amsterdam, NL: Rodopi.

Hannezo, E., and Heisenberg, C. P. (2019). Mechanochemical feedback loops in development and disease. *Cell* 178(1): 12-25. https://doi.org/10.1016/j.cell.2019.05.052.

Hansen, C. H., Endres, R. G., and Wingreen, N. S. (2008). Chemotaxis in *Escherichia coli*: A molecular model for precise adaptation. *PLoS Computational Biology* 4: 14-27. https://doi.org/10.1371/journal.pcbi.0040001.

Hanson, B. G. (1995). *General Systems Theory Beginning with Wholes*. Washington, DC: Taylor & Francis.

Hao, T., Ma, H. W., Zhao, X. M., and Goryanin, I. (2012). The reconstruction and analysis of tissue specific human metabolic networks. *Molecular BioSystems* 8(2): 663-670. https://doi.org/10.1039/C1MB05369H.

Hara, N., Solomon, P., Kim, S. L., and Sonnenwald, D. H. (2003). An emerging view of scientific collaboration: Scientists' perspectives on collaboration and factors that impact collaboration. *Journal of the American Society for Information Science and Technology* 54(10): 952-965. https://doi.org/10.1002/asi.10291.

Haraway, D. J. (1976). *Crystals, Fabrics, and Fields: Metaphors of Organicism in Twentieth-Century Developmental Biology*. New Haven, CT: Yale University Press.

Harel, D. (2003). A grand challenge for computing: Towards full reactive modeling of a multi-cellular animal. *Bulletin of the European Association for Theoretical Computer Science* 81: 226-235.

Hartgerink, J. D., Beniash, E., and Stupp, S. I. (2001). Self-assembly and mineralization of peptide-amphiphile nanofibers. *Science* 294: 1684-1688. https://doi.org/10.1126/science.1063187.

Harvey, W. (1989) *The Works of William Harvey*, R. Willis, trans. Philadelphia, PA: University of Pennsylvania Press.

Heams, T. (2014). Randomness in biology. *Mathematical Structures in Computer Science* 24(3): e240308. https://doi.org/10.1017/S096012951200076X.

Heil, J. (2017). Downward causation. In *Philosophical and Scientific Perspectives on Downward Causation* (pp. 42-53), M.P. Paoletti and F. Orilla (Eds.). New York: Routledge.

Hein, H. (1969). Molecular biology vs. organicism: The enduring dispute between mechanism and vitalism. *Synthese* 20: 238-253. https://doi.org/10.1007/BF00413789.

Heine, S. J., Dar-Nimrod, I., Cheung, B. Y., and Proulx, T. (2017). Essentially biased: Why people are fatalistic about genes. *Advances in Experimental Social Psychology* 55: 137-192. https://doi.org/10.1016/bs.aesp.2016.10.003.

Heine, S. J., Cheung, B. Y., and Schmalor, A. (2019). Making sense of genetics: The problem of essentialism. *Hastings Center Report* 49: S19-S26. https://doi.org/10.1002/hast.1013.

Hellman, G. P., and Thompson, F. W. (1975) Physicalism: Ontology, determinism, and reduction. *Journal of Philosophy* 72: 551-564. https://doi.org/10.2307/2025067.

Helmke, B. P., and Minerick, A. R. (2006). Designing a nano-interface in a microfluidic chip to probe living cells: Challenges and perspectives. *Proceedings of the National Academy of Sciences USA* 103: 6419-6424. https://doi.org/10.1073/pnas.0507304103.

Hemedan, A. A., Niarakis, A., Schneider, R., and Ostaszewski, M. (2022). Boolean modelling as a logic-based dynamic approach in systems medicine. *Computational and Structural Biotechnology Journal* 20: 3161-3172. https://doi.org/10.1016/j.csbj.2022.06.035.

Hempel, C. G. (1965). *Aspects of Scientific Explanation and Other Essays in the Philosophy of Science*. New York: Free Press.

Hempel, C. (1980). Comments on Goodman's *Ways of Worldmaking*. *Synthese* 45(2): 193–200. https://doi.org/10.1007/BF00413558.

Herrick, C. J. (1929). Mechanism and organism. *Journal of Philosophy* 26(22): 589-597. https://doi.org/10.2307/2015028.

Hespanha, J. P. (2018). *Linear Systems Theory*, 2nd edition. Princeton, NJ: Princeton University Press.

Hewa, S., and Hetherington, R. W. (1995). Specialists without spirit: Limitations of the mechanistic biomedical model. *Theoretical Medicine* 16(2): 129-139. https://doi.org/10.1007/BF00998540.

Higgins, J. P. (2002). Nonlinear systems in medicine. *Yale Journal of Biology and Medicine* 75(5-6): 247-260. https://www.ncbi.nlm.nih.gov/pmc/articles/PMC2588816/pdf/yjbm00009-0010.pdf.

Hilty, D. M., Torous, J., Parish, M. B., Chan, S. R., Xiong, G., Scher, L., and Yellowlees, P. M. (2021). A literature review comparing clinicians' approaches and skills to in-person, synchronous, and asynchronous care: Moving toward competencies to ensure quality care. *Telemedicine and e-Health*, *27*(4), 356-373. https://doi.org/10.1089/tmj.2020.0054.

Hirakawa, M. P., Krishnakumar, R., Timlin, J. A., Carney, J. P., and Butler, K. S. (2020). Gene editing and CRISPR in the clinic: Current and future perspectives. *Bioscience Reports* 40(4): BSR20200127. https://doi.org/10.1042/BSR20200127.

Hjelmeland, L. M. (2011). Dark matters in AMD genetics: Epigenetics and stochasticity. *Investigative Ophthalmology & Visual Science* 52(3): 1622-1631. https://doi.org/10.1167/iovs.10-6765.

Hodgson, D. (2012). *Rationality + Consciousness = Free Will*. New York: Oxford University Press. https://doi.org/10.1093/acprof:oso/9780199845309.001.0001.

Hoefer, C. (2003). Causal determinism. In *Stanford Encyclopedia of Philosophy,* E. N. Zalta (Ed.). https://plato.stanford.edu/entries/determinism-causal/.

Hofmeyr, J. H. S. (2007). The biological factory that autonomously fabricates itself: A system biological view of the living cell. In *Systems Biology: Philosophical Foundations* (pp. 217-242), F.C. Boogerd, F. J. Bruggeman, J. H. S. Hofmeyr, and H. V. Westerhoff (Eds.). Amsterdam, NL: Elsevier. https://doi.org/10.1016/B978-044452085-2/50012-7.

Holden, A. L. (2002). The SNP consortium: Summary of a private consortium effort to develop an applied map of the human genome. *Biotechniques* 32: S22-S26. https://doi.org/10.2144/jun0203.

Holland, J. H. (1998). *Emergence: From Chaos to Order*. New York: Oxford University Press.

Holliday, R. (2006). Epigenetics: A historical overview. *Epigenetics* 1: 76-80. https://doi.org/10.4161/epi.1.2.2762.

Holliday, R., and Pugh, J. E. (1975). DNA modification mechanisms and gene activity during development. *Science* 187(4173): 226-232. https://doi.org/10.1126/science.187.4173.226.

Holme, P. (2011). Metabolic robustness and network modularity: A model study. *PloS One* 6(2): e16605. https://doi.org/10.1371/journal.pone.0016605.

Hombach, S., and Kretz, M. (2016). Non-coding RNAs: Classification, biology and functioning. In *Non-Coding RNAs in Colorectal Cancer* (pp. 3-17), O. Slaby and G. A. Calin (Eds.). Cham, CH: Springer. https://doi.org/10.1007/978-3-319-42059-2_1.

Honderich, T. (1988). *A Theory of Determinism*. Oxford, UK: Clarendon Press.

Honegger, K., and de Bivort, B. (2018). Stochasticity, individuality and behavior. *Current Biology* 28(1): R8-R12. https://doi.org/10.1016/j.cub.2017.11.058.

Hongbao Ma, S. C. (2005). Nature of life. *Life Science Journal* 2: 7-15. http://www.lifesciencesite.com/lsj/life0201/life-0201-03.pdf.

Hood, L. (2003). Systems biology: Integrating technology, biology, and computation. *Mechanisms of Aging and Development* 124: 9-16. https://doi.org/10.1016/S0047-6374(02)00164-1.

Hood, L. (2013). Systems biology and p4 medicine: Past, present, and future. *Rambam Maimonides Medical Journal* 4(2): e0012. https://doi.org/10.5041/RMMJ.10112.

Hood, L., and Flores, M. (2012). A personal view on systems medicine and the emergence of proactive P4 medicine: Predictive, preventive, personalized and participatory. *New Biotechnology* 29(6): 613-624. https://doi.org/10.1016/j.nbt.2012.03.004.

Hood, L., Heath, J. R., Phelps, M. E., and Lin, B. (2004). Systems biology and new technologies enable predictive and preventive medicine. *Science* 306: 640-643. https://doi.org/10.1126/science.1104635.

Hood, L., Balling, R., and Auffray, C. (2012). Revolutionizing medicine in the 21st century through systems approaches. *Biotechnology Journal* 7: 992-1001. https://doi.org/10.1002/biot.201100306.

Horder, T. (2010). History of developmental biology. In *Encyclopedia of Life Sciences*. Chichester, UK: John Wiley & Sons. https://doi.org/10.1002/9780470015902.a0003080.pub2.

Horder, T. J., Witkowski, J. A., and Wylie, C. C. (Eds.) (1986). *A History of Embryology*. New York: Cambridge University Press.

Hornberg, J. J., Bruggeman, F. J., Westerhoff, H. V., and Lankelma, J. (2006). Cancer: A systems biology disease. *BioSystems* 83: 81-90. https://doi.org/10.1016/j.biosystems.2005.05.014.

Horwitz, R. I., Cullen, M. R., Abell, J., and Christian, J. B. (2013). (De)personalized medicine. *Science* 339(6124): 1155-1156https://doi.org/10.1126/science.1234106.

Hosseininejad, S. M., and Hashempour, M. R. (2017). Diseasome, A new fundamental genetic-based insight to diseases. *International Journal of Advanced Biotechnology and Research* 8: 639-644. https://srhcm.goums.ac.ir/files/balini/files/maghalat/maghalat_96/1oTPEzTgirBcsZUxYct040d0zFDFa5A7P.pdf.

Houser, J., and Oman, K. S. (Eds.). (2011). *Evidence-Based Practice: An Implementation Guide for Healthcare Organizations*. Sudbury, MA: Jones & Bartlett.

Howick, J. (2011). Exposing the vanities—and a qualified defense—of mechanistic reasoning in health care decision making. *Philosophy of Science* 78(5): 926-940. https://doi.org/10.1086/662561.

Howick, J. (2019). Exploring the asymmetrical relationship between the power of finance bias and evidence. *Perspectives in Biology and Medicine* 62(1): 159-187. https://doi.org/10.1353/pbm.2019.0009.

Hu, W., Camacho, E. F., and Xie, L. (2014). Feedforward and feedback control of dynamic systems. *IFAC Proceedings Volumes* 47(3): 7741-7748. https://doi.org/10.3182/20140824-6-ZA-1003.02313.

Hu, T., Chitnis, N., Monos, D., and Dinh, A. (2021). Next-generation sequencing technologies: An overview. *Human Immunology* 82(11): 801-811. https://doi.org/10.1016/j.humimm.2021.02.012.

Hucka, M., Finney, A., Bornstein, B.J., Keating, S. M., Shapiro, B. E., Matthews, J., Kovitz, B. L., Schilstra, M. J., Funahashi, A., Doyle, J. C., and Kitano, H. (2004). Evolving a lingua franca and associated software infrastructure for computational systems biology: The Systems Biology Markup Language (SBML) project. *Systems Biology* 1: 41-53. https://doi.org/10.1049/sb:20045008.

Hull, D. L. (1974). *Philosophy of Biological Science*. Englewood Cliffs, NJ: Prentice-Hall.

Hull, D. L., and Van Regenmortel, M.H.V. (2002). Introduction. In *Promises and Limits of Reductionism in the Biomedical Sciences*, (pp. 1-13), M. H. V. Van Regenmortel and D. L. Hull (Eds.). West Sussex, UK: John Wiley.

Hulswit, M. (2006). How causal is downward causation? *Journal for General Philosophy of Science* 36: 261-287. https://doi.org/10.1007/s10838-006-7153-3.

Humphreys, P. (2016). *Emergence: A Philosophical Account*. New York: Oxford University Press. https://doi.org/10.1093/acprof:oso/9780190620325.001.0001.

Hutchison, C. A., Chuang, R. Y., Noskov, V. N., Assad-Garcia, N., Deerinck, T. J., Ellisman, M. H., Gill, J., Kannan, K., Karas, B. J., Ma, L., and Pelletier, J. F. (2016). Design and synthesis of a minimal bacterial genome. *Science* 351(6280): aad6253. https://doi.org/101126/science.aad6253.

Ibrahim, R., Pasic, M., and Yousef, G. M. (2016). Omics for personalized medicine: Defining the current we swim in. *Expert Review of Molecular Diagnostics* 16(7): 719-722. https://doi.org/10.1586/14737159.2016.1164601.

Ideker, T., Bafna, V., and Lemberger, T. (2007). Integrating scientific cultures. *Molecular Systems Biology* 3: 105. https://doi.org/10.1038/msb4100145.

Iglesias, P. A., and Ingalls B. P. (2010). *Control Theory and Systems Biology*. Cambridge, MA: MIT Press.

Illari, P. M. (2011). Mechanistic evidence: Disambiguating the Russo–Williamson thesis. thesis. *International Studies in the Philosophy of Science* 25(2): 139-157. https://doi.org/10.1080/02698595.2011.574856.

International Human Genome Sequencing Consortium. (2004). Finishing the euchromatic sequence of the human genome. *Nature* 431: 931-945. https://doi.org/10.1038/nature03001.

Ioannidis, J. P. (2016). Evidence-based medicine has been hijacked: A report to David Sackett. *Journal of Clinical Epidemiology* 73: 82-86. https://doi.org/10.1016/j.jclinepi.2016.02.012.

Irizarry, R. A., Tankersley, C., Frank, R., and Flanders, S. (2001). Assessing homeostasis through circadian patterns. *Biometrics* 57: 1228-1237. https://doi.org/10.1111/j.0006-341X.2001.01228.x.

Isaza-Restrepo, A., Gómez, M. T., Cifuentes, G., and Argüello, A. (2018). The virtual patient as a learning tool: A mixed quantitative qualitative study. *BMC Medical Education* 18(1): 297. https://doi.org/10.1186/s12909-018-1395-8.

Ivanov, P. C., Liu, K. K., and Bartsch, R. P. (2016). Focus on the emerging new fields of network physiology and network medicine. *New Journal of Physics* 18(10): 100201. https://doi.org/10.1088/1367-2630/18/10/100201.

Jain, K. K. (2021). *Textbook of Personalized Medicine*, 3rd edition. New York: Springer. https://doi.org/10.1007/978-3-030-62080-6.

Jaiswal, J. K., Goldman, E. R., Mattoussi, H., and Simon, S. M. (2004). Use of quantum dots for live cell imaging. *Nature Methods* 1: 73-78. https://doi.org/10.1038/nmeth1004-73.

Jalili, M., Salehzadeh-Yazdi, A., Yaghmaie, M., Ghavamzadeh, A., and Alimoghaddam, K. (2016). Cancerome: A hidden informative subnetwork of the diseasome. *Computers in Biology and Medicine 76*: 173-177. https://doi.org/10.1016/j.compbiomed.2016.07.010.

Jameson, J. L., and Longo, D. L. (2015). Precision medicine—Personalized, problematic, and promising. *Obstetrical & Gynecological Survey 70*(10): 612-614. https://doi.org/10.1097/01.ogx.0000472121.21647.38.

Janiak, A. (2008). *Newton as Philosopher*. New York: Cambridge University Press.

Janjić, V., and Pržulj, N. (2012). The core diseasome. *Molecular Biosystems 8*(10): 2614-2625. https://doi.org/10.1039/C2MB25230A.

Janson, N. B. (2012). Non-linear dynamics of biological systems. *Contemporary Physics* 53(2): 137-168. https://doi.org/10.1080/00107514.2011.644441.

Jardine, L. (1974). *Francis Bacon: Discovery and the Art of Discourse*. Cambridge, UK: Cambridge University Press.

Jobes, D. A., and Chalker, S. A. (2019). One size does not fit all: A comprehensive clinical approach to reducing suicidal ideation, attempts, and deaths. *International Journal of Environmental Research and Public Health* 16(19): 3606. https://doi.org/10.3390/ijerph16193606.

Johannsen, W. (1909). *Elemente der exakten Erblichkeitslehre*. Jena: Gustav Fischer.

Johnson, M., and Gallagher, K. (2016). *One in a Billion: The story of Nic Volker and the Dawn of Genomic Medicine*. New York: Simon & Schuster.

Joly, Y., Saulnier, K. M., Osien, G., and Knoppers, B. M. (2014). The ethical framing of personalized medicine. *Current Opinion in Allergy and Clinical Immunology* 14(5): 404-408. https://doi.org/10.1097/ACI.0000000000000091.

Jones, R. H. (2000). *Reductionism: Analysis and the Fullness of Reality*. Lewisburg, PA: Bucknell University Press.

Jones, R. H. (2013). *Analysis & the Fullness of Reality: An Introduction to Reductionism & Emergence*. Lewisburg, PA: New York: Jackson Square Books.

Jörgenfelt, C., and Partington, H. (2019). A critical analysis of J. C. Smuts' theory of holism. *European Journal of Integrative Medicine* 31: 100980. https://doi.org/10.1016/j.eujim.2019.100980.

Joy, M. P., Elston, T. C., Lane, A. N., Macdonald, J. M., and Cascante, M. (2012). Introduction to metabolic control analysis (MCA). In *The Handbook of Metabolomics* (pp. 279-297), T. M. Fan, A. Lane, and R. Higashi (Eds.). Totowa, NJ: Humana Press. https://doi.org/10.1007/978-1-61779-618-0_9.

Juengst, E., McGowan, M. L., Fishman, J. R., and Settersten Jr, R. A. (2016). From "personalized" to "precision" medicine: The ethical and social implications of rhetorical reform in genomic medicine. *Hastings Center Report* 46(5): 21-33. https://doi.org/10.1002/hast.614.

Junker, B. H., and Schreiber, F. (Eds.). (2011). *Analysis of Biological Networks*. Hoboken, NY: John Wiley & Sons.

Kærn, M., Elston, T. C., Blake, W. J., and Collins, J. J. (2005). Stochasticity in gene expression: From theories to phenotypes. *Nature Reviews Genetics* 6(6): 451-464. https://doi.org/10.1038/nrg1615.

Kahlem, P., and Birney, E. (2006). Dry work in a wet world: Computation in systems biology. *Molecular Systems Biology* 4: 40. https://doi.org/10.1038/msb4100080.

Kahn, D., and Westerhoff, H. V. (1993). The regulatory strength: How to be precise about regulation and homeostasis. *Acta Biotheoretica* 41: 85-96. https://doi.org/10.1007/BF00712777.

Kaiser, M. I. (2011). The limits of reductionism in the life sciences. *History and Philosophy of the Life Sciences* 33(4): 453-476. http://www.jstor.org/stable/23335178.

Kaiser, M. I. (2015). *Reductive Explanation in Biological Sciences*. New York: Springer. https://doi.org/10.1007/978-3-319-25310-7.

Kalampokis, A., Kotsavasiloglou, C., Argyrakis, P., and Baloyannis, S. (2003). Robustness in biological neural networks. *Physica A: Statistical Mechanics and its Applications* 317(3-4): 581-590. https://doi.org/10.1016/S0378-4371(02)01340-7.

Kamada, T. (1991). System biomedicine: A new paradigm in bio-medical engineering. *Japanese Journal of Medical Electronics and Biological Engineering* 29(Supplement): 1. https://doi.org/10.11239/jsmbe1963.29.Supplement_1.

Kamada, T. (1992). System biomedicine: A new paradigm in biomedical engineering. *Frontiers of Medical and Biological Engineering* 4(1): 1-2.

Kamapantula, B. K., Abdelzaher, A. F., Mayo, M., Perkins, E. J., Das, S. K., and Ghosh, P. (2017). Quantifying robustness in biological networks using NS-2. In *Modeling, Methodologies and Tools for Molecular and Nano-scale Communications* (pp. 273-290), J. Suzuki, T. Nakano, and M. J. Moore (Eds.). Cham, CH: Springer. https://doi.org/10.1007/978-3-319-50688-3_12.

Kaminsky, D. A., Irvin, C. G., and Sterk, P. J. (2011). Complex systems in pulmonary medicine: A systems biology approach to lung disease. *Journal of Applied Physiology* 110(6): 1716-1722. https://doi.org/10.1152/japplphysiol.01310.2010.

Kampourakis, K. (2017). *Making Sense of Genes*. New York: Cambridge University Press.

Kaneko, K. (2012). Evolution of robustness and plasticity under environmental fluctuation: Formulation in terms of phenotypic variances. *Journal of Statistical Physics* 148(4): 687-705. https://doi.org/10.1007/s10955-012-0563-1.

Kaplan, D., and Glass, L. (1995). *Understanding Nonlinear Dynamics*. New York: Springer. https://doi.org/10.1007/978-1-4612-0823-5.

Kaptchuk, T. J. (2001). The double-blind, randomized, placebo-controlled trial: Gold standard or golden calf? *Journal of Clinical Epidemiology* 54(6): 541-549. https://doi.org/10.1016/S0895-4356(00)00347-4.

Kargozar, S., Hoseini, S. J., Milan, P. B., Hooshmand, S., Kim, H. W., and Mozafari, M. (2020). Quantum dots: A review from concept to clinic. *Biotechnology Journal* 15(12): 2000117. https://doi.org/10.1002/biot.202000117.

Karimi, M. R., Karimi, A. H., Abolmaali, S., Sadeghi, M., and Schmitz, U. (2022). Prospects and challenges of cancer systems medicine: From genes to disease networks. *Briefings in Bioinformatics* 23(1): bbab343. https://doi.org/10.1093/bib/bbab343.

Katsnelson, A. (2013). Momentum grows to make 'personalized' medicine more 'precise.' *Nature Medicine* 19(3), 249. https://doi.org/10.1038/nm0313-249.

Kazimierczyk, M., and Wrzesinski, J. (2021). Long non-coding RNA epigenetics. *International Journal of Molecular Sciences* 22(11): 6166. https://doi.org/10.3390/ijms22116166.

Kchouk, M., Gibrat, J.F., and Elloumi, M. (2017). Generations of sequencing technologies: From first to next generation. *Biology and Medicine* 9(3): 395. https://doi.org/10.4172/0974-8369.1000395.

Kegley, J. A. K. (1999). A new framework for the use of genetic information. In *Genetic Information: Acquisition, Access, and Control* (pp. 321-330), A. K. Thompson and R. F. Chadwick (Eds.). New York: Springer. https://doi.org/10.1007/978-0-585-34586-4_30.

Keller, E. F. (1994). Rethinking the meaning of genetic determinism. *Tanner Lectures on Human Values* 15: 113-139. https://tannerlectures.utah.edu/_resources/documents/a-to-z/k/keller94.pdf.

Keller, E. F. (2005). The century beyond the gene. *Journal of Biosciences* 30: 3-10. https://doi.org/10.1007/BF02705144.

Kelly, M. P., Kelly, R. S., and Russo, F. (2014). The integration of social, behavioral, and biological mechanisms in models of pathogenesis. *Perspectives in Biology and Medicine* 57(3): 308-328. https://doi.org/10.1353/pbm.2014.0026.

Kesić, S. (2016). Systems biology, emergence and antireductionism. *Saudi Journal of Biological Sciences* 23(5): 584-591. https://doi.org/10.1016/j.sjbs.2015.06.015.

Ketteler, R. (2012). On programmed ribosomal frameshifting: The alternative proteomes. *Frontiers in Genetics* 3: 242. https://doi.org/10.3389/fgene.2012.00242.

Khalil, I. G., and Hill, C. (2005). Systems biology for cancer. *Current Opinion in Oncology* 17: 44-48. https://doi.org/10.1097/01.cco.0000150951.38222.16.

Kherlopian, A. R., Song, T., Duan, Q., Neimark, A., Po, M. J., Gohagan, J. K., and Laine, A. F. (2008). A review of imaging techniques for systems biology. *BMC Systems Biology* 2: 74. https://doi.org/10.1186/1752-0509-2-74.

Khare, R., Good, B. M., Leaman, R., Su, A. I., and Lu, Z. (2016). Crowdsourcing in biomedicine: Challenges and opportunities. *Briefings in Bioinformatics* 17(1): 23-32. https://doi.org/10.1093/bib/bbv021.

Khoury, M. J., Gwinn, M. L., Glasgow, R. E., and Kramer, B. S. (2012). A population approach to precision medicine. *American Journal of Preventive Medicine* 42(6): 639-645. https://doi.org/10.1016/j.amepre.2012.02.012.

Kiberstis, P., and Roberts, L. (2002). It's not just the genes. *Science* 296: 685. https://doi.org/10.1126/science.296.5568.685.

Kiefer, J. C. (2007). Epigenetics in development. *Developmental Dynamics* 236: 1144-1156. https://doi.org/10.1002/dvdy.21094.

Kilpinen, H., and Barrett, J.C. (2013). How next-generation sequencing is transforming complex disease genetics. *Trends in Genetics* 29(1): 23-30. https://doi.org/10.1016/j.tig.2012.10.001.

Kim, J. (1993). *Supervenience and Mind: Selected Philosophical Essays*. New York: Cambridge University Press.

Kim, J. (1997). Explanation, prediction, and reduction in emergentism. *Intellectica* 25: 45-57.

Kim, J. (1999). Making sense of emergence. *Philosophical Studies* 95(1/2): 3-36. https://doi.org/10.1023/A:1004563122154.

Kim, J. (2006). Emergence: Core ideas and issues. *Synthese* 151(3): 547-559. https://doi.org/10.1007/s11229-006-9025-0.

Kim, Y. A., and Przytycka, T. M. (2013). Bridging the gap between genotype and phenotype via network approaches. *Frontiers in Genetics* 3: 227. https://doi.org/10.3389/fgene.2012.00227.

Kim, D., Kwon, Y. K., and Cho, K. H. (2006). Coupled positive and negative feedback circuits form an essential building block of cellular signaling pathways. *BioEssays* 29: 85-90. https://doi.org/10.1002/bies.20511.

Kim, E. S., Ahn, E. H., Chung, E., and Kim, D. H. (2013). Recent advances in nanobiotechnology and high-throughput molecular techniques for systems biomedicine. *Molecules and Cells* 36(6): 477-484. https://doi.org/10.1007/s10059-013-0304-6.

Kim, M., Paini, D., and Jurdak, R. (2019). Modeling stochastic processes in disease spread across a heterogeneous social system. *Proceedings of the National Academy of Sciences* 116(2): 401-406. https://doi.org/10.1073/pnas.1801429116.

Kimbrough, S. O. (1979). On the reduction of genetics to molecular biology. *Philosophy of Science* 46: 389-406. https://doi.org/10.1086/288883.

Kirkengen, A. L., Ekeland, T. J., Getz, L., Hetlevik, I., Schei, E., Ulvestad, E. and Vetlesen, A. J. (2016). Medicine's perception of reality–a split picture: Critical reflections on apparent anomalies within the biomedical theory of science. *Journal of Evaluation in Clinical Practice* 22(4): 496-501. https://doi.org/10.1111/jep.12369.

Kirschner, M. W. (2005). The meaning of systems biology. *Cell* 121: 503-504. https://doi.org/10.1016/j.cell.2005.05.005.

Kirschner, M. (2016). Systems medicine: Sketching the landscape. In *Systems Medicine* (pp. 3-15), U. Schmitz and O. Wolkenhauer (Eds.). New York: Humana Press. https://doi.org/10.1007/978-1-4939-3283-2_1.

Kirschner, M. W., and Gerhart, J. C. (1998). Evolvability. *Proceedings of the National Academy of Sciences USA* 95: 8420-8427. https://doi.org/10.1073/pnas.95.15.8420.

Kirschner, M. W., and Gerhart, J. C. (2005). *The Plausibility of Life: Resolving Darwin's Dilemma*. New Haven, CT: Yale University Press.

Kitano, H. (2002). Systems biology: A brief overview. *Science* 295: 1662-1664. https://doi.org/10.1126/science.1069492.

Kitano, H. (2004a). Biological robustness. *Nature Reviews Genetics* 5: 826-837. https://doi.org/10.1038/nrg1471.

Kitano, H. (2004b). Cancer as a robust system: Implications for anticancer therapy. *Nature Reviews Cancer* **4**: 227-235. https://doi.org/10.1038/nrc1300.

Kitano, H. (2007a). Towards a theory of biological robustness. *Molecular Systems Biology* 3: 137. https://doi.org/10.1038/msb4100179.

Kitano, H. (2007b). A robustness-based approach to systems-oriented drug design. *Nature Reviews Drug Discovery* 6(3): 202-210. https://doi.org/10.1038/nrd2195.

Kitano, H. (2010). Grand challenges in systems physiology. *Frontiers in Physiology* 1: 3. https://doi.org/10.3389/fphys.2010.00003.

Kitano, H., and Oda, K. (2006). Robustness trade-offs and host-microbial symbiosis in the immune system. *Molecular Systems Biology* 2: 0022. https://doi.org/10.1038/msb4100039.

Kitano, H., Oda, K., Kimura, T., Mastsuoka, Y., Csete, M., Doyle, J., and Muramatsu, M. (2004). Metabolic syndrome and robustness tradeoffs. *Diabetes* 53: S6-S15. https://doi.org/10.2337/diabetes.53.suppl_3.S6.

Kivelson, S., and Kivelson, S. A. (2016). Defining emergence in physics. *npj Quantum Materials* 1(1): 16024. https://doi.org/10.1038/npjquantmats.2016.24.

Kiviet, D. J., Nghe, P., Walker, N., Boulineau, S. (2014). Stochasticity of metabolism and growth at the single-cell level. *Nature* 514(7522): 376-379. https://doi.org/10.1038/nature13582.

Klipp, E., Liebermeister, W., Wierling, C., and Kowald, A. (2016). *Systems Biology: A Textbook*, 2nd edition. Weinheim, DE: Wiley-VCH.

Klonowski, W. (2006). The metaphor of "chaos." In *Systems Biology: Principles, Methods, and Concepts* (pp. 115-138), A. K. Konopka (Ed.). Boca Raton, FL: CRC Press.

Klonowski, W. (2007). From conformons to human brains: An informal overview of nonlinear dynamics and its implications in biomedicine. *Nonlinear Biomedical Physics* 1: 5. https://doi.org/10.1186/1753-4631-1-5.

Knox, S. S. (2010). From 'omics' to complex disease: A systems biology approach to gene-environment interactions in cancer. *Cancer Cell International* 10(1): 11. https://doi.org/10.1186/1475-2867-10-11.

Knüpfer, C., and Beckstein, C. (2013). Function of dynamic models in systems biology: Linking structure to behaviour. *Journal of Biomedical Semantics*, *4*(1): 24. https://doi.org/10.1186/2041-1480-4-24.

Koestler, A. (1970). Beyond atomism and holism—The concept of the holon. *Perspectives in Biology and Medicine* 13(2): 131-154. https://doi.org/10.1353/pbm.1970.0023.

Koestler A., and Smythies, J.R. (Eds.). (1969). *Beyond Reductionism: New Perspectives in the Life Sciences*. Boston, MA: Beacon Press.

Kohl, P., and Noble, D. (2009). Systems biology and the virtual physiological human. *Molecular Systems Biology* 5(1): 292. https://doi.org/10.1038/msb.2009.51.

Kohl, P., Crampin, E. J., Quinn, T. A., and Noble, D. (2010). Systems biology: An approach. *Clinical Pharmacology & Therapeutics* 88(1): 25-33. https://doi.org/10.1038/clpt.2010.92.

Kononowicz, A. A., Woodham, L. A., Edelbring, S., Stathakarou, N., Davies, D., Saxena, N., Car, L. T., Carlstedt-Duke, J., Car, J., and Zary, N. (2019). Virtual patient simulations in health professions education: Systematic review and meta-analysis by the digital health education collaboration. *Journal of Medical Internet Research* 21(7): e14676. https://doi.org/10.2196/14676.

Konopka, A. K. (2007). Basic concepts in systems biology. In *Systems Biology: Principles, Methods, and Concepts* (pp. 1-26), A. K. Konopka (Ed.). Boca Raton, FL: CRC Press.

Kontos, N. (2011). Biomedicine—menace or straw man? Reexamining the biopsychosocial argument. *Academic Medicine* 86(4): 509-515. https://doi.org/10.1097/ACM.0b013e31820e0d16.

Kosorok, M. R., and Laber, E. B. (2019). Precision medicine. *Annual Review of Statistics and Its Application* 6: 263-286. https://doi.org/10.1146/annurev-statistics030718-105251.

Kostyukov, A. I. (1987). Muscle dynamics: Dependence of muscle length on changes in external load. *Biological Cybernetics* 56: 375-387. https://doi.org/10.1007/BF00319517.

Kraft, V. (1953). *The Vienna Circle: The Origins of Neo-Positivism*. New York: Philosophical Library.

Krakauer, D. C. (2006). Robustness in biological systems: A provisional taxonomy. In *Complex Systems Science in Biomedicine* (pp. 183-205), T. S. Deisboeck and J. Y. Kresh (Eds.). New York: Springer. https://doi.org/10.1007/978-0-387-33532-2_6.

Krakauer, D. C., and Plotkin, J. B. (2002). Redundancy, antiredundancy, and the robustness of genomes. *Proceedings of the National Academy of Sciences* 99(3): 1405-1409. https://doi.org/10.1073/pnas.032668599.

Kraushaar, L. E., and Bauer, P. (2021). Dismantling anti-ageing medicine: Why age-relatedness of cardiovascular disease is proof of robustness rather than of ageing-associated vulnerability. *Heart, Lung and Circulation* 30(11): 1702-1709. https://doi.org/10.1016/j.hlc.2021.05.105.

Kraushaar, L. E., Dressel, A., and Maßmann, A. (2018). Vascular robustness: The missing parameter in cardiovascular risk prediction. *Preventive Medicine Reports* 9: 107-113. https://doi.org/10.1016/j.pmedr.2018.01.008.

Krauss, M., Schaller, S., Borchers, S., Findeisen, R., Lippert, J., and Kuepfer, L. (2012). Integrating cellular metabolism into a multiscale whole-body model. *PLoS Computational Biology* 8(10): e1002750. https://doi.org/10.1371/journal.pcbi.1002750.

Krieger, N. (1994). Epidemiology and the web of causation: Has anyone seen the spider? *Social Science & Medicine* 39(7): 887-903. https://doi.org/10.1016/0277-9536(94)90202-X.

Kriete, A. (2013). Robustness and aging—a systems-level perspective. *Biosystems* 112(1): 37-48. https://doi.org/10.1016/j.biosystems.2013.03.014.

Krimsky, S. (2013). Introduction: Evolving narratives of genetic explanation across disciplines. In *Genetic Explanations* (pp. 1-14), S. Krimsky and J. Gruber (Eds.). Cambridge, MA: Harvard University Press.

Kroedel, T. (2015). A simple argument for downward causation. *Synthese* 192(3): 841-858. https://doi.org/10.1007/s11229-014-0600-5.

Krohs, U., and Callebaut, W. (2007). Data without models merging with models without data. In *Systems Biology: Philosophical Foundations* (pp. 181-213), F. C. Boogerd, F. J. Bruggeman, J. H. S. Hofmeyr, and H. V. Westerhoff (Eds.). Amsterdam, NL: Elsevier. https://doi.org/10.1016/B978-044452085-2/50011-5.

Kruse, C. S., Goswamy, R., Raval, Y. J., and Marawi, S. (2016). Challenges and opportunities of big data in health care: A systematic review. *JMIR Medical Informatics* 4(4): e5359. https://doi.org/10.2196/medinform.5359.

Kubĵk, A. (2003). Toward a formalization of emergence. *Artificial Life* 9: 41-65. https://doi.org/10.1162/106454603321489518.

Kulikowski, C. A. (2019). Beginnings of artificial intelligence in medicine (AIM): Computational artifice assisting scientific inquiry and clinical art–with reflections on present aim challenges. *Yearbook of Medical Informatics* 28(01): 249-256. https://doi.org/10.1055/s-0039-1677895.

Kumar, D. (2008). Disorders of the genome architecture: A review. *Genomic Medicine* 2(3-4): 69-76. https://doi.org/10.1007/s11568-009-9028-2.

Kumar, S., Singh, A. K., and Mohapatra, T. (2017). Epigenetics: History, present status and future perspective. *Indian Journal of Genetics and Plant Breeding* 77(4): 445-463. https://doi.org/10.5958/0975-6906.2017.00061.X.

Kurreck, J., and Stein, C. A. (2016). *Molecular Medicine: An Introduction*. Weinheim, DE: Wiley-VCH.

Laird, J. E., Lebiere, C., and Rosenbloom, P. S. (2017). A standard model of the mind: Toward a common computational framework across artificial intelligence, cognitive science, neuroscience, and robotics. *AI Magazine* 38(4): 13-26. https://doi.org/10.1609/aimag.v38i4.2744.

Laland, K. N., Uller, T., Feldman, M. W., Sterelny, K., Müller, G. B., Moczek, A., Jablonka, E., and Odling-Smee, J. (2015). The extended evolutionary synthesis: Its structure, assumptions and predictions. *Proceedings of the Royal Society B: Biological Sciences* 282(1813): 20151019. https://doi.org/10.1098/rspb.2015.1019.

La Mettrie, J. O., de. (1996). *Machine Man and Other Writings*. New York: Cambridge University Press.

Lande, R., Engen, S., and Saether, B. E. (2003). *Stochastic Population Dynamics in Ecology and Conservation*. New York: Oxford University Press. https://doi.org/10.1093/acprof:oso/9780198525257.001.0001.

Landucci, F., and Volpe, G. (2020). The Covid-19 challenge to EBM. *Minerva Medica* https://doi.org/10.23736/s0026-4806.20.07140-2.

Laszlo, E. (1972). *Introduction to Systems Philosophy: Toward a New Paradigm of Contemporary Thought*. New York: Harper.

Latterich, M. (2005). Molecular systems biology at the crossroads: To know less about more, or to know more about less? *Proteome Science* 3: 8. https://doi.org/10.1186/1477-5956-3-8.

Layek, G. C. (2015). *An Introduction to Dynamical Systems and Chaos*. New Delhi: Springer India. https://doi.org/10.1007/978-81-322-2556-0.

Lecca, P., Laurenzi, I., and Jordan, F. (2013). *Deterministic versus Stochastic Modelling in Biochemistry and Systems Biology*. Amsterdam, NL: Elsevier.

Lederberg, J. (1994). The transformation of genetics by DNA: An anniversary celebration of Avery, MacLeod and McCarty (1944). *Genetics* 136: 423–426. https://doi.org/10.1093/genetics/136.2.423.

Lederberg, J. (2001). The meaning of epigenetics. *The Scientist* 15(18): 6.

Lee, Y., Rivera, J. G. L., and Liao, J. C. (2014). Ensemble modeling for robustness analysis in engineering non-native metabolic pathways. *Metabolic Engineering* 25: 63-71. https://doi.org/10.1016/j.ymben.2014.06.006.

Lehár, J., Krueger, A., Zimmerman, G., and Borisy, A. (2008). High-order combination effects and biological robustness. *Molecular Systems Biology* 4: 215. https://doi.org/10.1038/msb.2008.51.

Lemberger, T. (2007). Systems biology in human health and disease. *Molecular Systems Biology* 3: 136. https://doi.org/10.1038/msb4100175.

Lemke, T. (2021). *The Government of Things: Foucault and the New Materialism*. New York: New York University Press.

Lemmen, C., Woopen, C., and Stock, S. (2021). Systems medicine 2030: A Delphi study on implementation in the German healthcare system. *Health Policy* 125(1): 104-114. https://doi.org/10.1016/j.healthpol.2020.11.01.

Lenoir, T. (1999). Shaping biomedicine as an information science. In *Science Information Systems* (pp. 27-45), M. E. Bowden, T. B. Hahn, and R. V. Williams (Eds.). Medford, MJ: Information Today, Inc.

Lenormand, T., Roze, D., and Rousset, F. (2009). Stochasticity in evolution. *Trends in Ecology & Evolution* 24(3): 157-165. https://doi.org/10.1016/j.tree.2008.09.014.

Lenski, R. E., Barrick, J. E., and Ofria, C. (2006). Balancing robustness and evolvability. *PLoS Biology* 4: e428. https://doi.org/10.1371/journal.pbio.0040428.

Leonardo, R. (2018). PICO: Model for clinical questions. *Evidence Based Medical Practice* 3(2), 115. https://doi.org/10.4172/2471-9919.1000115.

Leonelli, S. (2019). *Data-Centric Biology: A Philosophical Study*. Chicago, IL: University of Chicago Press.

Lesne, A. (2008). Robustness: Confronting lessons from physics and biology. *Biological Reviews* 83: 509-532. https://doi.org/10.1111/j.1469-185X.2008.00052.x.

Levins, R. (2014). The road to wholeness in medicine and public health. *International Critical Thought* 4(2): 221-240. https://doi.org/10.1080/21598282.2014.906807.

Lewes, G. H. (1875). *Problems of the Life and Mind*, 2nd series, volume 2. London: Trübner.

Lewis, T. G. (2011). *Network Science: Theory and Applications*. New York: John Wiley & Sons.

Lewontin, R. C. (1983). Biological determinism. *Tanner Lectures on Human Values* 4: 147-183. https://tannerlectures.utah.edu/_resources/documents/a-to-z/l/lewontin83.pdf.

Li, G., and Reinberg, D. (2011). Chromatin higher-order structures and gene regulation. *Current Opinion in Genetics & Development* 21(2): 175-186. https://doi.org/10.1016/j.gde.2011.01.022.

Liang, M., Cowley Jr, A. W., Greene, A. S., Geurts, A. M., Liu, P., Liu, Y., and Rao, S. (2022). Advancing physiology with expanded multi-omics. *Function* 3(4): p.zqac031. https://doi.org/10.1093/function/zqac031.

Lidgard, S., and Hopkins, M. (2015). Stasis. In *Oxford Bibliographies on Evolutionary Biology*, J. B. Losos (Ed.). New York: Oxford University Press. https://doi.org/10.1093/OBO/9780199941728-0067.

Lightman, A. (2005). *The Discoveries: Great Breakthroughs in 20th-Century Science, Including the Original Papers*. New York: Vintage Books.

Li-Pook-Than, J., and Snyder, M. (2013). iPOP goes the world: Integrated personalized omics profiling and the road toward improved health care. *Chemistry & Biology* 20(5): 660-666. https://doi.org/10.1016/j.chembiol.2013.05.001.

Lippman, A. (1991). Prenatal genetic testing and screening: Constructing needs and reinforcing inequities. *American Journal of Law & Medicine* 17(1-2): 15-50. https://doi.org/10.1017/S0098858800007917.

Lipworth, W., Mason, P. H., Kerridge, I., Ioannidis, J. P. A. (2017). Ethics and epistemology in big data research. *Bioethical Inquiry* 14: 489–500. https://doi.org/10.1007/s11673-017-9771-3.

Lisacek, F., and Appel, R. D. (2007). Systems biology: A loose definition. *Proteomics* 7: 825-827. https://doi.org/10.1002/pmic.200790020.

Liu, E. T. (2005). Systems biology, integrative biology, predictive biology. *Cell* 121: 505-506. https://doi.org/10.1016/j.cell.2005.04.021.

Liu, E. T. (2010). Foundations of systems biomedicine: An introduction. In *Systems Biomedicine: Concepts and Perspectives* (pp. 3-13), E. T. Liu and D. A. Lauffenberger

(Eds.). New York: Academic Press. https://doi.org/10.1016/B978-0-12-372550-9.00001-8.

Liu, E. T., and Lauffenburger, D. A. (Eds.). (2010). *Systems Biomedicine: Concepts and Perspectives*. San Diego, CA: Academic Press. https://doi.org/10.1016/B978-0-12-372550-9.X0001-6.

Liu, N., and Pan, T. (2015). RNA epigenetics. *Translational Research* 165: 28-35. https://doi.org/10.1016/j.trsl.2014.04.003.

Livingstone, D. N. (2011). Environmental determinism. In *The SAGE Handbook of Geographical Knowledge* (pp. 368-380), J. A. Agnew and D. N. Livingstone (Eds.). London: SAGE.

Lloyd, D., Aon, M. A., and Cortassa, S. (2001). Why homeodynamics, not homeostasis? *The Scientific World Journal* 1: 133-145. https://doi.org/10.1100/tsw.2001.20.

Lock, M., and Gordon, D. (Eds.). (1988). *Biomedicine Examined*. Dordrecht, NL: Kluwer. https://doi.org/10.1007/978-94-009-2725-4.

Lock, M. M., and Nguyen, V. K. (2018). *An Anthropology of Biomedicine*, 2nd edition. John Wiley & Sons.

Loeb, J. (1912). *The Mechanistic Conception of Life: Biological Essays*. Chicago, IL: University of Chicago Press.

Loew, L. M., Schaff, J. C., Slepchenko, B. M., and Moraru, I. I. (2010). The virtual cell project. In *Systems Biomedicine: Concepts and Perspectives* (pp. 273-288), E. T. Liu and D. A. Lauffenberger (Eds.). New York: Academic Press. https://doi.org/10.1016/B978-0-12-372550-9.00011-0.

Loewer, B. (2001). From physics to physicalism. In *Physicalism and its Discontents* (pp. 37-56), C. Gillett and B. Loewer (Eds.). New York: Cambridge University Press. https://doi.org/10.1017/CBO9780511570797.003.

Lonergan, B. (1972). *Method in Theology*. New York: Herder & Herder.

Long, E. R. (1965). *A History of Pathology*. New York: Dover Publications.

Longino, C. F., Murphy, J. W., and Hendricks, J. (1995). *The Old Age Challenge to the Biomedical Model: Paradigm Strain and Health Policy*. New York: Routledge.

Longoni, M., Marangi, G., and Zollino, M. (2014). Utility and challenges of next generation sequencing in pediatric disorders. *Current Pediatrics Reports* 2(2): 82-92. https://doi.org/10.1007/s40124-014-0039-7.

Looijen, R. C. (2000). *Holism and Reductionism in Biology and Ecology: The Mutual Dependence of Higher and Lower Level Research Programmes*. Dordrecht, NL: Kluwer. https://doi.org/10.1007/978-94-015-9560-5.

López-Otín, C., Blasco, M. A., Partridge, L., Serrano, M., and Kroemer, G. (2023). Hallmarks of aging: An expanding universe. *Cell* 186(2): 243-278. https://doi.org/10.1016/j.cell.2022.11.001.

Loscalzo, J., and Barabasi, A. L. (2011). Systems biology and the future of medicine. *Systems Biology and Medicine* 3(6): 619-627. https://doi.org/10.1002/wsbm.144.

Loscalzo, J., Barabási, A. L., Siverman, E. K. (2017). *Network Medicine: Complex Systems in Human Disease and Therapeutics*. Cambridge, MA: Harvard University.

Losick, R., and Desplan, C. (2008). Stochasticity and cell fate. *Science* 320(5872): 65-68. https://doi.org/10.1126/science.1147888.

Lourida, K. G., and Louridas, G. E. (2021). Constraints in clinical cardiology and personalized medicine: Interrelated concepts in clinical cardiology. *Cardiogenetics* 11(2): 50-67. https://doi.org/10.3390/cardiogenetics11020007.

Louridas, G. E., and Lourida, K. G. (2017). Conceptual foundations of systems biology explaining complex cardiac diseases. *Healthcare* 5(1): 10. https://doi.org/10.3390/healthcare5010010.

Lowrance, W. W., and Collins, F. S. (2007). Identifiability in genomic research. *Science* 317(5838), 600-602. https://doi.org/10.1126/science.1147699.

Löwy, I. (2011). The historiography of biomedicine: "Bio," "medicine," and in between. *Isis* 102: 116-122. https://doi.org/10.1086/658661.

Luan, D., Zai, M., and Varner, J. D. (2007). Computationally derived points of fragility of a human cascade are consistent with current therapeutic strategies. *PLoS Computational Biology* 3: 1347-1359. https://doi.org/10.1371/journal.pcbi.0030142.

Lucas, J. R. (1970) *The Freedom of the Will*. Oxford, UK: Clarendon Press.

Luenberger, D. G. (1979). *Introduction to Dynamic Systems: Theory, Models, and Applications*. New York: John Wiley & Sons.

Ma, H., Sorokin, A., Mazein, A., Selkov, A., Selkov, E., Demin, O., and Goryanin, I. (2007). The Edinburgh human metabolic network reconstruction and its functional analysis. *Molecular Systems Biology* 3: 135. https://doi.org/10.1038/msb4100177.

Maar, A. (2019). Kinds of determinism in science. *Principia* 3(3), 503-528. https://doi.org/10.5007/1808-1711.2019v23n3p503.

Ma'ayan, A. (2017). Complex systems biology. *Journal of the Royal Society Interface* 14(134): 20170391. https://doi.org/10.1098/rsif.2017.0391.

MacArthur, B. D., Please, C. P., and Oreffo, R. O. (2008). Stochasticity and the molecular mechanisms of induced pluripotency. *PloS One* 3(8): e3086. https://doi.org/10.1371/journal.pone.0003086.

Macdonald, C., and Macdonald, G. (2010). Emergence and downward causation. In *Emergence in Mind* (pp. 139-168). C. Macdonald and G. Macdonald (Eds). New York: Oxford University Press. https://doi.org/10.1093/acprof:oso/9780199583621.003.0010.

Machamer, R., Darden, L., and Craver, C. F. (2000). Thinking about mechanisms. *Philosophy of Science* 67: 1-25. https://doi.org/10.1086/392759.

MacKay, D. M. (1974). *A Clock Work Image: A Christian Perspective on Science*. Downers Grove, IL: InterVarsity Press.

MacRae, C. A., Roden, D. M., and Loscalzo, J. (2016). The future of cardiovascular biomedicine. *Circulation* 133: 2610-2617. https://doi.org/10.1161/CIRCULATIONAHA.115.020553.

Magner, L. N. (2009). *The History of Infectious Diseases and the Microbial World*. London: Praeger.

Mahmood, S., Nona, P., Villablanca, P., Nunez-Gil, I., and Ramakrishna, H. (2021). The meta-analysis in evidence-based medicine: High-quality research when properly performed. *Journal of Cardiothoracic and Vascular Anesthesia* 35(9): 2556-2558. https://doi.org/10.1053/j.jvca.2021.05.025.

Maienschein, J. (2005). Epigenesis and preformationism. In In *Stanford Encyclopedia of Philosophy, E. N. Zalta (Ed.). https://plato.stanford.edu/entries/epigenesis/.*

Maier, D. (2017). Applying systems medicine in the clinic. *Current Opinion in Systems Biology* 3: 77-87. https://doi.org/10.1016/j.coisb.2017.04.014.

Maiorino, E., Baek, S. H., Guo, F., Zhou, X., Kothari, P. H., Silverman, E. K., Barabási, A. L., Weiss, S. T., Raby, B. A., and Sharma, A. (2020). Discovering the genes mediating the interactions between chronic respiratory diseases in the human interactome. *Nature Communications* 11(1): 811. https://doi.org/10.1038/s41467-020-14600-w.

Maltsev, A. V., and Stern, M. D. (2021). Social heterogeneity drives complex patterns of the COVID-19 pandemic: Insights from a novel Stochastic Heterogeneous Epidemic Model (SHEM). *Frontier in Physics* 8: 609224. https://doi.org/10.1101/2020.07.10.20150813.

Mandelkern, M., and Rothschild, D. (2021). Roads to necessitarianism. *Journal of Philosophical Logic* 50(1): 89-96. https://doi.org/10.1007/s10992-020-09562-9.

Mann, J. (1999). *The Elusive Magic Bullet: The Search for the Perfect Drug*. New York: Oxford University Press.

Mansel, H. L. (1851). *Prolegomena Logica: An Inquiry into the Psychological Character of Logical Processes*. Oxford, UK: William Graham.

Mapes, B. M., Foster, C. S., Kusnoor, S. V., Epelbaum, M. I., AuYoung, M., Jenkins, G., Lopez-Class, M., Richardson-Heron, D., Elmi, A., Surkan, K. and Cronin, R. M. (2020). Diversity and inclusion for the All of Us research program: A scoping review. *PloS One* 15(7): e0234962. https://doi.org/10.1371/journal.pone.0234962.

March, R., and Schott, C. (2017). Personalized/precision medicine/personalized healthcare: The art of giving different names to the same thing? *Personalized Medicine* 14(6): 463-466. https://doi.org/10.2217/pme-2017-0073.

Marcum, J. A. (1998). Defending the priority of "remarkable researches": The discovery of fibrin ferment. *History and Philosophy of the Life Sciences* 20: 51-76. http://www.jstor.org/stable/23332141.

Marcum, J. A. (2004). Biomechanical and phenomenological models of the body, the meaning of illness and quality of care. *Medicine, Health Care and Philosophy* 7(3): 311-320. https://doi.org/10.1007/s11019-004-9033-0.

Marcum, J. A. (2005). From the molecular genetics revolution to gene therapy: Translating basic research into medicine. *Journal of Laboratory and Clinical Medicine* 146(6): 312-316. https://doi.org/10.1016/j.lab.2005.07.009.

Marcum, J. A. (2008a). *An Introductory Philosophy of Medicine: Humanizing Modern Medicine*. New York: Springer. https://doi.org/10.1007/978-1-4020-6797-6.

Marcum, J. A. (2008b). Whitehead's philosophy of organism and systems biology. In *Chromatikon IV. Annuaire de la Philosophie en Process* (pp. 143-152), M. Weber (Ed.). Louvain: Presses Universitaires de Louvain. https://doi.org/10.5840/chromatikon2008413.

Marcum, J. A. (2008c). Does systems biology represent a Kuhnian paradigm shift? *New Phytologist* 179(3): 587-589. https://doi.org/10.1111/j.1469-8137.2008.02486.x.

Marcum, J. A. (2009). *The Conceptual Foundations of Systems Biology: An Introduction* New York: Nova Science Publishers.

Marcum, J. A. (2013). *Tampering with Nature: Empirical Methodology and Experimental Onto-Epistemology*. Hauppauge, NY: Nova Science Publishers.

Marcum, J. A. (2014). Philosophy of contemporary medicine. Oxford Bibliographies, Oxford University Press. https://www.oxfordbibliographies.com/view/document/obo-9780195396577/obo-9780195396577-0216.xml.

Marcum, J. A. (2017a). Kuhn's science and does medicine really care about patients? 3:16 (Richard Marshall interviewer). https://www.3-16am.co.uk/articles/kuhn-s-science-and-does-medicine-really-care-about-patients?c=end-times-archive.

Marcum, J. A. (Ed.). (2017b). *The Bloomsbury Companion to Contemporary Philosophy of Medicine*. London: Bloomsbury.

Marcum, J. A. (2019). The cancer epigenome: A review. *Journal of Biotechnology and Biomedicine* 2(3): 67-83. https://doi.org/10.26502/jbb.2642-91280011.

Marcum, J. A. (2020). *From Systems Biology to Systems Medicine*. New York: Nova Science Publishers.

Marcum, J. A. (2021). P7 medicine: Humanizing systems medicine. *Teorema: Revista Internacional de Filosofía* 40: 213-231. https://www.jstor.org/stable/27094761.

Marcum, J. A., and Rosenberg, R. D. (1989). Anticoagulantly active proteoheparan sulfate from vascular endothelium. *Annals of the New York Academy of Sciences* 556: 81-94. https://doi.org/10.1055/s-2007-1003523.

Marcum, J. A., and Tretter, F. (2023). From evidence-based corona medicine to organismic systems corona medicine. *Philosophy of Medicine*. 4(1): 1-16. https://doi.org/10.5195/pom.2023.138.

Marcum, J. A., and Verschuuren, G. M. N. (1986). Hemostatic regulation and Whitehead's philosophy of organism. *Acta Biotheoretica* 35: 123-133. https://doi.org/10.1007/BF00118370.

Marcum, J. A., Highsmith, R. F., and Kline, D. L. (1982). Streptokinase-dependent delayed activation of horse plasminogen. *Biochimica et Biophysica Acta* 709(1): 19-27. https://doi.org/10.1016/0167-4838(82)90416-2.

Marcum, J. A., Levin, J., and Prendergast, R. A. (1984). Clotting enzyme activity derived from the coelomocytes of the sea star *Asterias forbesi*. *Thrombosis and Haemostasis* 52: 1-3. https://doi.org/10.1055/s-0038-1661122.

Mardinoglu, A., and Nielsen, J. (2012). Systems medicine and metabolic modelling. *Journal of Internal Medicine* 271(2): 142-154. https://doi.org/10.1111/j.1365-2796.2011.02493.x.

Markič, O. (2004). Causal emergentism. *Acta Analytica* 19: 65-81. https://doi.org/10.1007/s12136-004-1013-8.

Martin, C. B. (2008). *The Mind in Nature*. New York: Oxford University Press. https://doi.org/10.1093/acprof:oso/9780199234103.001.0001.

Martini, C. (2021). What "evidence" in evidence-based medicine? *Topoi* 40(2): 299-305. https://doi.org/10.1086/341855.

Mason, P. H. (2015). Degeneracy: Demystifying and destigmatizing a core concept in systems biology. *Complexity* 20(3): 12-21. https://doi.org/10.1002/cplx.21534.

Masel, J., and Siegal, M. L. (2009). Robustness: Mechanisms and consequences. *Trends in Genetics* 25(9): 395-403. https://doi.org/10.1016/j.tig.2009.07.005.

Masel, J., and Trotter, M. V. (2010). Robustness and evolvability. *Trends in Genetics* 26(9): 406-414. https://doi.org/10.1016/j.tig.2010.06.002.

Mayer, G., Marcus, K., Eisenacher, M., and Kohl, M. (2016). Boolean modeling techniques for protein co-expression networks in systems medicine. *Expert Review of Proteomics* 13(6): 555-569. https://doi.org/10.1080/14789450.2016.1181546.

Mayr, E. (1998). *This is Biology: Science of the Living World*. Cambridge, MA: Harvard University Press.

Mazein, A., Ostaszewski, M., Kuperstein, I., Watterson, S., Le Novère, N., Lefaudeux, D., De Meulder, B., Pellet, J., Balaur, I., Saqi, M., and Nogueira, M. M. (2018). Systems medicine disease maps: Community-driven comprehensive representation of disease mechanisms. *NPJ Systems Biology and Applications* 4(1): 21. https://doi.org/10.1038/s41540-018-0059-y.

Mazzocchi, F. (2012). Complexity and the reductionism–holism debate in systems biology. *Wiley Interdisciplinary Reviews: Systems Biology and Medicine* 4(5): 413-427. https://doi.org/10.1002/wsbm.1181.

McBride, R. C., Ogbnugafor, C. B., and Turner, P. E. (2008). Robustness promotes evolvability of thermotolerance in an RNA virus. *BMC Evolutionary Biology* 8: 231. https://doi.org/10.1186/1471-2148-8-231.

McDaniel, K. (2010). Parts and wholes. *Philosophy Compass* 5(5): 412-425. https://doi.org/10.1111/j.1747-9991.2009.00238.x.

McEwen, B. S., and Wingfield, J. C. (2003). The concept of allostasis in biology and biomedicine. *Hormones and Behavior* 43: 2-15. https://doi.org/10.1016/S0018-506X(02)00024-7.

McGregor, K. (2020). Toward a phenomenology of the material. *Qualitative Inquiry* 26(5): 507-513. https://doi.org/10.1177/1077800419836690.

McGuire, A. L., and Gibbs, R. A. (2006). No longer de-identified. *Science* 312: 370-371. https://doi.org/10.1126/science.1125339.

McKewan, J. (2009). Predeterminism. In *Encyclopedia of Time: Science, Philosophy, Theology, & Culture*, volume 2 (pp. 1034-1035), H. J. Birx (Ed.). London: SAGE.

McLaughlin, B. P. (1992). The rise and fall of British Emergentism. In *Emergence or Reduction? Essays on the Prospects of Nonreductive Physicalism* (pp. 49-93), A. Beckermann, H. Flohr and J. Kim (Eds.). New York: Walter de Gruyter.

McLaughlin, B. P. (2019). British Emergentism. In *The Routledge Handbook of Emergence* (pp. 23-35), S. Gibb, R. F. Hendry, and T. Lancaster (Eds.). New York: Routledge.

Mebius, A., Kennedy, A. G., and Howick, J. (2016). Research gaps in the philosophy of evidence-based medicine. *Philosophy Compass* *11*(11): 757-771. https://doi.org/10.1111/phc3.12352.

Medawar, P. B. (1984). A view from the left. *Nature* 310(5974): 255-256. https://doi.org/10.1038/310255a0.

Medina, M. Á. (2013). Systems biology for molecular life sciences and its impact in biomedicine. *Cellular and Molecular Life Sciences* 70(6): 1035-1053. https://doi.org/10.1007/s00018-012-1109-z.

Megahed, F. A. K., Addissouky, T. A., Zhou, X., Sun, P., and El Sayed, I. E. T. (2020). Personalized or precision medicine: Current vision, challenges and future prospectives. *International Journal of Medical Science and Health Research* 4(4): 104-106.

Megason, S. G., and Fraser, S. E. (2007). Imaging in systems biology. *Cell* 130: 784-795. https://doi.org/10.1016/j.cell.2007.08.031.

Meidanis, J. (2021). Network science: A primer. *Matemática Contemporânea* 48: 167-180. https://doi.org/10.21711/231766362021/rmc4817.

Meincke, A. S. (2019). Autopoiesis, biological autonomy and the process view of life. *European Journal for Philosophy of Science* 9: 5. https://doi.org/10.1007/s13194-018-0228-2.

Meireles, A., and Simões, M. (2014). Metabolic control analysis and its applications. *Current Bioinformatics* 9(5): 490-498.

Meisenberg, B. R. (2015). The implications of "random chance" in cancer genesis: Why stochastic can be a dirty word. *JAMA Oncology* 1(5): 575-576. https://doi.org/10.1001/jamaoncol.2015.0786.

Melnyk, A. (1997). How to keep the 'physical' in physicalism. *Journal of Philosophy* 94(12): 622-637. https://doi.org/10.2307/2564597.

Meloni, M., and Testa, G. (2014). Scrutinizing the epigenetics revolution. *BioScocieties* 9(4): 431-456. https://doi.org/10.1057/biosoc.2014.22.

Melzer, D., Pilling, L.C., and Ferrucci, L. (2020). The genetics of human ageing. *Nature Reviews Genetics* 21(2): 88-101. https://doi.org/10.1038/s41576-019-0183-6.

Mendel, G. (1950). *Experiments in Plant Hybridization*. Cambridge, MA: Harvard University Press.

Mendonça, W. (2002). Supervenience and the problem of downward causation. In *Mental Causation, Proceedings of the Third International Colloquium in Philosophy of Mind* (pp. 251-270), A. Leclerc, G. De Queiroz, and M. B. Wrigley (Eds.). San Paulo, Brazil: State University of Campinas.

Merchant, C. (1980). *The Death of Nature: Women, Ecology, and the Scientific Revolution*. San Francisco, CA: Harper & Row.

Mercuri, M. (2020). Just follow the science: A government response to a pandemic. *Journal of Evaluation in Clinical Practice* 26: 1575-1578. https://doi.org/10.1111/jep.13491.

Mesarović, M. D., Sreenath, S. N., and Keene, J. D. (2004). Search for organising principles: Understanding in systems biology. *Systems Biology* 1: 19–27. https://doi.org/10.1049/sb:20045010.

Mesarović, M. D., and Sreenath, S. N. (2005). Beyond the flat earth perspective in systems biology. *Biological Theory* 1: 33-34. https://doi.org/10.1162/biot.2006.1.1.33.

Metzcar, J., Wang, Y., Heiland, R., and Macklin, P. (2019). A review of cell-based computational modeling in cancer biology. *JCO Clinical Cancer Informatics* 2: 1-13. https://doi.org/10.1200/CCI.18.00069.

Michael, J., Cliff, W., McFarland, J., Modell, H., and Wright, A. (2017). *The Core Concepts of Physiology: A New Paradigm for Teaching Physiology*. New York: Springer. https://doi.org/10.1007/978-1-4939-6909-8.

Mifsud, J., and Gavrilovici, C. (2019). Big data in healthcare and the life sciences. In *Ethics and Integrity in Health and Life Sciences Research*, volume 4 (pp. 63-83). Z. Koporc (Ed.). Bingley, UK: Emerald Publishing Limited. https://doi.org/10.1108/S2398-601820180000004005.

Miglani, G. S. (2006). Mendelian genetics. In *Plant Cell Biology* (pp. 259-348), W. V. Dashek and M. Harrison (Eds.). Enfield, NH: Science Publishers.

Mill, J. S. (1865). *A System of Logic: Ratiocinative and Inductive*, 6th edition, volume 1. London: Longmans, Green, & Co.

Miller Jr, W. B. (2018). Biological information systems: Evolution as cognition-based information management. *Progress in Biophysics and Molecular Biology* 134: 1-26. https://doi.org/10.1016/j.pbiomolbio.2017.11.005.

Mode, C. J., Durrett, R., Klebaner, F., and Olofsson, P. (2013). Applications of stochastic processes in biology and medicine. *International Journal of Stochastic Analysis* 2013: 790625. https://doi.org/10.1155/2013/790625.

Modell, H., Cliff, W., Michael, J., McFarland, J., Wenderoth, M. P., and Wright, A. (2015). A physiologist's view of homeostasis. *Advances in Physiology Education* 39(4): 259-266. https://doi.org/10.1152/advan.00107.2015.

Moncrieff, J. (2008). *The Myth of the Chemical Cure: A Critique of Psychiatric Drug Treatment*. New York: Palgrave Macmillan. https://doi.org/10.1007/978-0-230-58944-5.

Montero, B. (2003). Varieties of causal closure. In *Physicalism and Mental Causation: The Metaphysics of Mind and Action* (pp. 173-187), S. Walter and H. D. Heckmann (Eds.). Exeter, UK: Imprint Academic.

Moore, D. S. (2003). *The Dependent Gene: The Fallacy of "Nature vs. Nurture."* New York: Henry Holt & Company.

Moore, D. S. (2015). *The Developing Genome: An Introduction to Behavioral Epigenetics*. New York: Oxford University Press.

Moore Jr., J. E., and Maitland, D. J. (Eds.). (2014). *Biomedical Technology and Devices*, 2nd edition. Boca Raton, FL: CRC Press.

Morange, M. (2006). Post-genomics, between reduction and emergence. *Synthese* 151: 355-360. https://doi.org/10.1007/s11229-006-9029-9.

Morange, M. (2020). *The Black Box of Biology: A History of the Molecular Revolution*, M. Cobb, tans. Cambridge, MA: Harvard University Press. https://doi.org/10.4159/9780674245280.

Moraru, I. I., Schaff, J. C., Slepchenko, B. M., Blinov, M. L., Morgan, F., Lakshminarayana, A., Gao, F., Li, Y., and Loew, L. M. (2008). Virtual cell modeling and simulation software environment. *IET Systems Biology* 2: 352-362. https://doi.org/10.1049/iet-syb:20080102.

Morchio, R. (2003). Reductionism and history: The biology between Scylla and Charybdis. In *Determinism, Holism, and Complexity* (pp. 231-239), V. Benci, P. Cerrai, P. Freguglia, G. Israel, and C. Pellegrini (Eds.). New York: Plenum. https://doi.org/10.1007/978-1-4757-4947-2_21.

Morel, N. M., Holland, J. M., Van Der Greef, J., Marple, E. W., Clish, C., Loscalzo, J., and Naylor, S. (2004). Primer on medical genomics. Part XIV: Introduction to systems biology—A new approach to understanding disease and treatment. *Mayo Clinic Proceedings* 79: 651-658. https://doi.org/10.4065/79.5.651.

Morens, D. M., Taubenberger, J. K., and Fauci, A. S. (2022). Universal coronavirus vaccines—an urgent need. *New England Journal of Medicine* 386(4): 297-299. https://doi.org/10.1056/NEJMp2118468.

Morgan, C. L. (1927). *Emergent Evolution*, 2nd edition. London: Williams & Norgate.

Morgan, T. H. (1934). *Embryology and Genetics*. New York: Columbia University Press.

Morrison-Smith, S., Boucher, C., Sarcevic, A., Noyes, N., O'Brien, C., Cuadros, N., and Ruiz, J. (2022). Challenges in large-scale bioinformatics projects. *Humanities and Social Sciences Communications* 9(1): 125. https://doi.org/10.1057/s41599-022-01141-4.

Moss, L. (2003). *What Genes Can't Do*. Cambridge, MA: MIT Press.

Moss, L. (2007). From describing to performing the socioethical engagement with systems biology. *American Journal of Bioethics* 7: 86-87. https://doi.org/10.1080/15265160701221400.

Moss, L. (2012). Is the philosophy of mechanism philosophy enough? *Studies in History and Philosophy of Science Part C: Studies in History and Philosophy of Biological and Biomedical Sciences* 43(1): 164-172. https://doi.org/10.1016/j.shpsc.2011.05.015.

Müller, U. R., and Nicolau, D. V. (Eds.). (2005). *Microarray Technology and Its Applications*. Berlin: Springer. https://doi.org/10.1007/b137842.

Mulvihill, J. J., Capps, B., Joly, Y., Lysaght, T., Zwart, H. A., Chadwick, R., and International Human Genome Organisation (HUGO) Committee of Ethics, Law, and Society (CELS). (2017). Ethical issues of CRISPR technology and gene editing through the lens of solidarity. *British Medical Bulletin* 122(1): 17-29. https://doi.org/10.1093/bmb/ldx002.

Mumford, S., and Anjum, R. L. (2013). *Causation: A Very Short Introduction*. New York: Oxford University Press. https://doi.org/10.1093/actrade/9780199684434.001.0001.

Murad, M. H., Asi, N., Alsawas, M., and Alahdab, F. (2016). New evidence pyramid. *BMJ Evidence-Based Medicine* 21(4): 125-127. http://dx.doi.org/10.1136/ebmed-2016-110401.

Musen, M. A., Noy, N. F., Shah, N. H., Whetzel, P. L., Chute, C. G., Story, M. A., Smith, B., and NCBO team. (2012). The National Center for Biomedical Ontology. *Journal of the American Medical Informatics Association* 19(2): 190-195. https://doi.org/10.1136/amiajnl-2011-000523.

Mykhalovskiy, E., and Weir, L. (2004). The problem of evidence-based medicine: directions for social science. *Social Science & Medicine* 59(5): 1059-1069. https://doi.org/10.1016/j.socscimed.2003.12.002.

Nagamune, T. (2017). Biomolecular engineering for nanobio/bionanotechnology. *Nano Convergence* 4(1): 9. https://doi.org/10.1186/s40580-017-0103-4.

Nagel, E. (1961). *The Structure of Science: The Problems in the Logic of Scientific Explanation*. New York: Harcourt, Brace.

Nagel, T. (1965). Physicalism. *Philosophical Review* 74: 339-356. https://doi.org/10.2307/2183358.

Nair, S. R. (2010). Personalized medicine: Striding from genes to medicines. *Perspectives in Clinical Research* 1(4): 146. https://doi.org/10.4103/2229-3485.71775.

Nassar, S. F., Raddassi, K., Ubhi, B., Doktorski, J., and Abulaban, A. (2020). Precision medicine: Steps along the road to combat human cancer. *Cells* 9(9): 2056. https://doi.org/10.3390/cells9092056.

National Institutes of Health. (2016). Precision medicine initiative cohort program. https://allofus.nih.gov/.

National Research Council. (2011). *Toward Precision Medicine: Building a knowledge Network for Biomedical Research and a New Taxonomy of Disease*. Washington, DC: The National Academies Press. https://doi.org/10.17226/13284.

Nebbioso, A., Tambaro, F. P., Dell'Aversana, C., and Altucci, L. (2018). Cancer epigenetics: Moving forward. *PLoS genetics* 14(6): e1007362. https://doi.org/10.1371/journal.pgen.1007362.

Needham, J. (1928). Organicism in biology. *Journal of Philosophical Studies* 3(9): 29-40. https://doi.org/10.1017/S0031819100012602.

Needham, J., and Hughes, A. (1959). *A History of Embryology*, 2nd edition. Cambridge, UK: Cambridge University Press.

Nehaniv, C. L. (2003). Evolvability. *BioSystems* 69: 77-81. https://doi.org/10.1016/s0303-2647(02)00130-2.

Nelkin, D., and Lindee, M. S. (2004). *The DNA Mystique: The Gene as a Cultural Icon*. Ann Arbor, MI: University of Michigan Press.

Nelson, N. C. (2015). A knockout experiment: Disciplinary divides and experimental skill in animal behaviour genetics. *Medical History* 59(3): 465-485. https://doi.org/10.1017/mdh.2015.30.

Neurath, O. (1931). Physicalism: The philosophy of the Viennese circle. *Monist* 41(4): 618-623. http://www.jstor.org/stable/27901327.

Newman, S. (1999). Epigenetics vs. genetic determinism. *Wild Duck Review* 5(2): 8-12. https://doi.org/10.1590/S0104-59702006000400004.

Newman, M. (2018). *Networks*, 2nd edition. New York: Oxford University Press. https://doi.org/10.1093/oso/9780198805090.001.0001.

Newman, M., Barabási, A. L., and Watts, D. J. (Eds.). (2006). *The Structure and Dynamics of Networks*. Princeton, NJ: Princeton University Press. https://doi.org/10.1515/9781400841356.

Newton, I. (1730). *Opticks: Or, A Treatise of the Reflections, Refractions, Inflections and Colours of Light*, 4th edition, corrected. London: William Innys. https://ia600903.us.archive.org/23/items/opticksortreatis1730newt/opticksortreatis1730newt.pdf.

Ney, A. (2008). Defining physicalism. *Philosophy Compass* 3(5): 1033-1048. https://doi.org/10.1111/j.1747-9991.2008.00163.x.

Ng, Y. L., Salim, C. K., and Chu, J. J. H. (2021). Drug repurposing for COVID-19: Approaches, challenges and promising candidates. *Pharmacology & Therapeutics* 228: 107930. https://doi.org/10.1016/j.pharmthera.2021.107930.

Nicholson, D. J. (2012). The concept of mechanism in biology. *Studies in History and Philosophy of Science Part C: Studies in History and Philosophy of Biological and Biomedical Sciences* 43(1): 152-163. https://doi.org/10.1016/j.shpsc.2011.05.014.

Nicholson, D. J. (2014). The return of the organism as a fundamental explanatory concept in biology. *Philosophy Compass* 9(5): 347-359. https://doi.org/10.1111/phc3.12128.

Nicholson, D. J., and Gawne, R. (2015). Neither logical empiricism nor vitalism, but organicism: What the philosophy of biology was. *History and Philosophy of the Life Sciences* 37(4): 345-381. https://doi.org/10.1007/s40656-015-0085-7.

Nicoglou, A., and Merlin, F. (2017). Epigenetics: A way to bridge the gap between biological fields. *Studies in History and Philosophy of Biological and Biomedical Sciences* 66: 73-82. https://doi.org/10.1016/j.shpsc.2017.10.002.

Nicoglou, A., and Wolfe, C. T. (2018). Introduction: Sketches of a conceptual history of epigenesis. *History and Philosophy of the Life Sciences* 40(4): 64. https://doi.org/10.1007/s40656-018-0230-1.

Niederer, S. A., Aboelkassem, Y., Cantwell, C. D., Corrado, C., Coveney, S., Cherry, E. M., Delhaas, T., Fenton, F. H., Panfilov, A. V., Pathmanathan, P. and Plank, G. (2020). Creation and application of virtual patient cohorts of heart models. *Philosophical Transactions of the Royal Society A* 378(2173): 20190558. https://doi.org/10.1098/rsta.2019.0558.

Nielsen, J., and Keasling, J. D. (2016). Engineering cellular metabolism. *Cell* 164(6): 1185-1197. https://doi.org/10.1016/j.cell.2016.02.004.

Nijhout, H. F., Sadre-Marandi, F., Best, J., and Reed, M. C. (2017). Systems biology of phenotypic robustness and plasticity. *Integrative and Comparative Biology* 57(2): 171-184. https://doi.org/10.1093/icb/icx076.

Nijhout, H. F., Best, J. A., and Reed, M. C. (2019). Systems biology of robustness and homeostatic mechanisms. *Systems Biology and Medicine* 11(3): e1440. https://doi.org/10.1002/wsbm.1440.

Nikolov, S., Yankulova, E., Wolkenhauer, O., and Petrov, V., (2007). Principle difference between stability and structural stability (robustness) as used in systems biology. *Nonlinear Dynamics, Psychology, and Life Sciences* 11: 413-433.

Nikolova, I. (2020). On stochastic models in biology and medicine. *Asian-European Journal of Mathematics* 13(08): 2050168. https://doi.org/10.1142/S17935571 20501685.

Nishimura, M., Jung, E. J., Shah, M. Y., Lu, C., Spizzo, R., Shimizu, M., Han, H. D., Ivan, C., Rossi, S., Zhang, X., and Nicoloso, M. S. (2013). Therapeutic synergy between microRNA and siRNA in ovarian cancer treatment. *Cancer Discovery* 3(11): 1302-1315. https://doi.org/10.1158/2159-8290.CD-13-0159.

Noble, D. (2003). The future: Putting Humpty-Dumpty together again. *Biochemical Society Transactions* 31: 156-158. https://doi.org/10.1042/bst0310156.

Noble, D. (2006). *The Music of Life: Biology Beyond Genes*. New York: Oxford University Press.

Noble, D. (2008). Genes and causation. *Philosophical Transactions* 366A: 3001-3015. https://doi.org/10.1098/rsta.2008.0086.

Noble, D. (2012). A theory of biological relativity: No privileged level of causation. *Interface Focus* 2(1): 55-64. https://doi.org/10.1098/rsfs.2011.0067.

Noble, D. (2017). *Dance to the Tune of Life: Biological Relativity*. New York: Cambridge University Press.

Noble, R., Tasaki, K., Noble, P. J., and Noble, D. (2019). Biological relativity requires circular causality but not symmetry of causation: So, where, what and when are the boundaries? *Frontiers in Physiology* 10: 827. https://doi.org/10.3389/fphys.2019.00827.

Noell, G., Faner, R., and Agustí, A. (2018). From systems biology to P4 medicine: Applications in respiratory medicine. *European Respiratory Review* 27(147): 170110. https://doi.org/10.1183/16000617.0110-2017.

Novack, G. (1965). *The Origins of Materialism: The Evolution of a Scientific View of the World*. New York: Pathfinder.

November, J. A. (2012). *Biomedical Computing: Digitizing Life in the United States*. Baltimore, MD: The Johns Hopkins University Press.

Nunn, R. (2012). Many-models medicine: Diversity as the best medicine. *Journal of Evaluation in Clinical Practice* 18: 974-978. https://doi.org/10.1111/j.1365-2753.2012.01903.x.

Nye, R. A. (2003). The evolution of the concept of medicalization in the late twentieth century. *Journal of the History of the Behavioral Sciences 39*(2): 115-129. https://doi.org/10.1002/jhbs.10108.

O'Connor, D. J. (1971). *Free Will*. London: Macmillan.

O'Connor, T. (1994). Emergent properties. *American Philosophical Quarterly* 31(2): 91-104. https://www.jstor.org/stable/20014490.

O'Connor, T. (2020). Emergent properties. In *Stanford Encyclopedia of Philosophy, E. N. Zalta (Ed.). https://plato.stanford.edu/entries/properties-emergent/.*

Olby, R. C. (1974). *The Path to the Double Helix*. Seattle, WA: University of Washington Press.

Olby, R. C. (1985). *Origins of Mendelism*, 2nd edition. Chicago, IL: University of Chicago Press.

Olivier, B. G., Swat, M. J., and Moné, M. J. (2016). Modeling and simulation tools: From systems biology to systems medicine. In *Systems Medicine: Methods in Molecular Biology*, volume 1386 (pp. 441-463), U. Schmitz and O. Wolkenhauer (Eds.). New York: Humana Press. https://doi.org/10.1007/978-1-4939-3283-2_19.

Olofsson, P., and Andersson, M. (2012). *Probability, Statistics, and Stochastic Processes*, 2nd edition. New York: John Wiley & Sons.

Olson, M. V. (2017). A behind-the-scenes story of precision medicine. *Genomics, Proteomics & Bioinformatics* 15(1): 3-10. https://doi.org/10.1016/j.gpb.2017.01.002.

O'Malley, M. A., and Dupré, J. (2005). Fundamental issues in systems biology. *BioEssays* 27: 1270-1276. https://doi.org/10.1002/bies.20323.

O'Malley, M. A., Calvert, J., and Dupré, J. (2007). The study of socioethical issues in systems biology. *American Journal of Bioethics* 7: 67-78. https://doi.org/10.1080/15265160701221285.

Orsucci, F. F. (2003). *Changing Mind: Transitions in Natural and Artificial Environments*. Singapore: World Scientific Publishing. https://doi.org/10.1142/4991.

O'Shea, P. (2012). Future medicine shaped by an interdisciplinary new biology. *Lancet* 379(9825), 1544-1550. https://doi.org/10.1016/S0140-6736(12)60476-0.

Ovaskainen, O., de Knegt, H. J., and del Mar Delgado, M. (2016). *Quantitative Ecology and Evolutionary Biology: Integrating Models with Data*. New York: Oxford University Press. https://doi.org/10.1093/acprof:oso/9780198714866.001.0001.

Ozata, D. M., Gainetdinov, I., Zoch, A., O'Carroll, D., and Zamore, P. D. (2019). PIWI-interacting RNAs: Small RNAs with big functions. *Nature Reviews Genetics* 20(2): 89-108. https://doi.org/10.1038/s41576-018-0073-3.

Palaparthi, S. (2017). Role of homeostasis in human physiology: A review. *Journal of Medical Physiology & Therapeutics* 1(2): 101.

Palsson, B. O. (2006). *Systems Biology: Properties of Reconstructed Networks*. New York: Cambridge University Press.

Palsson, B. O. (2015). *Systems Biology: Constraint-based Reconstruction and Analysis*. New York: Cambridge University Press.

Pan, D., Rampal, R., and Mascarenhas, J. (2020). Clinical developments in epigenetic-directed therapies in acute myeloid leukemia. *Blood Advances* 4(5): 970-982. https://doi.org/10.1182/bloodadvances.2019001245.

Panzeri, I., and Pospisilik, J. A. (2018). Epigenetic control of variation and stochasticity in metabolic disease. *Molecular Metabolism* 14: 26-38. https://doi.org/10.1016/j.molmet.2018.05.010.

Paoletti, M. P. (2018). Formulating emergence. *Ratio*, *31*, 1-18. https://doi.org/10.1111/rati.12160.

Paoletti, M. P., and Orilia, F. (Eds.). (2017). *Philosophical and Scientific Perspectives on Downward Causation*. New York: Routledge.

Papineau, D. (2001). The rise of physicalism. In *Physicalism and its Discontents* (pp. 3-36), C. Gillett and B. Loewer (Eds.). New York: Cambridge University Press.

Papineau, D. (2009). The causal closure of the physical and naturalism. In *The Oxford Handbook of Philosophy of Mind* (pp. 53-65), B. McLaughlin, A. Beckermann, and S. Walter (Eds.). New York: Oxford University Press. https://doi.org/10.1093/oxfordhb/9780199262618.003.0003.

Parkkinen, V. P., Wallmann, C., Wilde, M., Clarke, B., Illari, P., Kelly, M. P., Norell, C., Russo, F., Shaw, B., and Williamson, J. (2018). *Evaluating Evidence of Mechanisms in Medicine: Principles and Procedures*. Cham, CH: Springer. https://doi.org/10.1007/978-3-319-94610-8.

Patel, M., and Nagl, S. (2006). Mathematical models of cancer. In *Cancer Bioinformatics from Therapy Design to Treatment* (pp. 59-93), S. Nagl (Ed.). New York: John Wiley & Sons. https://doi.org/10.1002/0470032898.ch4.

Patton, K. T., and Thibodea, J. A. (2014). *The Human Body in Health and Disease*, 6th edition. Amsterdam, NL: Elsevier.

Pauling, L., Itano, H. A., Singer, S. J., and Wells, I. C. (1949). Sickle cell anemia, a molecular disease. *Science* 110(2865): 543-548. https://doi.org/10.1126/science.110.2865.543.

Paus, T. (2013). *Population Neuroscience*. Berlin: Springer. https://doi.org/10.1007/978-3-642-36450-1_3.

Pearl, J. (2009). *Causality: Models, Reasoning, and Inference*, 2nd edition. New York: Cambridge University Press.

Peggs, K. (2012). *Animals and Sociology*. London: Palgrave Macmillan. https://doi.org/10.1057/9780230377271_2.

Pennazio, S. (2009). Homeostasis: A history of biology. *Rivista di Biologia* 102(2): 253-271.

Pepper, S. C. (1926). Emergence. *Journal of Philosophy* 23: 241-245. https://doi.org/10.2307/2014779.

Pereboom, D. (1995). Determinism al dente. *Noûs* 29(1): 21-45. https://doi.org/10.2307/2215725.

Perls, T., Kunkel, L., and Puca, A. (2002). The genetics of aging. *Current Opinion in Genetics & Development* 12(3): 362-369. https://doi.org/10.1016/S0959-437X(02)00310-6.

Perryman, C.L. (2018). Credit due: Multiple author attribution for interdisciplinary informatics research groups. *Hypothesis* 30(1): 21-32. https://doi.org/10.18060/25174.

Peters, T. (2003). *Playing God? Genetic Determinism and Human Freedom*, 2nd edition New York: Routledge.

Peterson, E. L. (2016). *The Life Organic: The Theoretical Biology Club and the Roots of Epigenetics*. Pittsburgh, PA: University of Pittsburgh Press.

Petrazzuoli, F., Morin, L., Angioni, D., Pecora, N., and Cherubini, A. (2022). Polypharmacy, overdiagnosis and overtreatment. In *The Role of Family Physicians in Older People Care* (pp. 325-340), J. Demurtas and N. Veronese (Eds.). Cham, CH: Springer. https://doi.org/10.1007/978-3-030-78923-7_19.

Pfaff, H., and Schmitt, J. (2021). The organic turn: Coping with pandemic and non-pandemic challenges by integrating evidence-, theory-, experience-, and context-based knowledge in advising health policy. *Frontiers in Public Health* 9: 727427. https://doi.org/10.3389/fpubh.2021.727427.

Philips, M. (2003). What is materialism? *Philosophy Now* 42: 18-19.

Phillips, D. C. (1970). Organicism in the late nineteenth and early twentieth centuries. *Journal of the History of Ideas* 31(3): 413-432. https://doi.org/10.2307/2708514.

Pickup, M. W., Mouw, J. K., and Weaver, V. M. (2014). The extracellular matrix modulates the hallmarks of cancer. *EMBO Reports* 15(12): 1243-1253. https://doi.org/10.15252/embr.201439246.

Piechocinska, B. (2004). Wholeness as a conceptual foundation of physical theories. *Physics Essays* 17(4): 505-517. https://doi.org/10.4006/1.3025712.

Pinkston, J. A. (2020). *Evidence and Hypothesis in Clinical Medical Science*. Cham: CH: Springer. https://doi.org/10.1007/978-3-030-44270-5.

Pisco, A. O., d'Hérouël, A. F., and Huang, S. (2016). Conceptual confusion: The case of epigenetics. *BioRxiv* 2016: 053009. https://doi.org/10.1101/053009.

Placek, T. (2004). Quantum state holism: A case for holistic causation. *Studies in the History and Philosophy of Modern Physics* 35: 671-692. https://doi.org/10.1016/j.shpsb.2004.06.001.

Plomin, R. (2018). *Blueprint: How DNA Makes Us Who We Are*. Cambridge, MA: MIT Press.

Pokorska-Bocci, A., Stewart, A., Sagoo, G. S., Hall, A., Kroese, M., and Burton, H. (2014). 'Personalized medicine': what's in a name? *Personalized Medicine* 11(2): 197-210. https://doi.org/10.2217/pme.13.107.

Polanyi, M. (1968). Life's irreducible structure. *Science* 160: 1308-1312. https://doi.org/10.1126/science.160.3834.1308.

Poli, R. (2011). Analysis-synthesis. In *Ontological Landscapes: Recent Thought on Conceptual Interfaces Between Science and Philosophy* (pp. 19-42), V. Petrov (Ed.). Frankfurt, DE: Ontos Verlag.

Popp, M., Reis S, Schießer S, Hausinger R. I., Stegemann M, Metzendorf M. I, Kranke P, Meybohm P, Skoetz N, Weibel S. (2022). Ivermectin for preventing and treating COVID-19. *Cochrane Database of Systematic Reviews* Issue 6: CD015017. https://doi.org/10.1002/14651858.CD015017.pub3.

Portin, P., and Wilkins, A. (2017). The evolving definition of the term "gene." *Genetics* 205(4): 1353-1364. https://doi.org/10.1534/genetics.116.196956.

Powathil, G. G., Swat, M., and Chaplain, M. A. (2015). Systems oncology: Towards patient-specific treatment regimes informed by multiscale mathematical modelling. *Seminars in Cancer Biology* 30: 13-20. https://doi.org/10.1016/j.semcancer.2014.02.003.

Powell, K. (2004). All systems go. *Journal of Cell Biology* 165(3): 299-303. https://doi.org/10.1083/jcb.200404013.

Prainsack, B. (2017). *Personalized Medicine: Empowered Patients in the 21st century?* New York: New York University Press. https://doi.org/10.18574/nyu/9781479814879.001.0001.

Pravettoni, G., and Triberti, S. (2020). A "P5" Approach to healthcare and health technology. In *P5 eHealth: An Agenda for the Health Technologies of the Future* (pp. 3-17), G. Pravettoni and S. Triberti (Eds.). Cham, CH: Springer. https://doi.org/10.1007/978-3-030-27994-3_1.

Preuer, K., Lewis, R. P., Hochreiter, S., Bender, A., Bulusu, K. C., and Klambauer, G. (2018). DeepSynergy: Predicting anti-cancer drug synergy with Deep Learning. *Bioinformatics* 34(9): 1538-1546. https://doi.org/10.1093/bioinformatics/btx806.

Price, N. D., Edelman, L. B., Lee, I., Yoo, H., Hwang, D., Carlson, G., Galas, D. J., Heath, J. R., and Hood, L. (2010). Systems biology and systems medicine. In *Essentials of Genomic and Personalized Medicine* (pp. 131-141), G. S. Ginsburg and H. F. Willard (Eds.). London: Academic Press. https://doi.org/10.1016/B978-0-12-374934-5.00011-8.

Prosser, S. (2012). Emergent causation. *Philosophical Studies* 159(1): 21-39. https://doi.org/10.1007/s11098-010-9685-y.

Quina, A. S., Buschbeck, M., and Di Croce, L. (2006). Chromatin structure and epigenetics. *Biochemical Pharmacology* 72(11): 1563-1569. https://doi.org/10.1016/j.bcp.2006.06.016.

Rahim, F., Soltani, A., and Haghpanah, V. (2012). Developing organized level of biomedical evidence: Evidence-based biomedicine. *Frontiers in Physiology* 3: 428. https://doi.org/10.3389/fphys.2012.00428.

Raj, A., and Van Oudenaarden, A. (2008). Nature, nurture, or chance: Stochastic gene expression and its consequences. *Cell* 135(2): 216-226. https://doi.org/10.1016/j.cell.2008.09.050.

Ramirez, A. H., Sulieman, L., Schlueter, D. J., Halvorson, A., Qian, J., Ratsimbazafy, F., Loperena, R., Mayo, K., Basford, M., Deflaux, N., and Muthuraman, K. N. (2022). The All of Us Research Program: Data quality, utility, and diversity. *Patterns* 3(8): 100570. https://doi.org/10.1016/j.patter.2022.100570.

Ramsay, D. S., and Woods, S. C. (2014). Clarifying the roles of homeostasis and allostasis in physiological regulation. *Psychological Review* 121(2): 225-247. https://doi.org/10.1037/a0035942.

Ranea, J. A., Perkins, J., Chagoyen, M., Díaz-Santiago, E., and Pazos, F. (2022). Network-based methods for approaching human pathologies from a phenotypic point of view. *Genes* 13(6): 1081. https://doi.org/10.3390/genes13061081.

Rangel, U., and Keller, J. (2011). Essentialism goes social: Belief in social determinism as a component of psychological essentialism. *Journal of Personality and Social Psychology 100*(6): 1056–1078. https://doi.org/10.1037/a0022401.

Rao, G. H. R. (2021). Biomedicine in the COVID age: Opportunities, responses, and challenges. *International Journal of Biomedicine* 11: 241-249. https://doi.org/10.21103/Article11(3)_RA1.

Raposo, V. L. (2019). Gene editing, the mystic threat to human dignity. *Journal of Bioethical Inquiry* 16(2): 249-257. https://doi.org/10.1007/s11673-019-09906-4.

Rasband, S. N. (2015). *Chaotic Dynamics of Nonlinear Systems*. Mineola, NY: Dover Publications.

Rather, L. J. (1988). Virchow and the mechanistic concept of life in 1845. *Bulletin of the History of Medicine* 62(1): 107-111. https://www.jstor.org/stable/44449298.

Rattan, S. I. S. (2020). Biological health and homeodynamic space. In *Explaining Health Across the Sciences* (pp. 43-51), J. Sholl and S. I. S. Rattan (Eds.). Cham, CH: Springer. https://doi.org/10.1007/978-3-030-52663-4_4.

Rehman, S. U., Rehman, S. U., and Yoo, H. H. (2021). COVID-19 challenges and its therapeutics. *Biomedicine & Pharmacotherapy* 142: 112015. https://doi.org/10.1016/j.biopha.2021.112015.

Reid, R. G. B. (2007). *Biological Emergences: Evolution by Natural Experiment*. Cambridge, MA: MIT Press.

Resnik, D. B., and Vorhaus, D. B. (2006). Genetic modification and genetic determinism. *Philosophy, Ethics, and Humanities in Medicine* 1: 9. https://doi.org/10.1186/1747-5341-1-9.

Revel, M. (2005). Are genes our destiny? Implications and ethical limitations of genetic determinism in medicine and behavioral sciences. In *The Embryo: Scientific Discovery and Medical Ethics* (pp. 143-165), S. Blazar and E. Z. Zimmer (Eds.). New York: Karger.

Rheinberger, H. J., and Gaudillière, J. P. (2004). *Classical Genetic Research and Its Legacy: The Mapping Cultures of Twentieth-Century Genetics*. New York: Routledge.

Ribrault, C., Sekimoto, K., and Triller, A. (2011). From the stochasticity of molecular processes to the variability of synaptic transmission. *Nature Reviews Neuroscience* 12(7): 375-387. https://doi.org/10.1038/nrn3025.

Rice, S. H., Papadopoulos, A., and Harting, J. (2011). Stochastic processes driving directional evolution. In *Evolutionary Biology–Concepts, Biodiversity, Macroevolution and Genome Evolution* (pp. 21-33), P. Pontarotti (Ed.). Berlin: Springer. https://doi.org/10.1007/978-3-642-20763-1_2.

Richardson, R. C., and Stephan, A. (2007a). Mechanism and mechanical philosophy in systems biology. In *Systems Biology: Philosophical Foundations* (pp. 123-144), F. C. Boogerd, F. J. Bruggeman, J. H. S. Hofmeyr, and H. V. Westerhoff (Eds.). Amsterdam, NL: Elsevier. https://doi.org/10.1016/B978-044452085-2/50008-5.

Richardson, R. C., and Stephan, A. (2007b). Emergence. *Biological Theory* 2: 91-96. https://doi.org/10.1162/biot.2007.2.1.91.

Rickles, D., Hawe, P., and Shiell, A. (2007). A simple guide to chaos and complexity. *Journal of Epidemiology & Community Health* 61(11): 933-937. http://dx.doi.org/10.1136/jech.2006.054254.

Riggs, A. D. (1975). X inactivation, differentiation, and DNA methylation. *Cytogenetic and Genome Research* 14(1): 9-25. https://doi.org/10.1159/000130315.

Riggs, A. D., Martienssen, R. A., and Russo, V. E. A. (1996). Introduction. In *Epigenetic Mechanisms of Gene Regulation* (pp. 1-4), V. E. A. Russo, R. A. Martienssen, and A. D. Riggs (Eds.). Woodbury, NY: Cold Spring Harbor Laboratory Press.

Rijke, R. (1993). Health in medicine science: From determinism towards autonomy. In *Towards a New Science of Health* (pp. 58-65), R. Lafaille and S. Fulder (Eds.). New York: Routledge.

Ristić, A. J., Zaharijević, A., and Miličić, N. (2021). Foucault's concept of clinical gaze today. *Health Care Analysis* 29: 99-112. https://doi.org/10.1007/s10728-020-00402-0.

Ritchey, T. (1991). Analysis and synthesis: On scientific method–Based on a study by Bernhard Riemann. *Systems Research* 8(4): 21-41. https://doi.org/10.1002/sres.3850080402.

Ritter, W. E., and Bailey, E. W. (1928). The organismal conception: Its place in science and its bearing on philosophy. *University of California Publications in Zoology* 31: 307-358.

Robert, J. S. (2007). Systems bioethics. *American Journal of Bioethics* 7: 80-82. https://doi.org/10.1080/15265160701221467.

Robert, J. S., and Plantikow, T. (2005). Genetics, neuroscience and psychiatric classification. *Psychopathology* 38(4): 215-218. https://doi.org/10.1159/000086095.

Roberts, T. (2014). From things to events: Whitehead and the materiality of process. *Environment and Planning D: Society and Space* 32(6): 968-983. https://doi.org/10.1068/d13195p.

Robinson, J. D. (1992). Aims and achievements of the reductionist approach in biochemistry/molecular biology/cell biology: A response to Kincaid. *Philosophy of Scienc*e 59: 465-470. https://doi.org/10.1086/289683.

Rocca, E., and Anjum, R. L. (2020). Complexity, reductionism and the biomedical model. In *Rethinking Causality, Complexity and Evidence for the Unique Patient* (pp. 75-94), R. L. Anjum, S. Copeland, and E. Rocca (Eds.). Cham, CH: Springer. https://doi.org/10.1007/978-3-030-41239-5_5.

Rockhold, F., Nisen, P., and Freeman, A. (2016). Data sharing at a crossroads. *New England Journal of Medicine* 375(12): 1115-1117. https://doi.org/10.1056/NEJMp1608086.

Roco, M. C. (2003). Nanotechnology: Convergence with modern biology and medicine. *Current Opinion in Biotechnology* 14: 337-346. https://doi.org/10.1016/S0958-1669(03)00068-5.

Rodenhiser, D., and Mann, M. (2006). Epigenetics and human disease: Translating basic biology into clinical applications. *Canadian Medical Association Journal* 174(3): 341-348. https://doi.org/10.1503/cmaj.050774.

Roell, K. R., Reif, D. M., and Motsinger-Reif, A. A. (2017). An introduction to terminology and methodology of chemical synergy—perspectives from across disciplines. *Frontiers in pharmacology* 8: 158. https://doi.org/10.3389/fphar.2017.00158.

Rohani, P., Keeling, M. J., and Grenfell, B. T. (2002). The interplay between determinism and stochasticity in childhood diseases. *American Naturalist* 159(5): 469-481. https://doi.org/10.1086/339467.

Röhl, J. (2012). Mechanisms in biomedical ontology. *Journal of Biomedical Semantics* 3(2): S9. https://doi.org/10.1186/2041-1480-3-S2-S9.

Rosen, W. (2017). *Miracle Cure: The Creation of Antibiotics and the Birth of Modern Medicine*. New York: Viking.

Rosenberg, W., and Donald, A. (1995). Evidence based medicine: An approach to clinical problem-solving. *British Medical Journal* 310(6987): 1122-1126. https://doi.org/10.1136/bmj.310.6987.

Rosner, A. L. (2012). Evidence-based medicine: Revisiting the pyramid of priorities. *Journal of Bodywork and Movement Therapies* 16(1): 42-49. https://doi.org/10.1016/j.jbmt.2011.05.003.

Rosslenbroich, B. (2016). The significance of an enhanced concept of the organism for medicine. *Evidence-Based Complementary and Alternative Medicine* 2016: 1587652. https://doi.org/10.1155/2016/1587652.

Rothman, K. J. (1974). Synergy and antagonism in cause-effect relationships. *American Journal of Epidemiology* 99: 385-388. https://doi.org/10.1093/oxfordjournals.aje.a121626.

Rothschild, L. J. (2006). The role of emergence in biology. In *The Re-Emergence of Emergence: The Emergentist Hypothesis from Science to Religion* (pp. 151-165), P. Clayton and P. Davies (Eds.). New York: Oxford University Press. https://doi.org/10.1093/acprof:oso/9780199544318.003.0006.

Roukos, D. H. (2012). Longevity with systems medicine? Epigenome, genome and environment interactions network. *Epigenomics* 4(2): 119-123. https://doi.org/10.2217/epi.12.1.

Rubeis, G. (2021). Guardians of humanity? The challenges of nursing practice in the digital age. *Nursing Philosophy* 22: e12331. https://doi.org/10.1111/nup.12331.

Runge, M. S., and Patterson, C. (Eds.). (2006). *Principles of Molecular Medicine*, 2nd edition. New York: Humana Press. https://doi.org/10.1007/978-1-59259-963-9.

Ruse, M. (1971). Reduction, replacement, and molecular biology. *Dialectica* 25: 38-72. https://doi.org/10.1111/j.1746-8361.1971.tb00591.x.

Ruse, M. (2013). From organicism to mechanism—and halfway back? In *Beyond Mechanism: Putting Life Back into Biology* (pp. 412-432), B. G. Henning and A. Scarfe (Eds.). Lanham, MD: Lexington Books.

Russell, L. (2014). *Sociology for Health Professionals*. London: SAGE.

Russell, R., and Superti-Furga, G. (2005). Systems biology: Understanding the biological mosaic. *FEBS Letters* 579: 1771. https://doi.org/10.1016/j.febslet.2005.02.029.

Russo, F., and Williamson, J. (2007). Interpreting causality in the health sciences. *International Studies in the Philosophy of Science* 21(2): 157-170. https://doi.org/10.1080/02698590701498084.

Sabatello, M., and Juengst, E. (2019). Genomic essentialism: Its provenance and trajectory as an anticipatory ethical concern. *Hastings Center Report* 49: S10-S18. https://doi.org/10.1002/hast.1012.

Sabino, A. U., Vasconcelos, M. F., Sittoni, M. Y., Lautenschlager, W. W., Queiroga, A. S., Morais, M. C., and Ramos, A. F. (2018). Lessons and perspectives for applications of stochastic models in biological and cancer research. *Clinics* 73: e536s. https://doi.org/10.6061/clinics/2018/e536s.

Sabra, A. I. (1981). *Theories of Light from Descartes to Newton*. New York: Cambridge University Press.

Sachse, C. (2007). *Reductionism in the Philosophy of Science*. Frankfurt: Ontos Verlag.

Sackett, D. L., Rosenberg, W. M., Gray, J. M., Haynes, R. B., and Richardson, W. S. (1996). Evidence based medicine: What it is and what it isn't. *British Medical Journal* 312(7023): 71-72. https://doi.org/10.1136/bmj.312.7023.71.

Salari, P., and Larijani, B. (2017). Ethical issues surrounding personalized medicine: A literature review. *Acta Medica Iranica* 209-217.

Saliba, A. E., Westermann, A. J., Gorski, S. A., and Vogel, J. (2014). Single-cell RNA-seq: Advances and future challenges. *Nucleic Acids Research* 42(14): 8845-8860. https://doi.org/10.1093/nar/gku555.

Sankar, P. L., and Parker, L. S. (2017). The Precision Medicine Initiative's All of Us Research Program: An agenda for research on its ethical, legal, and social issues. *Genetics in Medicine 19*(7): 743-750. https://doi.org/10.1038/gim.2016.183.

Santos, G. C. (2015). Upward and downward causation from a relational-horizontal ontological perspective. *Axiomathes* 25(1): 23-40. https://doi.org/10.1007/s10516-014-9251-x.

Santos, R. (2020). Patient care after COVID: Providers must correct 'one size fits all' approach, experts say. *Health Policy Watch* Dec 10. https://healthpolicy-watch.news/patient-care-after-covid-providers-must-address-unfit-one-size-fits-all-approach-experts-say/.

Saqi, M., Pellet, J., Roznovat, I., Mazein, A., Ballereau, S., De Meulder, B., and Auffray, C. (2016). Systems medicine: The future of medical genomics, healthcare, and wellness. In *Systems Medicine: Methods in Molecular Biology,* volume 1386 (pp. 43-60), U. Schmitz and O. Wolkenhauer (Eds.). New York: Humana Press. https://doi.org/10.1007/978-1-4939-3283-2_3.

Sarkar, S. (1998). *Genetics and Reductionism*. New York: Cambridge University Press.

Sastry, S. (1999). *Nonlinear Systems: Analysis, Stability, and Control*. New York: Springer. https://doi.org/10.1007/978-1-4757-3108-8.

Sastry, S., and Bodson, M. (2011). *Adaptive Control: Stability, Convergence and Robustness*. Mineola, NY: Dover Publications.

Saulsberry, L., and Olopade, O. I. (2021). Precision oncology: Directing genomics and pharmacogenomics toward reducing cancer inequities. *Cancer Cell* 39(6): 730-733. https://doi.org/10.1016/j.ccell.2021.04.013.

Savageau, M. A. (1969a). Biochemical systems analysis. I. Some mathematical properties of the rate law for the component enzymatic reactions. *Journal of Theoretical Biology* 25: 365-369. https://doi.org/10.1016/S0022-5193(69)80026-3.

Savageau, M. A. (1969b). Biochemical systems analysis. II. The steady-state solutions for an n-pool system using a power-law approximation. *Journal of Theoretical Biology* 25: 370-379. https://doi.org/10.1016/S0022-5193(69)80027-5.

Savageau, M. A. (1970). Biochemical systems analysis. III. Dynamic solutions using a power-law approximation. *Journal of Theoretical Biology* 26: 215-226. https://doi.org/10.1016/S0022-5193(70)80013-3.

Savageau, M. A. (1976). *Biochemical Systems Analysis: A Study of Function and Design in Molecular Biology*. Reading, MA: Addison–Wesley.

Savageau, M. A. (1991). Reconstructionist molecular biology. *New Biologist* 3: 190-197.

Schaffer, J. (2003). Overdetermining causes. *Philosophical Studies* 114(1/2): 23-45. http://www.jstor.org/stable/4321372.

Schaffner, K. F. (1967). Approaches to reduction. *Philosophy of Science* 34: 137-147. https://doi.org/10.1086/288137.

Schaffner, K. F. (2007). Theories, models, and equations in systems. In *Systems Biology: Philosophical Foundations* (pp. 145-162), F. C. Boogerd, F. J. Bruggeman, J. H. S. Hofmeyr, and H. V. Westerhoff (Eds.). Amsterdam, NL: Elsevier. https://doi.org/10.1016/B978-044452085-2/50009-7.

Schaffner, K. F. (2012). Ernest Nagel and reduction. *Journal of Philosophy* 109(8/9): 534-565. https://www.jstor.org/stable/43820725.

Schleidgen, S., Klingler, C., Bertram, T., Rogowski, W. H., and Marckmann, G. (2013). What is personalized medicine: Sharpening a vague term based on a systematic literature review. *BMC Medical Ethics* 14(1): 55. https://doi.org/10.1186/1472-6939-14-55.

Schleidgen, S., Fernau, S., Fleischer, H., Schickhardt, C., Oßa, A. K., and Winkler, E. C. (2017). Applying systems biology to biomedical research and health care: A précising definition of systems medicine. *BMC Health Services Research* 17(1): 761. https://doi.org/10.1186/s12913-017-2688-z.

Schmitz, U., and Wolkenhauer, O. (Eds.). (2016). *Systems Medicine: Methods in Molecular Biology*, volume 1386. New York: Humana Press.

Schouten, M., and De Jong, H. L. (2006). Mind matters: The roots of reductionism. In *The Matter of the Mind: Philosophical Essays on Psychology, Neuroscience, and Reduction* (pp. 1-28), M. Schouten and H. L. De Jong (Eds.). Malden, MA: Blackwell.

Schulkin, J. (2003). Allostasis: A neural behavioral perspective. *Hormones and Behavior* 43(1): 21-30. https://doi.org/10.1016/S0018-506X(02)00035-1.

Schuol, S. (2017). Epigenetics and genetic determinism (in popular science). In *Epigenetics: Ethical, Legal and Social Aspects* (pp. 41-54), R. Heil, S. B. Seitz, H. König, and J. Robienski (Eds.). Wiesbaden, DE: Springer. https://doi.org/10.1007/978-3-658-14460-9_4.

Schuster, P. (2007). A beginning of the end of the holism versus reductionism debate? *Complexity* 13: 10-13. https://doi.org/10.1002/cplx.20193.

Schuster, P. (2016). *Stochasticity in Processes: Fundamentals and Applications to Chemistry and Biology*. Berlin: Springer. https://doi.org/10.1007/978-3-319-39502-9.

Scott, A. C. (2007). *The Nonlinear Universe: Chaos, Emergence, Life*. New York: Springer. https://doi.org/10.1007/978-3-540-34153-6.

Seager, W. (2000). Physicalism. In *A Companion to the Philosophy of Science* (pp. 340-342), W. H. Newton-Smith (Ed.). Malden, MA: Blackwell.

Seager, W. (2018). The philosophical and scientific metaphysics of David Bohm. *Entropy* 20(7): 493. https://doi.org/10.3390/e20070493.

Searls, D. B. (2010). The roots of bioinformatics. *PLoS Computational Biology* 6(6): e1000809. https://doi.org/10.1371/journal.pcbi.1000809.

Segaliny, A. I., Li, G., Kong, L., Ren, C., Chen, X., Wang, J. K., Baltimore, D., Wu, G., and Zhao, W. (2018). Functional TCR T cell screening using single-cell droplet microfluidics. *Lab on a Chip* 18(24): 3733-3749. https://doi.org/10.1039/C8LC00818C.

Sehon, S. R., and Stanley, D. E. (2003). A philosophical analysis of the evidence-based medicine debate. *BMC Health Services Research* 3(1): 14. https://doi.org/10.1186/1472-6963-3-14.

Selinger, D. W., Wright, M. A., and Church, G. M. (2003). On the complete determination of biological systems. *TRENDS in Biotechnology* 21: 251-254. https://doi.org/10.1016/S0167-7799(03)00113-6.

Selye, H. (1973). Homeostasis and heterostasis. *Perspectives in Biology and Medicine* 16(3): 441-445. https://doi.org/10.1353/pbm.1973.0056.

Serre, R., Benzekry, S., Padovani, L., Meille, C., André, N., Ciccolini, J., Barlesi, F., Muracciole, X., and Barbolosi, D. (2016). Mathematical modeling of cancer immunotherapy and its synergy with radiotherapy. *Cancer Research* 76(17): 4931-4940. https://doi.org/10.1158/0008-5472.CAN-15-3567.

Sevimoglu, T., and Arga, K. Y. (2014). The role of protein interaction networks in systems biomedicine. *Computational and Structural Biotechnology Journal* 11(18): 22-27. https://doi.org/10.1016/j.csbj.2014.08.008.

Shamasunder, S., Holmes, S. M., Goronga, T., Carrasco, H., Katz, E., Frankfurter, R., and Keshavjee, S. (2020). COVID-19 reveals weak health systems by design: Why we must re-make global health in this historic moment. *Global Public Health* 15(7): 1083-1089. https://doi.org/10.1080/17441692.2020.1760915.

Shaneyfelt, T. (2016). Pyramids are guides not rules: The evolution of the evidence pyramid. *BMJ Evidence-Based Medicine* 21(4): 121-122. http://dx.doi.org/10.1136/ebmed-2016-110498.

Shapin, S. (1996). *The Scientific Revolution*. Chicago, IL: University of Chicago Press.

Shastry, B. S. (2003). SNPs and haplotypes: Genetic markers for disease and drug response. *International Journal of Molecular Medicine* 11(3): 379-382. https://doi.org/10.3892/ijmm.11.3.379.

Shastry, B. S. (2007). SNPs in disease gene mapping, medicinal drug development and evolution. *Journal of Human Genetics* 52(11): 871-880. https://doi.org/10.1007/s10038-007-0200-z.

Sheldrake, R. (1980). Three approaches to biology: Part I. The mechanistic theory of life. *Theoria to Theory* 14: 125-144.

Sheldrake, R. (1981a). Three approaches to biology: Part II. Vitalism. *Theoria to Theory* 14: 227-40.

Sheldrake, R. (1981b). Three approaches to biology: Part III: Organicism. *Theoria to Theory* 14: 301-311.

Sheldrake, R. (2013). Setting science free from materialism. *Explore* 9(4): 211-218. https://doi.org/10.1016/j.explore.2013.04.004.

Shereen, M. A., Khan, S., Kazmi, A., Bashir, N., and Siddique, R. (2020). COVID-19 infection: Emergence, transmission, and characteristics of human coronaviruses. *Journal of Advanced Research* 24: 91-98. https://doi.org/10.1016/j.jare.2020.03.005.

Shin, S. H., Bode, A. M., and Dong, Z. (2017). Precision medicine: The foundation of future cancer therapeutics. *NPJ Precision Oncology* 1(1): 12. https://doi.org/10.1038/s41698-017-0016-z.

Shoemaker, L. G., Sullivan, L. L., Donohue, I., Cabral, J. S., Williams, R. J., Mayfield, M. M., Chase, J. M., Chu, C., Harpole, W. S., Huth, A., and HilleRisLambers, J. (2020). Integrating the underlying structure of stochasticity into community ecology. *Ecology* 101(2): e02922. https://doi.org/10.1002/ecy.2922.

Schofield, T. (2015). *A Sociological Approach to Health Determinants*. New York: Cambridge University Press.

Siddiqi, S. H., Taylor, J. J., Horn, A., and Fox, M. D. (2023). Bringing human brain connectomics to clinical practice in psychiatry. *Biological Psychiatry* 93(5), 386-387. https://doi.org/10.1016/j.biopsych.2022.05.026.

Silberstein, M. (2002). Reduction, emergence and explanation. *The Blackwell Guide to the Philosophy of Science* (pp. 80-107), P. Machamer and M. Silberstein (Eds.). Malden, MA: Blackwell. https://doi.org/10.1002/9780470756614.ch5.

Silverman, P. H. (2004). Rethinking genetic determinism: With only 30,000 genes, What is it that makes humans human? *The Scientist* 18: 32-33.

Silverman, E. K., Schmidt, H. H., Anastasiadou, E., Altucci, L., Angelini, M., Badimon, L., Balligand, J. L., Benincasa, G., Capasso, G., Conte, F., and Di Costanzo, A. (2020). Molecular networks in Network Medicine: Development and applications. *Systems Biology and Medicine* 12(6), e1489. https://doi.org/10.1002/wsbm.1489.

Silvestri, E., Lombardi, A., de Lange, P., Glinni, D., Senese, R., Cioffi, F., Lanni, A., Goglia, F., and Moreno, M. (2011). Studies of complex biological systems with applications to molecular medicine: The need to integrate transcriptomic and proteomic approaches. *Journal of Biomedicine and Biotechnology* 2011: 810242. https://doi.org/10.1155/2011/810242.

Simonton, D. K. (2003). Scientific creativity as constrained stochastic behavior: The integration of product, person, and process perspectives. *Psychological Bulletin* 129(4): 475-494. https://doi.org/10.1037/0033-2909.

Singh, S. (Ed.). (2022). *Systems Biomedicine Approaches in Cancer Research*. Singapore: Springer. https://doi.org/10.1007/978-981-19-1953-4.

Singh, B., Ryan, H., Kredo, T., Chaplin, M., and Fletcher, T. (2021). Chloroquine or hydroxychloroquine for prevention and treatment of COVID-19. *Cochrane Database of Systematic Reviews* Issue 2: CD013587. https://doi.org/10.1002/14651858.CD013587.pub2.

Situma, C., Hashimoto, M., and Soper, S. A. (2006). Merging microfuidics with micro-array-based bioassays. *Biomolecular Engineering* 23: 213-231. https://doi.org/10.1016/j.bioeng.2006.03.002.

Slabbert, M. N. (2006). "Genes 'R' Us": A critique of genetic essentialism. *Stellenbosch Law Review* 17(2): 251-265. https://hdl.handle.net/10520/EJC54594.

Slater, O., Miller, B., and Kontoyianni, M. (2020). Decoding protein-protein interactions: An overview. *Current Topics in Medicinal Chemistry* 20(10), 855-882. https://doi.org/10.2174/1568026620666200226105312.

Slepchenko, B. M., Schaff, J. C., Macara, I., and Loew, L. M. (2003). Quantitative cell biology with the Virtual Cell. *TRENDS in Cell Biology* 13: 570-576. https://doi.org/10.1016/j.tcb.2003.09.002.

Slife, B. D., Yanchar, S. C., and Williams, B. (1999). Conceptions of determinism in radical behaviorism: A taxonomy. *Behavior and Philosophy* 27(2): 75-96. http://www.jstor.org/stable/27759394.

Smart, J. J. C. (1963). Materialism. *Journal of Philosophy* 60(22): 651-662. https://doi.org/10.2307/2023512.

Smith, C. U. M. (2002). Julien Offray de la Mettrie (1709-1751). *Journal of the History of the Neurosciences* 11: 110-124. https://doi.org/10.1076/jhin.11.2.110.15188.

Smuts, J. (1926). *Holism and Evolution*. New York: Macmillan.

Smith, J. C., and Goodhew, D. W. (2021). Personal observations on COVID-19 and the conduct and application of biomedical science. *Interface Focus* 11(6): 20210053. https://doi.org/10.1098/rsfs.2021.0053.

Smye, S. W., and Frangi, A. F. (2021). Interdisciplinary research: Shaping the healthcare of the future. *Future Healthcare Journal* 8(2): e218. https://doi.org/10.7861/fhj.2021-0025.

Sniegowski, P. D., and Murphy, H. A. (2006). Evolvability. *Current Biology* 16: R831-R834. https://doi.org/10.1016/j.cub.2006.08.080.

Snyder, M. (2016). *Genomics and Personalized Medicine: What Everyone Needs to Know®*. New York: Oxford University Press.

Socolar, J. E. S. (2006). Nonlinear dynamical systems. In *Complex Systems Science in Biomedicine* (pp. 115-140), T. S. Deisboeck and J. Y. Kresh (Eds.). New York: Springer. https://doi.org/10.1007/978-0-387-33532-2_3.

Solomon, M. (2015). *Making Medical Knowledge*. New York: Oxford University Press. https://doi.org/10.1093/acprof:oso/9780198732617.001.0001.

Solomon, M. (2021). "EBM or EBM+ when evaluating evidence for the effectiveness of Covid-19 therapies." https://www.youtube.com/watch?v=-WcBw23Jl0o.

Soltani, A., and Moayyeri, A. (2007). Deterministic versus evidence-based attitude towards clinical diagnosis. *Journal of Evaluation in Clinical Practice* 13(4): 533-537. https://doi.org/10.1111/j.1365-2753.2007.00716.x.

Sonawane, A. R., Weiss, S. T., Glass, K., and Sharma, A. (2019). Network medicine in the age of biomedical big data. *Frontiers in Genetics* 10: 294. https://doi.org/10.3389/fgene.2019.00294.

Sorbel, R. (2010). "(W)holistic": The coining and the connotations. *Hektoen International: A Journal of Medical Humanities* 2(1). https://hekint.org/2017/01/30/wholistic-the-coining-and-the-connotations/.

Sorger, P. (2005). A reductionist's systems biology: Opinion. *Current Opinion in Cell Biology* 17: 9-11. https://doi.org/10.1016/j.ceb.2004.12.012.

Soto, A. M., and Sonnenschein, C. (2014). One hundred years of somatic mutation theory of carcinogenesis: Is it time to switch? *BioEssays* 36(1), 118-120. https://doi.org/10.1002/bies.201300160.

Soto, A. M., and Sonnenschein, C. (2018). Reductionism, organicism, and causality in the biomedical sciences: A critique. *Perspectives in Biology and Medicine* 61(4): 489-502. https://doi.org/10.1353/pbm.2018.0059.

Sperry, R. W. (1980). Mind-brain interaction: Mentalism, yes; Dualism, no. *Neuroscience* 5: 195-206. https://doi.org/10.1016/0306-4522(80)90098-6.

Sporn, M. B. (2006). Dichotomies in cancer research: Some suggestions for a new synthesis. *Nature Clinical Practice Oncology* 3: 364-373. https://doi.org/10.1038/ncponc0536.

Srivastava, R., and Varner, J. (2007). Emerging technologies: Systems biology. *Biotechnology Progress* 23: 24-27. https://doi.org/10.1021/bp060352v.

Stadler, F. (2001). *The Vienna Circle: Studies in the Origins, Development, and Influence of Logical Empiricism*. New York: Springer. https://doi.org/10.1007/978-3-319-16561-5.

Stalidzans, E., Zanin, M., Tieri, P., Castiglione, F., Polster, A., Scheiner, S., Pahle, J., Stres, B., List, M., Baumbach, J. and Lautizi, M. (2020). Mechanistic modeling and multiscale applications for precision medicine: Theory and practice. *Network and Systems Medicine* 3(1): 36-56. https://doi.org/10.1089/nsm.2020.0002.

Starling, E. H. (1923). The wisdom of the body. *British Medical Journal* 2: 685-690. https://doi.org/10.1136/bmj.2.3277.685.

Starr, C., Taggart, R., Evers, C., and Starr, L. (2019). *Biology: The Unity and Diversity of Life*, 15th edition. Boston, MA: Cengage.

Stedman, E., and Stedman, E. (1950). Cell specificity of histones. *Nature* 166(4227): 780-781. https://doi.org/10.1038/166780a0.

Steel, M. (2005). Molecular medicine: Promises, promises? *Journal of the Royal Society of Medicine* 98(5): 197-199. https://doi.org/10.1177/014107680509800506.

Stegenga, J. (2018). *Medical Nihilism*. New York: Oxford University Press. https://doi.org/10.1093/oso/9780198747048.001.0001.

Stein, H. F. (1990). *American Medicine as Culture*. San Francisco, CA: Westfield Press.

Stelling, J., Sauer, U., Szallasi, Z., Doyle III, F. J., and Doyle, J. (2004). Robustness of cellular functions. *Cell* 118: 675-685. https://doi.org/10.1016/j.cell.2004.09.008.

Stephan, A. (1992). Emergence—A systematic view of its historical facets. In *Emergence or Reduction? Essays on the Prospects of Nonreductive Physicalism*, (pp. 25-48), A. Beckermann, H. Flohr, and J. Kim (Eds.). Berlin: Walter de Gruyter.

Stephan, A. (1999). Varieties of emergentism. *Evolutions and Cognition* 5: 49-59.

Stephan, A. (2002). Emergentism, irreducibility, and downward causation. *Grazer Philosophische Studien* 65: 77-93. https://doi.org/10.1163/18756735-90000794.

Stephan, A. (2006). Emergence. In *Encyclopedia of Cognitive Science* (pp. 1-7), L. Nadel (Ed.). Hoboken, NJ: Wiley InterScience.

Sterling, P. (2020). *What is Health? Allostasis and the Evolution of Human Design*. Cambridge, MA: MIT Press.

Sterling, P., and Eyer, J. (1988). Allostasis: a new paradigm to explain arousal pathology. pathology. In *Handbook of Life Stress, Cognition and Health*. (pp. 629-649), S. Fisher and J. Reason (Eds.). New York: John Wiley & Sons.

Stevens, A. (2020). Governments cannot just 'follow the science' on COVID-19. *Nature Human Behaviour* 4: 560-560. https://doi.org/10.1038/s41562-020-0894-x.

Stöckler, M. (1991). A short history of emergence and reductionism. In *The Problem of Reductionism in Science* (pp. 71-90), E. Agazzi (Ed.). Dordrecht, NL: Kluwer. https://doi.org/10.1007/978-94-011-3492-7_4.

Stoljar, D. (2010). *Physicalism.* New York: Routledge.

Strasser, B. J. (2008). Magic bullets and wonder pills: Making drugs and diseases in the twentieth century. *Historical Studies in the Natural Sciences* 38(2): 303–312. https://doi.org/10.1525/hsns.2008.38.2.303.

Strasser, B. J. (2014). *Biomedicine: Meanings, Assumptions, and Possible Futures. Report to the Swiss Science and Innovation Council (SSIC) 1/2014.* Bern, CH: Swiss Science and Innovation Council.

Strasser, B. J., and Fantini, B. (1998). Molecular diseases and diseased molecules: Ontological and epistemological dimensions. *History and Philosophy of the Life Sciences* 20: 189-214. http://www.jstor.org/stable/23332101.

Straus, S. E., Glasziou, P., Richardson, W. S., and Haynes, R. B. (2019). *Evidence-Based Medicine: How to Practice and Teach EBM*, 5th edition. New York: Elsevier.

Strebhardt, K., and Ullrich, A. (2008). Paul Ehrlich's magic bullet concept: 100 years of progress. *Nature Reviews Cancer* 8(6): 473-480. https://doi.org/10.1038/nrc2394.

Streelman, J. T., and Karl, S. A. (1997). Paradigms and the rise (or fall?) of molecular biology. *Nature Biotechnology* 15(8): 696-697. https://doi.org/10.1038/nbt0897-696.

Strogatz, S. H. (2018). *Nonlinear Dynamics and Chaos: With Applications to Physics, Biology, Chemistry, and Engineering*, 2nd edition. Boca Raton, FL: CRC Press.

Strohman, R. C. (1995). Linear genetics, non-linear epigenetics: Complementary approaches to understanding complex diseases. *Integrative Physiological and Behavioral Science* 30(4): 273-282. https://doi.org/10.1007/BF02691601.

Strohman, R. C. (2002). Maneuvering in the complex space between genotype and phenotype. *Science* 296: 701-703. https://doi.org/10.1126/science.1070534.

Strohman, R. C. (2003). Genetic determinism as a failing paradigm in biology and medicine: Implications for health and wellness. *Journal of Social Work Education* 39(2): 169-191. https://doi.org/10.1080/10437797.2003.10779130.

Sturmberg, J. P. (2016). "Returning to holism": An imperative for the twenty-first century. In *The Value of Systems and Complexity Sciences for Healthcare* (pp. 3-19), J. P. Sturmberg (Ed.). Cham, CH: Springer. https://doi.org/10.1007/978-3-319-26221-5_1.

Sturmberg, J. P. (2019). Evidence-based medicine—Not a panacea for the problems of a complex adaptive world. *Journal of Evaluation in Clinical Practice* 25(5): 706-716. https://doi.org/10.1111/jep.13122.

Sturtevant, A. H. (1965). *A History of Genetics*. New York: Harper & Row.

Sumari, A. D. W., and Ahmad, A. S. (2018). Cognitive artificial intelligence: Concept and applications for humankind. In *Intelligent System* (pp. 23-55), C. Wongehoosuk (Ed.). London: IntechOpen. https://doi.org/10.5772/intechopen.72764.

Sun, M., Xie, L., Liu, Y., Li, K., Jiang, B., Lu, Y., Yang, Y., Yu, H., Song, Y., Bai, C., and Yang, D. (2022). The metaverse in current digital medicine. *Clinical eHealth* 5: 52-57. https://doi.org/10.1016/j.ceh.2022.07.002.

Sur, R. L., and Dahm, P. (2011). History of evidence-based medicine. *Indian Journal of Urology 27*(4): 487-489. https://doi.org/10.4103/0970-1591.91438.

Swain, P. S., Elowitz, M. B., and Siggia, E. D. (2002). Intrinsic and extrinsic contributions to stochasticity in gene expression. *Proceedings of the National Academy of Sciences* 99(20): 12795-12800. https://doi.org/10.1073/pnas.162041399.

Swat, M., Kel, A., and Herzel, H. (2004). Bifurcation analysis of the regulatory modules of the mammalian in G1/S transition. *Bioinformatics* 20: 1506-1511. https://doi.org/10.1093/bioinformatics/bth110.

Swinburne, R. (2019). The implausibility of the causal closure of the physical. *Organon F* 26(1): 25-39. https://doi.org/10.31577/orgf.2019.26103.

Symons, J. (2018). Brute facts about emergence. In *Brute Facts* (pp. 177-196), E. Vintiadis and C. Mekios (Eds.). New York: Oxford University Press. https://doi.org/10.1093/oso/9780198758600.003.0010.

Szasz, T. (2007). *The Medicalization of Everyday Life: Selected Essays*. Syracuse, NY: Syracuse University Press.

Szentágothai, J. (1984). Downward causation? *Annual Review of Neuroscience* 7: 1-11. https://doi.org/10.1146/annurev.ne.07.030184.000245.

Tabaczek, M. (2013). The metaphysics of downward causation: Rediscovering the formal cause. *Zygon* 48(2): 380-404. https://doi.org/10.1111/zygo.12012.

Tabery, J. G. (2004). Synthesizing activities and interactions in the concept of mechanism. *Philosophy of Science* 71: 1-15. https://doi.org/10.1086/381409.

Takahashi, K., Yugi, K., Hashimoto, K., Yamada, Y., Pickett, C. J., and Tomita, M. (2002). Computational challenges in cell simulation: A software engineering approach. *IEEE Intelligent Systems & Their Applications* 17: 64-71. https://doi.org/10.1109/MIS.2002.1039834.

Tang, Z. F., and McMillen, D. R. (2016). Design principles for the analysis and construction of robustly homeostatic biological networks. *Journal of Theoretical Biology* 408: 274-289. https://doi.org/10.1016/j.jtbi.2016.06.036.

Taylor, R. (2006). Determinism, A historical survey. In *The Encyclopedia of Philosophy*, 2nd edition, volume 3 (pp. 4-23), D.M. Borchert (Ed.). New York: Macmillan.

Taylor, P., and Lewontin, R. (2021). The genotype/phenotype distinction. In *The Stanford Encyclopedia of Philosophy, E. N. Zalta (Ed.). https://plato.stanford.edu/archives/sum2021/entries/genotype-phenotype/.*

Taylor, J. G., Choi, E. H., Foster, C. B., and Chanock, S. J. (2001). Using genetic variation to study human disease. *Trends in Molecular Medicine* 7(11): 507-512. https://doi.org/10.1016/S1471-4914(01)02183-9.

Teixeira, A. P., Dias, J. M., Carinhas, N., Sousa, M., Clemente, J. J., Cunha, A. E., von Stosch, M., Alves, P. M., Carrondo, M. J., and Oliveira, R. (2011). Cell functional enviromics: Unravelling the function of environmental factors. *BMC Systems Biology* 5: 92. https://doi.org/10.1186/1752-0509-5-92.

Teschendorff, A. E., Jones, A., and Widschwendter, M. (2016). Stochastic epigenetic outliers can define field defects in cancer. *BMC Bioinformatics* 17(1): 178. https://doi.org/10.1186/s12859-016-1056-z.

Testa, C. M., and Jankovic, J. (2019). Huntington disease: A quarter century of progress since the gene discovery. *Journal of the Neurological Sciences* 396: 52-68. https://doi.org/10.1016/j.jns.2018.09.022.

Teufel, T. (2011). Wholes that cause their parts: Organic self-reproduction and the reality of biological teleology. *Studies in History and Philosophy of Science Part C: Studies in History and Philosophy of Biological and Biomedical Sciences* 42(2), 252-260. https://doi.org/10.1016/j.shpsc.2010.12.002.

The International HapMap Consortium. (2003). The International HapMap Project. Nature Project. *Nature* 426(6968): 789-796. http://doi.org/10.1038/nature02168.

The International HapMap Consortium (2005). A haplotype map of the human genome. *Nature* 437: 1299–1320. https://doi.org/10.1038/nature04226.

The White House. (2015). Remarks by the President on precision medicine. https://obamawhitehouse.archives.gov/the-press-office/2015/01/30/remarks-president-precision-medicine.

Thibault, D., Jensen, P. A., Wood, S., Qabar, C., Clark, S., Shainheit, M. G., Isberg, R. R., and van Opijnen, T. (2019). Droplet Tn-Seq combines microfluidics with Tn-Seq for identifying complex single-cell phenotypes. *Nature Communications* 10(1): 5729. https://doi.org/10.1038/s41467-019-13719-9.

Thieffry, D. (2007). Dynamic roles of biological regulatory circuits. *Briefings in Bioinformatics* 8: 220-225. https://doi.org/10.1093/bib/bbm028.

Thieffry, D., and Sarkar, S. (1998). Forty years under the central dogma. *Trends in Biochemical Sciences* 23: 312-316. https://doi.org/10.1016/s0968-0004(98)01244-4.

Thomas, R. (1996). Feedback loops: The wheels of regulatory networks. In *Integrative Approached to Molecular Biology* (pp. 167-178), J. Collado-Vides, B. Magasanik, and T. F. Smith (Eds.). Cambridge, MA: MIT Press.

Thomas, R., and D'Ari, R. (1990). *Biological Feedback*. Boca Raton, FL: CRC Press.

Thomas, P., Terradot, G., Danos, V., and Weiße, A. Y. (2018). Sources, propagation and consequences of stochasticity in cellular growth. *Nature Communications* 9(1): 4528. https://doi.org/10.1038/s41467-018-06912-9.

Thorisson, G. A., and Stein, L. D. (2003). The SNP Consortium website: past, present and future. *Nucleic Acids Research* 31(1): 124-127. https://doi.org/10.1093/nar/gkg052.

Thorisson, G. A., Smith, A. V., Krishnan, L., and Stein, L. D. (2005). The International HapMap Project web site. *Genome Research* 15(11): 1592-1593. https://doi.org/10.1101/gr.4413105.

Thyagarajan, T., and Kalpana, D. (2021). *Linear and Non-Linear System Theory*. Boca Raton, FL: CRC Press.

Tian, T., Olson, S., Whitacre, J. M., and Harding, A. (2011). The origins of cancer robustness and evolvability. *Integrative Biology* 3(1): 17-30. https://doi.org/10.1039/c0ib00046a.

Tiehen, J. (2015). Explaining causal closure. *Philosophical Studies* 172(9): 2405-2425. https://doi.org/10.1007/s11098-014-0418-5.

Tiehen, J. (2018). Physicalism. *Analysis* 78(3): 537-551. https://doi.org/10.1093/analys/any037.

Timmermans, S., and Kolker, E. S. (2004). Evidence-based medicine and the reconfiguration of medical knowledge. *Journal of Health and Social Behavior* 45: 177-193. http://www.jstor.org/stable/3653831.

Tomasetti, C., and Vogelstein, B. (2015). Variation in cancer risk among tissues can be explained by the number of stem cell divisions. *Science* 347(6217): 78-81. https://doi.org/10.1126/science.1260825.

Tomita, M. (2001). Whole cell simulation: A grand challenge of the 21st century. *Trends in Biotechnology* 19: 205-210. https://doi.org/10.1016/S0167-7799(01)01636-5.

Tonelli, G. (1976). Analysis and synthesis in XXVIIIth century philosophy prior to Kant. *Archiv für Begriffsgeschichte*, *20*, 178-213. http://www.jstor.org/stable/24359045.

Torday, J. S. (2015). Homeostasis as the mechanism of evolution. *Biology* 4(3), 573-590. https://doi.org/10.3390/biology4030573.

Torok, M. A., Evans, S. A. S., and Marcum, J. A. (1993). cDNA sequence for bovine biglycan (PGI) protein core. *Biochimica et Biophysica Acta* 1173: 81-84. https://doi.org/10.1016/0167-4781(93)90247-B.

Townsend, J. T., and Ashby, F. G. (1983). *Stochastic Modeling of Elementary Psychological Processes*. New York: Cambridge University Press.

Trachana, K., Bargaje, R., Glusman, G., Price, Huang, S., and Hood, L. E. (2018). Taking systems medicine to heart. *Circulation Research* 122(9): 1276-1289. https://doi.org/10.1161/CIRCRESAHA.117.310999.

Tranquillo, J. (2019). *An Introduction to Complex Systems: Making Sense of a Changing World*. Cham, CH: Springer. https://doi.org/10.1007/978-3-030-02589-2.

Treadwell, J., and McCartney, M. (2016). Overdiagnosis and overtreatment: Generalists—It's time for a grassroots revolution. *British Journal of General Practice:* 66(644): 116-117. https://doi.org/10.3399/bjgp16X683881.

Trent, R. (2012). *Molecular Medicine: Genomics to Personalized Healthcare*, 4th edition. London: Academic Press.

Tretter, F. (2019). "Systems medicine" in the view of von Bertalanffy's "organismic biology" and systems theory. *Systems Research and Behavioral Science* 36(3): 346-362. https://doi.org/10.1002/sres.2588.

Tretter, F., and Löffler-Stastka, H. (2019). Medical knowledge integration and "systems medicine": Needs, ambitions, limitations and options. *Medical Hypotheses* 133: 109386. https://doi.org/10.1016/j.mehy.2019.109386.

Tretter, F., and Franz-Balsen, A. (2020). COVID-19: Science, politics, media, and the public—A systemic view. *Human Ecology Review* 26(1): 31-46. https://doi.org/10.22459/HER.26.01.2020.04.

Tretter, F., and Marcum, J. (2023). 'Medical Corona Science': Philosophical and systemic issues: Re-thinking medicine? On the epistemology of Corona medicine. *Journal of Evaluation in Clinical Practice* 29(3): 405-414. https://doi.org/10.1111/jep.13734.

Tretter, F., Wolkenhauer, O., Meyer-Hermann, M., Dietrich, J. W., Green, S., Marcum, J., and Weckwerth, W. (2021). The quest for system-theoretical medicine in the COVID-19 era. *Frontiers in Medicine* 8: 640974. https://doi.org/10.3389/fmed.2021.640974.

Tretter, F., Peters, E. M. J., Sturmberg, J., Bennett, J., Voit, E., Dietrich, J. W., Smith, G., Weckwerth, W., Grossman, Z., Wolkenhauer, O., and Marcum, J. A. (2023). Perspectives of (/memorandum for) systems thinking on COVID-19 pandemic and pathology. *Journal of Evaluation in Clinical Practice* 29: 415-429. https://doi.org/10.1111/jep.13772.

Trewavas, A. (2006). A brief history of systems biology. *The Plant Cell* 18: 2420-2430. https://doi.org/10.1105/tpc.106.042267.

Trinder, L, and Reynolds, S. (Eds.). (2000). *Evidence-Based Practice: A Critical Appraisal*. Malden, MA: Blackwell Science.

Trotter, G. (2007). Enough about Rawls already: Systems theory and bioethics in the 21st century. *American Journal of Bioethics* 7: 83-85. https://doi.org/10.1080/15265160701221491.

Tu, Y., Zhao, Z., Lam, J. W., and Tang, B. Z. (2021). Aggregate science: Much to explore in the meso world. *Matter* 4(2): 338-349. https://doi.org/10.1016/j.matt.2020.12.005.

Tucker, A., Wang, Z., Rotalinti, Y., and Myles, P. (2020). Generating high-fidelity synthetic patient data for assessing machine learning healthcare software. *npj Digital Medicine* 3(1): 147. https://doi.org/10.1038/s41746-020-00353-9.

Tuckwell, H. C. (1989). *Stochastic Processes in the Neurosciences*. Philadelphia, PA: Society for Industrial and Applied Mathematics.

Tuena, C., Semonella, M., Fernández-Álvarez, J., Colombo, D., and Cipresso, P. (2020). Predictive precision medicine: Towards the computational challenge. In *P5 eHealth: An Agenda for the Health Technologies of the Future* (pp. 71-86), G. Pravettoni and S. Triberti (Eds.). Cham, CH: Springer. https://doi.org/10.1007/978-3-030-27994-3_5.

Tuffin, R. (2016). Implications of complexity theory for clinical practice and healthcare organization. *BJA Education* 16(10): 349-352. https://doi.org/10.1093/bjaed/mkw013.

Turanli, B., Gulfidan, G., and Arga, K. Y. (2017). Systems biomedicine: From genome scale molecular networks to efficacious biomarkers and therapeutic targets. In *Researches on Science and Art in 21st Century Turkey*, volume 2 (pp. 2380-2388), H. Arapligirlioglu, A. Atik, R. L. Elliott, and E. Turgeon E. (Eds.). Ankara, TR: Gece Kitapligi.

Uecker, H., and Hermisson, J. (2011). On the fixation process of a beneficial mutation in a variable environment. *Genetics* 188(4): 915-930. https://doi.org/10.1534/genetics.110.124297.

Ueda, K. (2001). Synthesis and emergence—Research overview. *Artificial Intelligence in Engineering* 15(4): 321-327. https://doi.org/10.1016/S0954-1810(01)00022-X.

Ueda, K., Fujii, N., and Inoue, R. (2007). An emergent synthesis approach to simultaneous process planning and scheduling. *CIRP Annals* 56(1): 463-466. https://doi.org/10.1016/j.cirp.2007.05.111.

Ueltzhöffer, K., Armbruster-Genç, D. J., and Fiebach, C. J. (2015). Stochastic dynamics underlying cognitive stability and flexibility. *PLoS Computational Biology* 11(6): e1004331. https://doi.org/10.1371/journal.pcbi.1004331.

Umlauf, D., and Mourad, R. (2018). The 3D genome: From fundamental principles to disease and cancer. *Seminars in Cell and Developmental Biology* 90: 128-137. https://doi.org/10.1016/j.semcdb.2018.07.002.

Valles, S. (2020). Philosophy of biomedicine. In *The Stanford Encyclopedia of Philosophy, E. N. Zalta (Ed.). https://plato.stanford.edu/archives/sum2020/entries/biomedicine/.*

Vandamme, D., Fitzmaurice, W., Kholodenko, B., and Kolch, W. (2013). Systems medicine: Helping us understand the complexity of disease. *QJM: An International Journal of Medicine* 106(10): 891-895. https://doi.org/10.1093/qjmed/hct163.

Van De Vijver, G., Van Speybroeck, L., and De Waele, D. (2002). Epigenetics: A challenge for genetics evolution, and development? *Annals of the New York Academy of Sciences* 981: 1-6. https://doi.org/10.1111/j.1749-6632.2002.tb04909.x.

Van Den Tweel, J. G., and Taylor, C. R. (2010). A brief history of pathology. *Virchows Archiv* 457(1): 3-10. https://doi.org/10.1007/s00428-010-0934-4.

Van Der Greef, J. (2011). Perspective: All systems go. *Nature* 480(7378): S87. https://doi.org/10.1038/480S87a.

Van Dijk, W., Meinders, M. J., Tanke, M. A., Westert, G. P., and Jeurissen, P. P. (2020). Medicalization defined in empirical contexts–A scoping review. *International Journal of Health Policy and Management* 9(8): 327-334. https://doi.org/10.15171/ijhpm.2019.101.

Van Gulick, R. (2001). Reduction, emergence and other recent options on the mind/body problem. A philosophic overview. *Journal of Consciousness Studies* 8(9-10): 1-34.

Van Kampen, N. G. (1992). *Stochastic Processes in Physics and Chemistry*, revised edition. Amsterdam, NL: Elsevier.

Van Regenmortel, M. H. V. (2004). Reductionism and complexity in molecular biology. *EMBO Reports* 5: 1016-1020. https://doi.org/10.1038/sj.embor.7400284.

Van Regenmortel, M. H. V., and Hull, D. L. (Eds.). (2002). *Promises and Limits of Reductionism in the Biomedical Sciences*. West Sussex, UK: John Wiley.

Van Riel, R. (2011). Nagelian reduction beyond the Nagel model. *Philosophy of Science* 78(3): 353-375. https://doi.org/10.1086/660300.

Van Speybroeck, L., De Backer, P., Van Poucke, J., and De Waele, D. (2005). The conceptual challenge of systems biology. *BioEssays* 27: 1305-1307. https://doi.org/10.1002/bies.20333.

Varela, M., Ruiz-Esteban, R., and De Juan, M. J. M. (2010). Chaos, fractals, and our concept of disease. *Perspectives in Biology and Medicine* 53(4): 584-595. https://doi.org/10.1353/pbm.2010.0003.

Vasconcelos, V. V., Santos, F. P., Santos, F. C., and Pacheco, J. M. (2017). Stochastic dynamics through hierarchically embedded Markov chains. *Physical Review Letters* 118(5): 058301. https://doi.org/10.1103/PhysRevLett.118.058301.

Vaughn, L. K., Veale, W. L., and Cooper, K. E. (1980). Antipyresis: Its effect on mortality rate of bacterially infected rabbits. *Brain Research Bulletin* 5(1): 69-73. https://doi.org/10.1016/0361-9230(80)90285-3.

Vaux, D. L. (2011). In defense of the somatic mutation theory of cancer. *BioEssays* 33(5): 341-343. https://doi.org/10.1002/bies.201100022.

Vegter, M. W. (2018). Towards precision medicine; A new biomedical cosmology. *Medicine, Health Care and Philosophy* 21: 443-456. https://doi.org/10.1007/s11019-018-9828-z.

Velchiti, V., and Punekar, S. R. (Eds.). (2022). *Handbook of Cancer-Treatment-Related Symptoms and Toxicities*. Philadelphia, PA: Elsevier.

Ventriglia, G., and Murgia, V. (2011). *The Homeostasis Model: Health, Illness, Disease*. Sansepolcro, IT: Aboca Edizioni.

Verma, M., and Barh, D. (Eds.). (2017). *Progress and Challenges in Precision Medicine*. New York: Academic Press.

Verschuuren, G. M. (1995). *Life Scientists: Their Convictions, Their Activities, and Their Values*. North Andover, MA: Genesis Publishing Company.

Verschuuren, G. M. (2017). *Holism-Redcutionism Debate: In Physics, Genetics, Biology, Neuroscience, Ecology, and Sociology*. Virginia Beach, VA: Createspace Publishing.

Viceconti, M., and Hunter, P. (2016). The virtual physiological human: Ten years after. *Annual Review of Biomedical Engineering* 18: 103-123. https://doi.org/10.1146/annurev-bioeng-110915-114742.

Vicente, A. (2006). On the causal completeness of physics. *International Studies in the Philosophy of Science* 20(2): 149-171. https://doi.org/10.1080/02698590600814332.

Vickers, B. (1992). Francis Bacon and the progress of knowledge. *Journal of the History of Ideas* 53(3): 495-518. https://doi.org/10.2307/2709891.

Vidal, M., Cusick, M.E., and Barabási, A.L. (2011). Interactome networks and human disease. *Cell* 144(6): 986-998. https://doi.org/10.1016/j.cell.2011.02.016.

Vintiadis, E. (2013). Emergence. In *Internet Encyclopedia of Philosophy*, J. Fieser and B. Dowden (Eds.). https://philpapers.org/archive/VINE.pdf.

Vlahou, A., Mischak, H., Zoidakis, J., and Magni, F. (Eds.). (2018). *Integration of Omics Approaches and Systems Biology for Clinical Applications*. Hoboken, NJ: John Wiley & Sons.

Vogt, H., Ulvestad, E., Eriksen, T. E., and Getz, L. (2014). Getting personal: Can systems medicine integrate scientific and humanistic conceptions of the patient? *Journal of Evaluation in Clinical Practice* 20(6): 942-952. https://doi.org/10.1111/jep.12251.

Vogt, H., Hofmann, B., and Getz, L. (2016). The new holism: P4 systems medicine and the medicalization of health and life itself. *Medicine, Health Care and Philosophy* 19(2): 307-323. https://doi.org/10.1007/s11019-016-9683-8.

Volkov, I., Radchenko, G., and Tchernykh, A. (2021). Digital twins, internet of things and mobile medicine: a review of current platforms to support smart healthcare. *Programming and Computer Software* 47: 578-590. https://doi.org/10.1134/S0361768821080284.

Voisey, J., and Morris, C. P. (2008). SNP technologies for drug discovery: A current review. *Current Drug Discovery Technologies* 5(3): 230-235. https://doi.org/10.2174/157016308785739811.

Voit, E. O. (2013). Biochemical systems theory: A review. *ISRN Biomathematics* 2013: 897658. https://doi.org/10.1155/2013/897658.

Wachbroit, R. (2002). Genetic determinism, genetic reductionism, and genetic essentialism. In *Encyclopedia of Ethical, Legal and Policy Issues in Biotechnology* (pp. 352-356), T. H. Murray and J. Mehlman (Eds.). New York: Wiley-Interscience. https://doi.org/10.1002/0471250597.mur069.

Waddington, C. H. (1942). Canalization of development and the inheritance of acquired characteristics. *Nature* 150: 563-565. https://doi.org/10.1038/150563a0.

Waddington, C. H. (2012). The epigenotype. *International Journal of Epidemiology* 41(1): 10-13. https://doi.org/10.1093/ije/dyr184.

Waddington, C. H. (2014). *The Strategy of the Genes*. New York: Routledge.

Waddington, C. H. (2016). *An Introduction to Modern Genetics*. New York: Routledge.

Wade, D. T., and Halligan, P. W. (2004). Do biomedical models of illness make for good healthcare systems? *British Medical Journal* 329(7479): 1398–1401. https://doi.org/10.1136/bmj.329.7479.1398.

Waggoner, D. (2007). Mechanisms of disease: Epigenesis. *Seminars in Pediatric Neurology* 14: 7-14. https://doi.org/10.1016/j.spen.2006.11.004.

Waggoner, M. R., and Uller, T. (2015). Epigenetic determinism in science and society. *New Genetics and Society* 34(2): 177-195. https://doi.org/10.1080/14636778.2015.1033052.

Wagner, A. (1999). Causality in complex systems. *Biology and Philosophy* 14: 83-101. https://doi.org/10.1023/A:1006580900476.

Wagner, A. (2005). *Robustness and Evolvability in Living Systems*. Princeton, NJ: Princeton University Press.

Wagner, A. (2008). Robustness and evolvability: A paradox resolved. *Proceedings of the Royal Society B* 275: 91-100. https://doi.org/10.1098/rspb.2007.1137.

Wagner, G. P., and Altenberg, L. (1996). Complex adaptations and the evolution of evolvability. *Evolution* 50: 967-976. https://doi.org/10.2307/2410639.

Wagner, G. P., Pavlicev, M., and Cheverud, J. M. (2007). The road to modularity. *Nature Reviews Genetics* 8(12): 921-931. https://doi.org/10.1038/nrg2267.

Waldrop, M. M. (1992). *Complexity: The Emerging Science at the Edge of Order and Chaos*. New York: Simon & Schuster.

Walker, C., Mojares, E., and del Río Hernández, A. (2018). Role of extracellular matrix in development and cancer progression. *International Journal of Molecular Sciences* 19(10): 3028. https://doi.org/10.3390/ijms19103028.

Walsh, M. M., Einstein, E. H., and Gluck, K. A. (2013). A quantification of robustness. *Journal of Applied Research in Memory and Cognition* 2(3): 137-148. https://doi.org/10.1016/j.jarmac.2013.07.002.

Wang, E., Lenferink, A., and O'Connor-McCourt, M. (2007). Cancer systems biology: Exploring cancer-associated genes on cellular networks. *Cellular and Molecular Life Science* 64: 1752-1762. https://doi.org/10.1007/s00018-007-7054-6.

Wang, R. S., Maron, B. A., and Loscalzo, J. (2015). Systems medicine: Evolution of systems biology from bench to bedside. *Systems Biology and Medicine* 7(4): 141-161. https://doi.org/10.1002/wsbm.1297.

Waters, K. M., Pounds, J. G., and Thrall, B. D. (2006). Data merging for integrated microarray and proteomic analysis. *Briefings in Functional Genomics and Proteomics* 5: 261-272. https://doi.org/10.1093/bfgp/ell019.

Watson, J. D., and Crick, F. (1953). Molecular structure of nucleic acids: A structure for deoxyribose nucleic acid. *Nature* 171: 737-738. https://doi.org/10.1038/171737a0.

Watson, J. D., Davies, K., and Berry, A. (2017). *DNA: The Story of the Genetic Revolution*, revised edition. New York: Knopf.

Wazny, K. (2018). Applications of crowdsourcing in health: An overview. *Journal of Global Health* 8(1): 010502. https://doi.org/10.7189/jogh.08.010502.

Weatherford, R. C. (1995). Determinism. In *The Oxford Companion to Philosophy* (pp. 194-195), T. Honderich (Ed.). New York: Oxford University Press.

Weber, B. (2018). Life. In *The Stanford Encyclopedia of Philosophy, E. N. Zalta (Ed.). https://plato.stanford.edu/entries/life/.*

Wei, J. W., Huang, K., Yang, C., and Kang, C. S. (2017). Non-coding RNAs as regulators in epigenetics. *Oncology Reports* 37(1): 3-9. https://doi.org/10.3892/or.2016.5236.

Weiner, M. P., and Hudson, T. J. (2002). Introduction to SNPs: Discovery of markers for disease. *Biotechniques* 32: S4-S13. https://doi.org/10.2144/jun0201.

Weiner, K., Martin, P., Richards, M., and Tutton, R. (2017). Have we seen the geneticisation of society? Expectations and evidence. *Sociology of Health & Illness* 39(7): 989-1004. https://doi.org/10.1111/1467-9566.12551.

Weinert, F. (2016). *The Demons of Science: What They Can and Cannot Tell Us About Our World*. Cham, CH: Springer. https://doi.org/10.1007/978-3-319-31708-3.

Welshon, R. (2002). Emergence, supervenience, and realization. *Philosophical Studies* 108(1): 39-51. https://doi.org/10.1023/A:1015755913389.

Wennekamp, S., and Hiiragi, T. (2012). Stochastic processes in the development of pluripotency in vivo. *Biotechnology Journal* 7(6): 737-744. https://doi.org/10.1002/biot.201100357.

West, B. J. (2103). *Fractal Physiology and Chaos in Medicine*, 2nd edition. Singapore: World Scientific Publishing.

Westerhoff, H. V., and Alberghina, L. (2005). Systems biology: Did we know it all along? In *Systems Biology: Definitions and Perspectives* (pp. 3-9), L. Alberghina and H. Westerhoff (Eds.). Berlin: Springer. https://doi.org/10.1007/b137744.

Westerhoff, H. V., and Hofmeyr, J H. S. (2005). What is systems biology? From genes to function and back. *Topics in Current Genetics* 13: 119-141. https://doi.org/10.1007/b137122.

Westerhoff, H. V., and Kell, D. B. (2007). The methodologies of systems biology. In *Systems Biology: Philosophical Foundations* (pp. 23-70), F. C. Boogerd, F. J. Bruggeman, J. H. S. Hofmeyr, and H. V. Westerhoff (Eds.). Amsterdam: Elsevier. https://doi.org/10.1016/B978-044452085-2/50004-8.

Westfall, R. S. (1977). *The Construction of Modern Science: Mechanisms and Mechanics*. New York: Cambridge University Press.

Whitacre, J. M. (2012). Biological robustness: Paradigms, mechanisms, and systems principles. *Frontiers in Genetics* 3: 67. https://doi.org/10.3389/fgene.2012.00067.

Whitehead, A. N. (1925). *Process and Reality: An Essay in Cosmology*, corrected edition. New York: Free Press.

Whitehead, A. N. (1979). *Science and the Modern World*. New York: Macmillan.

Whitesides, G. M. (2006). The origins and the future of microfluidics. *Nature* 442(7101), 368-373. https://doi.org/10.1038/nature05058.

Wikswo, J. P. (2004). Instrumentation challenges for systems biology. *Sensors* 2: 558-559. https:/doi.org/10.1109/ICSENS.2004.1426225.

Wikswo, J. P., Prokop, A., Baudenbacher, F., Cliffel, D., Csukas, B., and Velkovsky, M. (2006). Engineering challenges of BioNEMS: The integration of microfluidics, micro- and nanodevices, models and external control for systems biology. *Proceedings-Nanobiotechnology* 153(4): 81-101. https:/doi.org/10.1049/ip-nbt:20050045.

Wildermuth, M. C. (2000). Metabolic control analysis: Biological applications and insights. *Genome Biology* 1: 1031.1–1031.5. https://doi.org/10.1186/gb-2000-1-6-reviews1031.

Wilkes, K. V. (1978). *Physicalism*. New York: Humanities Press.

Williamson, J. (2021). The feasibility and malleability of EBM+. *Theoria* 36(2): 191-209. https://doi.org/10.1387/theoria.21244.

Wilson, C. (1995). *The Invisible World: Early Modern Philosophy and the Invention of the Microscope*. Princeton, NJ Princeton University Press.

Wilson, R. A. (2005). *Genes and the Agents of Life: The Individual in the Fragile Sciences.* New York: Cambridge University Press.

Wilson, J. M. (2021). *Metaphysical Emergence.* New York: Oxford University Press. https://doi.org/10.1093/oso/9780198823742.001.0001.

Wimsatt, W. C. (2000). Emergence as non-aggregativity and the biases of reductionisms. *Foundations of Science* 5(3): 269-297. https://doi.org/10.1023/A:1011342202830.

Wimsatt, W. C. (2006). Reductionism and its heuristics: Making methodological reductionism honest. *Synthese* 151: 445–475. https://doi.org/10.1007/s11229-006-9017-0.

Winau, F., Westphal, O., and Winau, R. (2004). Paul Ehrlich—In search of the magic bullet. *Microbes and Infection* 6(8): 786-789. https://doi.org/10.1016/j.micinf.2004.04.003.

Woehle, R. (2007). Complexity theory, nonlinear dynamics, and change: Augmenting systems theory. *Advances in Social Work* 8(1): 141-151. https://doi.org/10.18060/137.

Wolfe, C. T. (2012). Chance between holism and reductionism: Tensions in the conceptualisation of life. *Progress in Biophysics and Molecular Biology* 110(1): 113-120. https://doi.org/10.1016/j.pbiomolbio.2012.05.005.

Wolfe, C. T. (2016). *Materialism: A Historico-Philosophical Introduction.* New York: Springer. https://doi.org/10.1007/978-3-319-24820-2.

Wolfe, C. T. (2017). Materialism new and old. *Anthropología Experimental* 17: 215-224. https://doi.org/10.17561/rae.v0i17.3510.

Wolfe, E. L., Barger, A. C., and Benison, S. (2000). *Walter B. Cannon, Science and Society.* Boston, MA: Boston Medical Library.

Wolkenhauer, O. (Ed.). (2020). *Systems Medicine: Integrative, Qualitative and Computational Approaches*, 3 volumes. New York: Academic Press.

Wolkenhauer, O., and Green, S. (2013). The search for organizing principles as a cure against reductionism in systems medicine. *The FEBS Journal* 280(23): 5938-5948. https://doi.org/10.1111/febs.12311.

Wolkenhauer, O., Mesarović, M., and Wellstead, P. (2007). A plea for more theory in molecular biology. In *Systems Biology: Ernst Schering Research Foundation Workshop*, volume 61 (pp. 117-137), P. Bringmann, E. C. Butcher, G. Parry, and B. Weiss (Eds.). Berlin: Springer. https://doi.org/10.1007/978-3-540-31339-7_6.

Wolkenhauer, O., Fell, D., De Meyts, P., Bluthgen, N., Herzel, H., Le Novere, N., Höfer, T., Schürrle, K., and Van Leeuwen, I. (2009). SysBioMed report: Advancing systems biology for medical applications. *IET Systems Biology* 3(3): 131-136. https://doi.org/10.1049/iet-syb.2009.0005.

Wolkenhauer, O., Auffray, C., Jaster, R., Steinhoff, G., and Dammann, O. (2013). The road from systems biology to systems medicine. *Pediatric Research* 73(2): 502-507. https://doi.org/10.1038/pr.2013.4.

Wolkenhauer, O., Auffray, C., Brass, O., Clairambault, J., Deutsch, A., Drasdo, D., Gervasio, F., Preziosi, L., Maini, P., Marciniak-Czochra, A., and Kossow, C. (2014).

Enabling multiscale modeling in systems medicine. *Genome Medicine* 6: 1-3. https://doi.org/10.1186/gm538.

Wong, K. C. (Ed.). (2016). *Big Data Analytics in Genomics*. Cham, CH: Springer. https://doi.org/10.1007/978-3-319-41279-5.

Woodger, J. H. (1930). The "concept of organism" and the relation between embryology and genetics. Part I. *Quarterly Review of Biology* 5(1): 1-22. https://doi.org/10.1086/394349.

Worrall, J. (2002). What evidence in evidence-based medicine? *Philosophy of Science* 69(S3): S316-S330. https://doi.org/10.1086/341855.

Wu, C. T., and Morris, J. R. (2001). Genes, genetics, and epigenetics: A correspondence. *Science* 293: 1103-1105.

Wu, D., Sanin, D. E., and Wang, X. (2016). Clinical applications and systems biomedicine. In *Application of Clinical Bioinformatics* (pp. 323-335), X. Wang, C. Baumgartner, D. Shields, H. W. Deng, J. Beckmann (Eds). Dordrecht, NL: Springer. https://doi.org/10.1007/978-94-017-7543-4_13.

Yadav, D. K., Yadav, N., and Khurana, S. M. P. (2013). -Environomics: Omics for the environment. In *OMICS* (pp. 660-693), D. Barh, V. Zambare, and V. Azevedo (Eds.). Boca Raton, FL: CRC Press.

Yan, Q. (2011). Toward the integration of personalized and systems medicine: Challenges, opportunities and approaches. *Personalized Medicine* 8(1): 1-4. https://doi.org/10.2217/pme.10.77.

Yan, Q. (2017). Toward dynamical systems medicine: Personalized and preventive strategies. *Personalized Medicine* 14(5): 551-554. https://doi.org/10.2217/pme-2017-0030.

Yang, Y., Chen, Y., Tang, H., Zong, N., and Jiang, X. (2020). Microfluidics for biomedical analysis. *Small Methods* 4(4): 1900451. https://doi.org/10.1002/smtd.201900451.

Yates, D. (2013). Emergence. In *Encyclopaedia of the Mind* (pp. 283-287), H. Pashler (Ed.). London: SAGE.

Yau, T. O. (2019). Precision treatment in colorectal cancer: Now and the future. *JGH Open* 3(5): 361-369. https://doi.org/10.1002/jgh3.12153.

You, L. (2004). Toward computational systems biology. *Cell Biochemistry and Biophysics* 40: 167-184. https://doi.org/10.1385/CBB:40:2:167.

Yu, K. D., Cai, Y. W., Wu, S. Y., Shui, R. H., and Shao, Z. M. (2021). Estrogen receptor-low breast cancer: Biology chaos and treatment paradox. *Cancer Communications* 41(10): 968-980. https://doi.org/10.1002/cac2.12191.

Yuan, B. (2019). Toward holistic medicine and holistic biology: Life sciences after precision medicine and systems biology. *Frontiers in Life Science* 12(1): 14-26. https://doi.org/10.1080/21553769.2019.1682064.

Zagris, N. (2022). Aristotle (384-322 BC): The beginnings of embryology. *International Journal of Developmental Biology* 66(1-3): 5-8. https://doi.org/10.1387/ijdb.220040nz.

Zanin, M., Aitya, N. A., Basilio, J., Baumbach, J., Benis, A., Behera, C. K., Bucholc, M., Castiglione, F., Chouvarda, I., Comte, B., and Dao, T. T. (2021). An early stage researcher's primer on systems medicine terminology. *Network and Systems Medicine* 4(1): 2-50. https://doi.org/10.1089/nsm.2020.0003.

Zechner, C., Nerli, E., and Norden, C. (2020). Stochasticity and determinism in cell fate decisions. *Development* 147(14): dev181495. https://doi.org/10.1242/dev.181495.

Zeng, Y., Chen, X., and Wang, X. (2018). Roles of single cell systems biomedicine in lung diseases. In *Single Cell Biomedicine* (pp. 177-185), J. Gu and X. Wang (Eds.). Singapore: Springer. https://doi.org/10.1007/978-981-13-0502-3_15.

Zernicka-Goetz, M., and Huang, S. (2010). Stochasticity versus determinism in development: a false dichotomy? *Nature Reviews Genetics* 11(11): 743-744. https://doi.org/10.1038/nrg2886.

Zhang, W. J. (2018). *Fundamentals of Network Biology*. Singapore: World Scientific Publishing.

Zhang, C., and Hua, Q. (2016). Applications of genome-scale metabolic models in biotechnology and systems medicine. *Frontiers in Physiology* 6: 413. https://doi.org/10.3389/fphys.2015.00413.

Zhang, H., and Mace, R. (2021). Cultural extinction in evolutionary perspective. *Evolutionary Human Sciences* 3: e30. https://doi.org/10.1017/ehs.2021.25.

Zhang, S., Davidson, D. D., Zhang, D. Y., Parks, J. A., and Cheng, L. (2008). Principles of clinical molecular biology. In *Molecular Genetic Pathology* (pp. 3-32), L. Cheng and D. Y. Zhang (Eds.). Totown, NJ: Humana Press. https://doi.org/10.1007/978-1-59745-405-6_1.

Zhang, Z., Zhao, Z., Liu, B., Li, D., Zhang, D., Chen, H., and Liu, D. (2013). Systems biomedicine: It's your turn—Recent progress in systems biomedicine. *Quantitative Biology* 1(2): 140-155. https://doi.org/10.1007/s40484-013-0009-z.

Zhang, H., Zhao, Z., Turley, A. T., Wang, L., McGonigal, P. R., Tu, Y., Li, Y., Wang, Z., Kwok, R. T., Lam, J. W., and Tang, B. Z. (2020). Aggregate science: From structures to properties. *Advanced Materials* 32(36): 2001457. https://doi.org/10.1002/adma.202001457.

Zhao, J., Tao, L., Yu, H., Luo, J. H., Cao, Z., and Li, Y. (2007). Bow-tie topological features of metabolic networks and the functional significance. *Chinese Science Bulletin* 52(8): 1036-1045. https://doi.org/10.1007/s11434-007-0143-y.

Zhou, W., Wang, T., Cheng, X., Han, L., Zhang, Y. (2016). Techniques for molecular network construction in network pharmacology study. *Journal of International Pharmaceutical Research* 43: 797-812. https://doi.org/10.13220/j.cnki.jipr.2016.05.001.

Zhu, M., Yu, M., and Zhao, S. (2009). Understanding quantitative genetics in the systems biology era. *International journal of biological sciences* 5(2): 161. https://doi.org/10.7150/ijbs.5.161.

Zhukov, D., Khvatova, T., Millar, C., and Zaltcman, A. (2020). Modelling the stochastic dynamics of transitions between states in social systems incorporating self-organization and memory. *Technological Forecasting and Social Change* 158: 120134. https://doi.org/10.1016/j.techfore.2020.120134.

Zoghbi, H. Y., and Beaudet, A. L. (2016). Epigenetics and human disease. *Cold Spring Harbor Perspectives in Biology* 8(2): a019497. https://doi.org/10.1101/cshperspect.a019497.

Zwart, H. (2009). Genomics metaphors and genetic determinism. In *New Visions of Nature: Complexity and Authenticity* (pp. 155-172), M. Drenthen, F. Keulartz, and J. Proctor (Eds.). New York: Springer. https://doi.org/10.1007/978-90-481-2611-8_12.

Zwart, H. (2014). Genetic determinism. In: *Encyclopedia of Global Bioethics*, H. Ten Have (Ed.). Berlin: Springer. https://doi.org/10.1007/978-3-319-05544-2_208-1.

Index

A

agential realism, 65
aggregativity, 77, 277
All of Us, 18, 19, 162, 204, 205, 226, 247, 258, 262
allopoiesis, 65
allostasis, 113, 122, 123, 124, 137, 209, 249, 258, 263, 267
analysis, xi, 6, 17, 19, 20, 21, 34, 44, 46, 49, 52, 61, 75, 77, 82, 84, 86, 89, 90, 91, 110, 118, 121, 124, 136, 141, 142, 147, 149, 151, 160, 169, 170, 171, 172, 173, 174, 175, 176, 182, 183, 187, 194, 196, 199, 203, 204, 208, 211, 216, 217, 218, 220, 221, 224, 225, 230, 231, 232, 237, 241, 243, 246, 250, 251, 256, 257, 260, 262, 263, 264, 269, 270, 271, 275, 276, 278
Aristotle, 59, 78, 79, 98, 205, 230, 278
artificial intelligence, 152, 178, 215, 216, 242, 243, 268, 272
atomism, 13, 42, 59, 241
autonomy, 8, 38, 169, 197, 208, 250, 260
autopoiesis, 65, 225, 250

B

Bacon, F., 60, 89, 206, 237, 274
big data, 13, 176, 185, 188, 189, 195, 204, 216, 221, 242, 244, 266, 278
bioinformatics, 11, 12, 13, 33, 159, 176, 196, 206, 213, 219, 221, 222, 225, 238, 239, 250, 252, 255, 256, 258, 264, 269, 270, 278
biological system, 40, 88, 114, 125, 126, 128, 134, 136, 159, 205, 214, 225, 237, 241, 264, 265
biomarker, 169
biomedical model, ix, xi, 1, 2, 3, 4, 5, 9, 26, 27, 33, 49, 50, 54, 63, 65, 68, 75, 76, 78, 89, 96, 110, 130, 131, 133, 135, 136, 137, 142, 184, 188, 220, 233, 245, 260, 275
biomedicine, v, x, 1, 2, 3, 4, 9, 12, 13, 14, 15, 28, 29, 33, 34, 46, 49, 52, 53, 59, 66, 69, 72, 73, 74, 75, 88, 89, 90, 93, 97, 102, 103, 105, 106, 124, 130, 133, 145, 154, 155, 158, 164, 165, 177, 178, 179, 180, 182, 183, 186, 189, 190, 196, 199, 205, 206, 211, 214, 217, 223, 224, 227, 238, 239, 241, 243, 244, 245, 246, 248, 249, 258, 259, 265, 266, 268, 272, 279
biomes, 23, 136
biopsychosocial model, 4, 179, 184, 185, 195, 209, 211, 228
biostatistical theory, 2
biostatistics, 11, 200
Bouillaud, J., 35
bow-tie architecture, 128, 129, 140, 227
Boyle, R., 27, 29, 205
British Emergentism, 79, 80, 81, 82, 249

C

cancerome, 21, 169, 236
carcinogenesis, ix, 19, 21, 70, 101, 109, 133, 136, 166, 169, 266
causal closure, 68, 69, 70, 223, 228, 251, 256, 269, 270
causation, x, 8, 27, 41, 59, 60, 66, 67, 68, 69, 70, 71, 72, 73, 74, 87, 92, 103, 104, 166, 169, 171, 180, 187, 189, 191, 197, 206, 208, 214, 218, 223, 228, 229, 233, 242, 250, 251, 252, 254, 257, 258, 269
central dogma of molecular biology, 32, 33
chaos, 82, 87, 134, 135, 136, 156, 169, 203, 213, 215, 217, 224, 229, 234, 241, 243, 260, 263, 268, 273, 275, 276, 278

chronic diseases, 1, 20, 66, 69, 78, 90, 101, 135, 158, 189, 190, 193, 198, 212
circular causality, 71, 74, 254
clinical expertise, 7
cognition, 79, 170, 225, 251, 267, 275
cognomics, 23, 149, 170
complex adaptive system, 76
complex system, 31, 44, 83, 84, 125, 134, 135, 141, 155, 169, 170, 190, 213, 241, 245, 266, 271, 275
complexity, 10, 11, 12, 14, 46, 57, 63, 73, 79, 82, 83, 91, 92, 114, 127, 134, 135, 136, 141, 146, 149, 150, 156, 166, 170, 178, 200, 203, 204, 209, 210, 214, 217, 218, 219, 223, 225, 226, 227, 228, 229, 230, 248, 249, 251, 260, 263, 268, 272, 273, 275, 277, 280
complexity theory, 79, 272
connectomics, 23, 149, 165, 170, 265
consciousness, x, 15, 79, 86, 91, 170, 175, 225, 228, 234, 273
constitutive reductionism, 57
constraints, 8, 69, 70, 72, 83, 127, 155, 170, 246
coronavirus (COVID-19), v, vii, x, 2, 8, 9, 10, 90, 109, 145, 153, 164, 165, 205, 214, 215, 224, 230, 231, 243, 247, 251, 253, 259, 264, 265, 266, 267, 271
CRISPR, 161, 203, 207, 220, 229, 234, 252
cure, 3, 106, 130, 170, 184, 191, 195, 197, 251, 261, 277

D

Descartes, R., 27, 30, 60, 61, 63, 76, 206, 221, 227, 262
determinism, vi, x, 3, 69, 75, 87, 94, 95, 103, 104, 105, 109, 110, 134, 170, 176, 204, 222, 224, 227, 231, 233, 234, 244, 245, 246, 251, 257, 259, 260, 261, 266, 268, 269, 274, 275, 279, 280
diagnosis, 5, 11, 12, 53, 89, 90, 105, 170, 173, 175, 178, 180, 183, 185, 188, 192, 197, 199, 223, 231, 266
digital health, 193, 241
dignity, 4, 22, 90, 162, 170, 226, 259
diseasome, 14, 21, 170, 229, 235, 236, 237
DNA methylation, ix, 99, 100, 102, 210, 260
downward causation, vi, ix, 27, 66, 69, 70, 72, 74, 84, 86, 87, 92, 214, 219, 223, 225, 226, 230, 233, 235, 242, 246, 250, 256, 262, 267, 269
drugome, 21, 171, 216
dualism, 50, 82, 171, 173, 267
dynamics, x, 20, 39, 84, 113, 131, 133, 134, 135, 136, 148, 150, 173, 174, 176, 204, 205, 211, 213, 226, 228, 239, 241, 243, 253, 259, 272, 273, 279

E

EBM+, 34, 164, 230, 266, 277
efficient cause, 62, 175
emergence, vi, ix, x, 2, 8, 10, 15, 39, 60, 67, 70, 74, 75, 76, 78, 80, 81, 82, 83, 84, 85, 86, 87, 88, 91, 92, 110, 111, 139, 154, 167, 171, 191, 203, 206, 207, 208, 209, 211, 214, 215, 216, 217, 218, 219, 220, 223, 225, 228, 229, 230, 234, 236, 237, 239, 240, 242, 246, 249, 251, 256, 259, 261, 263, 265, 267, 268, 269, 272, 273, 274, 276, 277, 278
emergent, vi, ix, x, 4, 52, 62, 69, 75, 76, 79, 80, 81, 82, 83, 84, 85, 86, 87, 88, 89, 91, 92, 93, 110, 111, 155, 161, 171, 175, 210, 218, 223, 229, 251, 255, 258, 272
emergent mechanism, 75, 111, 175, 229
emergent property, 76, 81, 84, 86, 88, 89, 91, 161
emergent synthesis, vi, ix, x, 52, 75, 88, 89, 91, 92, 93, 110, 155, 272
emergentism, 79, 80, 81, 82, 84, 228, 239, 248, 267
empiricism, 63, 171, 175, 226, 253, 267
entanglement, 25, 65, 66, 73, 88, 91, 93, 130, 131, 142, 154, 155, 163, 171, 207
entelechy, 31, 78, 79
enviromics, 23, 149, 165, 171, 205, 269

environment, 28, 59, 65, 83, 99, 105, 107, 113, 114, 116, 117, 119, 126, 133, 138, 139, 140, 141, 159, 161, 171, 172, 174, 175, 199, 241, 251, 260, 261, 272, 278
environomics, 23, 149, 165, 171, 278
epidemiology, 11, 23, 165, 171, 219, 221, 224, 236, 238, 242, 260, 261, 274
epigenesis, ix, x, 97, 98, 229, 230, 246, 254, 275
epigeneticism, vi, x, 75, 88, 93, 97, 98, 99, 101, 103, 110, 171
epigenetics, 98, 99, 100, 101, 102, 171, 206, 209, 210, 216, 220, 223, 225, 231, 234, 238, 239, 242, 243, 245, 250, 251, 253, 254, 257, 258, 260, 263, 268, 273, 276, 278, 279
epigenome, ix, 101, 208, 220, 248, 261
epigenomics, ix, 10, 23, 102, 154, 165, 261
epistemological reductionism, 42, 45
epistemological wholism, 52, 55
epistemology, 67, 171, 189, 198, 208, 213, 222, 244, 247, 271
evidence-based medicine (EBM), v, ix, xi, 1, 5, 6, 7, 8, 9, 10, 14, 26, 29, 34, 46, 49, 59, 63, 69, 78, 89, 90, 105, 133, 145, 164, 165, 183, 186, 187, 190, 191, 198, 205, 211, 214, 217, 230, 243, 246, 248, 252, 264, 266, 268, 277, 278
evolution, 37, 50, 80, 99, 101, 106, 107, 108, 125, 126, 129, 137, 140, 141, 154, 185, 190, 197, 206, 210, 213, 214, 216, 218, 220, 223, 224, 227, 228, 238, 244, 251, 255, 259, 264, 266, 267, 271, 273, 275
evolvability, vi, x, 113, 115, 125, 137, 138, 139, 140, 141, 142, 143, 171, 219, 240, 244, 248, 249, 253, 266, 270, 275
explanation, 42, 50, 56, 77, 85, 92, 94, 96, 141, 156, 171, 172, 173, 175, 180, 188, 206, 207, 208, 209, 226, 229, 233, 237, 239, 242, 252, 265
exposomics, 23, 149, 165, 172, 231

F

feedback, 72, 114, 115, 119, 120, 121, 125, 127, 131, 132, 133, 135, 169, 170, 205, 218, 221, 227, 232, 235, 239, 270
formal cause, 60, 269
fragility, x, 113, 115, 125, 137, 141, 142, 172, 175, 246
fragmentation, 51, 172, 176
functionality, 114, 150, 172

G

genetic determinism, 93, 94, 95, 96, 101, 102, 103, 104, 239, 253, 257, 259, 263, 265, 280
genetic essentialism, 19, 95, 96, 265, 274
genetic fatalism, 95, 96
genetic reductionism, 95, 96, 274
geneticism, vi, x, 3, 75, 93, 94, 95, 96, 97, 99, 101, 103, 110, 172, 212, 226
genome, 10, 16, 58, 72, 90, 93, 97, 101, 111, 138, 171, 172, 174, 203, 206, 207, 217, 220, 227, 231, 234, 236, 242, 251, 252, 259, 260, 261, 270, 272, 276, 278, 279
genomic medicine, 5, 185, 191, 196, 237, 242
genomics, 10, 15, 23, 46, 102, 148, 154, 162, 163, 165, 172, 182, 185, 189, 196, 199, 203, 204, 206, 225, 229, 251, 255, 262, 266, 271, 275, 278, 280
genotype, 33, 41, 43, 47, 48, 56, 58, 93, 94, 95, 96, 97, 98, 104, 125, 130, 138, 139, 142, 156, 229, 239, 268, 269
GRADE, 6, 7, 230, 231
graph theory, 20

H

haplotype, 270
Harvey, W., 98, 229, 233
healing, 53, 74, 115, 172, 181, 185, 189, 191, 200

health, x, 1, 2, 3, 11, 12, 15, 17, 18, 19, 24, 27, 38, 39, 53, 66, 75, 88, 89, 92, 96, 97, 102, 114, 115, 123, 131, 154, 158, 159, 162, 164, 165, 167, 170, 172, 177, 178, 179, 180, 181, 185, 186, 187, 188, 189, 190, 191, 192, 193, 195, 196, 197, 198, 199, 200, 201, 206, 210, 211, 212, 216, 217, 218, 221, 224, 225, 227, 229, 234, 235, 241, 242, 243, 244, 245, 247, 249, 250, 252, 256, 257, 258, 259, 260, 261, 262, 263, 264, 265, 267, 268, 270, 272, 273, 274, 275, 276, 289
heterostasis, 113, 122, 264
holism, 13, 49, 50, 197, 204, 214, 220, 223, 224, 225, 227, 237, 241, 245, 249, 251, 257, 263, 266, 268, 274, 277
holon, 12, 241
homeodynamics, 113, 122, 124, 143, 245
homeostasis, vi, x, 3, 113, 114, 115, 116, 117, 118, 119, 120, 121, 122, 123, 126, 129, 130, 131, 135, 137, 138, 143, 209, 210, 214, 218, 220, 222, 223, 224, 225, 226, 231, 236, 237, 245, 251, 256, 258, 264, 271, 273
Human Genome Project, 15, 21, 36, 97, 100, 101, 161, 172, 181, 227

I

idealism, 61, 172, 175
illness, 2, 4, 22, 24, 38, 39, 54, 56, 66, 72, 90, 92, 97, 105, 106, 110, 112, 124, 130, 136, 137, 150, 159, 160, 172, 177, 179, 180, 181, 182, 189, 191, 192, 195, 198, 199, 201, 204, 213, 214, 217, 225, 247, 273, 275, 276
information, 5, 6, 11, 16, 24, 33, 37, 44, 45, 47, 49, 55, 56, 57, 58, 93, 94, 95, 97, 101, 102, 104, 107, 127, 148, 156, 158, 161, 162, 165, 166, 167, 172, 174, 200, 206, 215, 225, 232, 238, 243, 251
integrated personalized omics profiling (iPOP), 13, 36, 244
integration, 7, 10, 11, 12, 24, 25, 28, 39, 55, 107, 149, 152, 153, 155, 156, 159, 172, 174, 221, 239, 265, 271, 274, 276, 278
integrity, 49, 51, 52, 53, 55, 56, 57, 64, 93, 114, 125, 126, 128, 129, 138, 140, 148, 161, 162, 163, 171, 173, 250
interactome, 20, 21, 148, 172, 203, 208, 228, 247, 274
interdisciplinary, 11, 13, 153, 156, 157, 169, 178, 194, 204, 227, 249, 255, 257, 266
International HapMap Consortium, 16, 270
intuition, 30, 80, 172, 179
irreducibility, 46, 85, 86, 92, 267

L

La Mettrie, J. O., 60, 63, 243
Laennec, R., 35, 222
Leucippus, 103
Lewes, G. H., 79, 80, 244
linear causality, 9
linear dynamics, vi, x, 3, 113, 114, 115, 131, 132, 133, 135, 136, 137, 143, 229, 237

M

machine, 27, 30, 36, 49, 61, 63, 66, 69, 73, 89, 90, 117, 173, 189, 194, 221, 243, 272
Mansel, H., 103, 247
material cause, 60, 61
materialism, v, x, 3, 27, 34, 59, 60, 61, 62, 63, 64, 65, 74, 82, 173, 174, 198, 207, 211, 213, 226, 231, 255, 257, 265, 266, 277
materiality, 65, 73, 260
mechanical philosophy, 27, 28, 29, 204, 212, 217, 227, 229, 259
mechanism, v, x, 3, 8, 12, 13, 21, 27, 28, 29, 30, 31, 32, 33, 34, 35, 36, 37, 73, 75, 76, 78, 81, 82, 92, 100, 111, 114, 117, 120, 121, 131, 132, 133, 138, 140, 164, 169, 170, 171, 173, 174, 175, 180, 189,

204, 219, 220, 221, 226, 229, 233, 252, 253, 259, 261, 269, 271
mechanistic evidence, 8
mechanistic explanation, 30, 32, 33, 212, 229
mechanistic resultant, 75, 110, 111
medicalization, 3, 218, 255, 269, 273, 274
Mendel, G., 46, 47, 57, 207, 250
metabolomics, 10, 16, 23, 102, 148, 154, 173, 206, 224, 237
metaphysics, 28, 34, 48, 59, 64, 173, 189, 198, 205, 208, 216, 218, 251, 264, 269
methodological reductionism, 43, 44, 53, 54, 277
methodological wholism, 53, 54
methodology, 34, 52, 54, 91, 145, 173, 194, 222, 247, 261
microbiomics, 10, 23, 173, 224
Mill, J. S., 79, 80, 251
molecular biology, 2, 12, 31, 32, 33, 35, 40, 46, 48, 57, 74, 75, 99, 206, 210, 212, 219, 223, 224, 240, 251, 255, 260, 261, 262, 263, 268, 270, 273, 277, 279
molecular genetics, 46, 48, 208, 247
molecular medicine, 14, 15, 26, 179, 195, 199, 205, 211, 215, 242, 261, 264, 265, 269, 271
molecular systems medicine, v, 1, 10, 14, 15, 20, 26, 38

N

nanotechnology, 147, 174, 223, 260
narrative, 46, 174, 179, 181, 191, 194, 212
naturalism, 69, 84, 174, 256
necessitarianism, 103, 247
network medicine, v, 1, 10, 20, 21, 190, 215, 236, 245, 265
network theory, 20, 124, 156, 194, 224
network topology, 20
new materialism, v, vi, ix, x, 23, 27, 50, 59, 64, 65, 66, 72, 73, 93, 155, 216, 221, 227, 243
Newton, I., 27, 89, 103, 221, 222, 231, 236, 253, 262, 264
next-generation sequencing, 17, 239
noncoding RNA (ncRNA), 100, 216
nondeducibility, 85, 86, 92
nonlinear dynamics, vi, x, 113, 114, 131, 134, 135, 136, 137, 143, 155, 203, 215, 221, 238, 241, 254, 268, 277
nosology, 19, 188
nutrigenomics, 23, 102, 154, 174

O

objectivity, 54, 174, 176, 192, 212
omics, ii, 10, 11, 13, 15, 17, 18, 19, 21, 22, 23, 26, 36, 38, 54, 136, 147, 148, 149, 154, 162, 163, 165, 166, 174, 175, 178, 200, 201, 206, 216, 221, 236, 241, 244, 274, 278
one size fits all, 90, 92, 217, 262
ontological reductionism, 42, 47, 57
ontological wholism, 57
ontologies, 34, 57, 174, 193
ontology, x, 32, 33, 50, 62, 67, 174, 184, 192, 204, 213, 216, 231, 233, 252, 261
organicism, v, ix, x, 27, 28, 29, 34, 35, 36, 37, 38, 72, 74, 164, 165, 167, 173, 174, 204, 208, 212, 228, 232, 233, 253, 257, 261, 264, 267
organism, x, 2, 13, 28, 35, 36, 37, 38, 40, 41, 43, 44, 47, 49, 53, 57, 58, 64, 65, 66, 68, 76, 79, 86, 90, 93, 94, 95, 97, 98, 99, 102, 107, 108, 113, 114, 115, 116, 117, 118, 119, 121, 123, 124, 138, 139, 148, 171, 172, 173, 174, 175, 176, 221, 222, 223, 233, 247, 248, 253, 261, 278
organismal systems medicine, 10
organismic biology, 35, 38, 271
organismic context, 35

P

P4 systems medicine, 21, 22, 88, 165, 274
P7 systems medicine, v, ix, x, 1, 10, 21, 23, 38, 50, 52, 53, 54, 55, 56, 57, 59, 72, 73, 74, 75, 76, 88, 92, 94, 102, 110, 112,

115, 130, 136, 142, 143, 145, 146, 148, 154, 155, 160, 163, 164, 165, 167
paradigm, 8, 13, 32, 33, 48, 73, 75, 113, 115, 123, 154, 155, 190, 212, 215, 224, 238, 243, 245, 247, 250, 267, 268
pathology, ix, 3, 4, 23, 88, 137, 151, 165, 172, 175, 180, 193, 218, 225, 245, 267, 271, 273, 279
pathome, 23, 136, 149, 174
pathophenome, 11
personal health, 27, 160, 163
personalism, 23, 175
personalized medicine, v, 1, 5, 10, 11, 15, 16, 17, 18, 23, 26, 36, 90, 158, 178, 181, 182, 185, 186, 188, 193, 196, 198, 199, 204, 207, 210, 211, 215, 216, 224, 225, 226, 229, 231, 235, 236, 237, 246, 247, 257, 258, 262, 263, 266, 278
personome, 23, 136, 149, 175
phenomenology, 65, 175, 177, 182, 183, 188, 192, 195, 198, 199, 201, 220, 249
phenotype, 13, 17, 20, 33, 41, 47, 48, 56, 58, 94, 95, 96, 97, 98, 100, 102, 104, 107, 125, 130, 138, 139, 140, 142, 156, 172, 229, 239, 268, 269
physical determinism, 104
physicalism, v, 27, 59, 62, 63, 64, 68, 69, 70, 175, 214, 218, 221, 223, 224, 228, 233, 245, 249, 250, 251, 252, 253, 256, 264, 267, 268, 270, 276
physiology, 3, 23, 83, 88, 94, 118, 151, 185, 191, 200, 209, 210, 213, 220, 223, 226, 229, 231, 232, 236, 238, 240, 244, 250, 251, 254, 256, 258, 276, 279, 289
physiome, 23, 136, 149, 175
PICO, 5, 244
plasticity, 38, 94, 115, 124, 137, 140, 171, 175, 238, 254
Plato, 28, 60
pluralism, 8, 44, 73, 173, 175, 188
population health, 171, 179, 189, 190, 192, 199, 200
precision medicine, v, 1, 10, 15, 17, 18, 19, 20, 25, 26, 89, 102, 178, 179, 181, 191, 192, 200, 204, 205, 209, 211, 216, 218, 219, 220, 222, 239, 247, 249, 253, 255, 262, 267, 270, 272, 273, 278
Precision Medicine Initiative Cohort Program, 18
prognosis, 5, 11, 175, 188
protein-protein interaction (PPI), 13, 20, 194, 266
proteomics, 10, 16, 23, 102, 154, 165, 175, 203, 206, 244, 249, 255, 275
psychiatome, 22, 23, 175, 212
psychology, 23, 38, 91, 94, 179, 207, 212, 220, 226, 232, 233, 254, 259, 263
public health, 22, 164, 165, 179, 183, 185, 187, 193, 197, 199, 200, 205, 213, 237, 244, 257, 264

R

randomness, 103, 106, 107, 109, 213, 214, 233
rationalism, 63, 171, 175
realism, 65, 172, 175, 197, 223
reductionism, v, x, 3, 27, 39, 40, 41, 42, 43, 44, 45, 46, 49, 50, 53, 54, 56, 57, 58, 70, 73, 74, 79, 80, 82, 83, 87, 95, 96, 154, 155, 170, 171, 173, 174, 175, 180, 197, 198, 203, 204, 206, 208, 209, 211, 212, 214, 216, 220, 225, 227, 235, 237, 241, 245, 249, 251, 260, 262, 263, 267, 268, 273, 277
resultant, vi, x, 1, 2, 31, 37, 75, 76, 77, 78, 80, 81, 88, 90, 92, 110, 111, 171, 175
resultant mechanism, 78, 171
revolution, 27, 33, 60, 98, 99, 100, 178, 181, 182, 193, 199, 210, 217, 224, 226, 247, 250, 251, 264, 271, 275
robustness, vi, ix, x, 112, 113, 114, 115, 124, 125, 126, 127, 128, 129, 130, 131, 137, 138, 139, 140, 141, 142, 143, 154, 167, 172, 175, 207, 209, 214, 219, 221, 222, 225, 228, 232, 234, 238, 240, 241, 242, 243, 244, 248, 249, 254, 262, 267, 270, 275, 276
Rostan, L., 35
Russo-Williamson thesis, 8, 34

S

Schmidt, A., 61, 158, 195, 207, 265
scientific determinism, 104, 105, 106, 219
scientific materialism, 61, 64, 213, 230
Severe Acute Respiratory Syndrome Coronavirus 2 (SARS-CoV-2), 9, 164, 165, 215
Single-Nucleotide Polymorphism (SNP), 16, 17, 234, 270, 274
SNP Consortium, 16, 270
socioethics, 160, 161, 163
stasis, vi, x, 113, 114, 115, 118, 122, 137, 142, 143, 175, 217, 244
stochastic process, 49, 103, 106, 107, 108, 109, 212, 221, 240, 251, 255, 272, 273
stochasticity, vi, ix, x, 75, 88, 103, 106, 107, 108, 109, 110, 170, 176, 210, 225, 227, 234, 237, 240, 244, 245, 246, 256, 259, 261, 263, 265, 269, 270, 279
subjectivity, 54, 174, 176, 182, 192, 212
suffering, 3, 4, 9, 17, 66, 90, 101, 117, 172, 176, 180, 182, 189, 198, 215
synergy, 75, 89, 91, 92, 93, 218, 254, 258, 261, 264
synthesis, vi, x, 40, 46, 48, 49, 64, 67, 75, 89, 90, 91, 92, 93, 110, 129, 169, 176, 215, 225, 226, 232, 236, 243, 257, 260, 267, 271, 272
systems biology, xi, 10, 11, 12, 13, 14, 15, 21, 33, 38, 48, 74, 114, 134, 141, 146, 147, 151, 153, 154, 155, 158, 160, 163, 174, 191, 203, 204, 205, 206, 207, 208, 210, 211, 213, 215, 216, 217, 218, 219, 221, 222, 225, 226, 228, 234, 235, 236, 237, 238, 239, 240,241, 242, 243, 245, 246, 247, 248, 249, 250, 251, 252, 254, 255, 256, 259, 263, 265, 266, 269, 272, 273, 274, 275, 276, 277, 278, 279, 289
Systems Biology Markup Language (SBML), 151, 152, 235
systems biomedicine, v, 1, 10, 12, 13, 14, 20, 26, 155, 205, 206, 207, 222, 223, 224, 240, 244, 245, 264, 265, 278, 279
systems pathology, ix
systems physiology, 165, 240
systems psychology, 165
systems science, 12, 13, 23, 82, 106, 154, 155, 176, 204, 226
systems theory, 4, 13, 20, 124, 155, 209, 232, 233, 271, 274, 277

T

Theoretical Biology Club, 36, 257
transcriptomics, 23, 102, 148, 154, 165, 176
translational medicine, 5, 149, 195, 200

U

unpredictability, 9, 86, 92, 214
upward causation, vi, x, 27, 52, 57, 67, 68, 69, 70, 71, 72, 74, 88

V

vaccine, 9
Vienna Circle, 62, 241, 267
Virchow, R., 35, 61, 259
virology, 165
vitalism, 29, 31, 34, 35, 36, 62, 65, 79, 81, 82, 84, 204, 220, 233, 253, 264

W

wellbeing, x, 92, 105, 176
wholeness, x, 50, 51, 52, 53, 54, 56, 57, 66, 80, 172, 176, 211, 244, 257
wholism, v, ix, x, 27, 39, 40, 49, 50, 51, 52, 53, 54, 56, 72, 73, 154, 155, 171, 173, 174, 175, 176, 224

About the Author

James A. Marcum, PhD
Professor
Department of Philosophy
Baylor University, Waco, Texas, USA
Email: james_marcum@baylor.edu

James A. Marcum earned doctorates in physiology from the University of Cincinnati Medical College and in philosophy from Boston College. He was a faculty member at Harvard Medical School as a molecular biologist for over a decade before joining Baylor's philosophy department. His current research interests include the philosophy and history of science and medicine. Examples of his recent publications appear in *Annals of Science, International Studies in the Philosophy of Science*, *Synthese*, *Perspectives on Science*, *History and Philosophy of the Life Sciences*, *Journal of the History of Medicine and Allied Sciences*, *Medicine, Health Care and Philosophy*, *Perspectives in Biology and Medicine*, and *Theoretical Medicine and Bioethics*. He is author of *The Conceptual Foundations of Systems Biology: An Introduction*. Hauppauge, NY: Nova Science Publishers, 2009, *An Introductory Philosophy of Medicine: Humanizing Modern Medicine*. New York: Springer, 2010, *Thomas Kuhn's Revolutions: A Historical and an Evolutionary Philosophy of Science*. London: Bloomsbury, 2015, and *From Systems Biology to Systems Medicine*, Hauppauge, NY: Nova Science Publishers, 2020.